WITHDRAWN

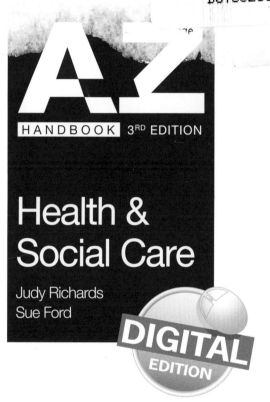

A-Z

HANDBOOK 3RD EDITION

Health & Social Care

Judy Richards
Sue Ford

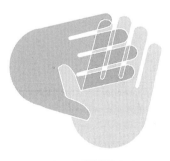

DIGITAL EDITION

Philip Allan Updates, an imprint of Hodder Education, an Hachette UK company, Market Place, Deddington, Oxfordshire OX15 0SE

Orders

Bookpoint Ltd, 130 Milton Park, Abingdon, Oxfordshire OX14 4SB
tel: 01235 827720
fax: 01235 400454
e-mail: uk.orders@bookpoint.co.uk

Lines are open 9.00 a.m.–5.00 p.m., Monday to Saturday, with a 24-hour message answering service. You can also order through the Philip Allan Updates website: www.philipallan.co.uk

ISBN 978-0-340-99108-4

First published 1999
Second edition 2003
Third edition 2010

Impression number   5   4   3   2   1
Year   2015   2014   2013   2012   2011   2010

Typeset by Macmillan, India.

Printed by CPI Antony Rowe, Chippenham, Wiltshire.

Environmental information
Hachette UK's policy is to use papers that are natural, renewable and recyclable products and made from wood grown in sustainable forests. The logging and manufacturing processes are expected to conform to the environmental regulations of the country of origin.

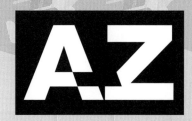

Contents

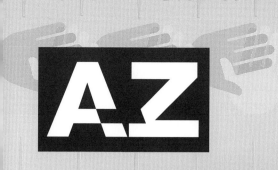

How to use this book

The *A–Z Health & Social Care Handbook* is an alphabetical glossary designed for easy use. As you can appreciate, health and social care covers a wide subject area and the major concepts that you will come across in your health and social care studies have been included. This handbook therefore constitutes an important reference work that will help you to understand the basic requirements for your study. Government legislation and reports which have been responsible for structural changes within health and social care services are included to support your research – a list of the relevant legislation and reports are included at the back of the book.

Each entry begins with a definition. This should help you to gain some understanding of what you are looking for. The length of an entry usually depends on how relevant the content is to the caring concepts within health and social care. Entries therefore try to provide some guidance or introduce you to the major points. Illustrations and tables have been provided to help you to understand the entry.

To support your research, you can make use of the cross-referenced entries. These are to be found in bold italics either in the main body of an entry or at the end of the entry. These cross-references direct you to related subjects.

The handbook is a glossary that will aid your study of health and social care; it is important to recognise that it is not a textbook. This means that you will need to carry out further reading to complete your grasp of the subject, but the handbook will provide you with a handy reference source when you come across terms of which you are unsure.

Samples of organisations have been included to support you and increase your understanding of the scope of voluntary organisations. These include the umbrella organisations in Northern Ireland, Scotland and Wales.

To help you in your revision, lists of terms have been provided at the end of the book. We have used the most popular AS and A-level courses to structure these lists. You should look up the exam board whose qualification you are studying and check which revision lists are relevant to the particular topics you are taking. You can also use the website that accompanies this handbook to access revision lists specific to your exam board unit. You should find these lists valuable when you come to do your revision.

A–Z Online

This new digital edition of the *A–Z Health & Social Care Handbook* includes free access to a supporting website and a free desktop widget to make searching for terms even quicker. Log on to **www.philipallan.co.uk/a-zonline** and create an account using the unique code provided on the inside front cover of this book.

Once you are logged on, you will be able to:

- search the entire database of terms in this handbook
- print revision lists specific to your exam board
- get expert advice from examiners on how to get an A* grade
- create a personal library of your favourite terms
- expand your vocabulary with our word of the week.

You can also add the other *A–Z Handbooks (digital editions)* that you own to your personal library on A–Z Online.

Finally, we hope that you enjoy using the handbook on a daily basis and that you find it is an invaluable resource in your studies. We have certainly enjoyed compiling it.

Acknowledgements

This has been an enormous task which we could not have achieved without our invaluable supporters.

Judy wishes to thank her husband Jeff, her daughters Jessica and Helen, her son-in-law Ian and her grand-daughter Georgia who kept her spirits up during the research and writing of the book. She also thanks Laura Odell and David Odell, as well as Carole Ford and Hilda Hans who contributed to the earlier editions of this book.

Sue wishes to thank her husband Graham and her children Chris, Charlotte and Georgia for their support and encouragement. She also thanks the health and social care team at North Hertfordshire College.

Judy Richards and Sue Ford

The authors and publishers would like to thank the following for permission to reproduce material in this volume:

The Controller of Her Majesty's Stationery Office for the use of Crown copyright material (PSI licence number C2007001851), and St. John Ambulance, St. Andrew's Ambulance Association and British Red Cross for the use of information in the *First Aid Manual*, published by Dorling Kindersley.

Every effort has been made to obtain necessary permission with reference to copyright material. The publishers apologise if inadvertently any sources remain unacknowledged and will be glad to make the necessary arrangements at the earliest opportunity.

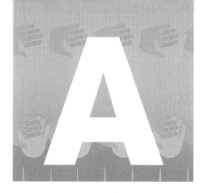

ABC of behaviour describes the process involved in *behaviour* patterns. It comprises:

- antecedent – what happens before the behaviour occurs. This can involve an incident or event which can trigger behaviour
- behaviour – the behaviour presents itself. It is either positive, which is acceptable, or negative, which is unacceptable
- consequence – the results of the behaviour which can have either positive or negative effects.

This is a useful model because it can be used in *behaviour modification*. By removing certain triggers during the antecedent phase one can reduce the possibility of some negative or *anti-social behaviour* presenting itself.

ABC of resuscitation: a method of resuscitation which can be applied in an emergency:

- A is for airway – tilting the casualty's head back and lifting the chin will 'open the airway'. The tilted position lifts the casualty's *tongue* from the back of the throat so that it does not block the air passage.
- B is for breathing – if the casualty is not breathing, another person can breathe for him or her and so oxygenate the *blood*, by giving 'artificial ventilation', blowing their expired air into the casualty's *lungs*.
- C is for circulation – if the *heart* has stopped, 'chest compressions' can be applied to force blood through the heart and around the body. These must be accompanied by artificial ventilation so that the blood is oxygenated. (See *artificial respiration*.)

(Source: *First Aid Manual.*)

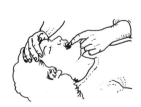 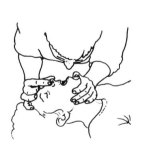 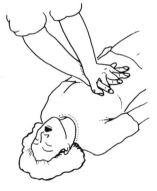

A is for Airway   *B is for Breathing*   *C is for Circulation*

ABC of resuscitation

A First Class Service 1998: a consultation document to ensure quality in the **NHS (National Health Service)** by inviting comment on the UK government's proposal for reorganisation in the NHS. This led to the creation of a modern service that delivers high standards of care for all. It stated that quality would be maintained by the setting of standards through **National Service Frameworks** and the **National Institute for Clinical Excellence** (NICE).

abdomen: the region of the body that contains all the internal organs except the **heart** and **lungs**. The abdomen is separated from the thorax or chest region by a partition called the **diaphragm**. The abdomen is lined with a membrane called the peritoneum.

abortion: the termination of **pregnancy**. Abortion can be either by natural means (spontaneous abortion), commonly known as **miscarriage**, or by artificial or surgical means. Abortion is increasingly viewed as the termination of an unplanned and unwanted pregnancy. Since 1967, following the **Abortion Act 1967**, it is legal to terminate a pregnancy up to 24 weeks in duration. However, most abortions are carried out in the first 12 weeks of pregnancy, via either the **NHS (National Health Service)** or private medicine. There are different views on abortion; for example:

- 'Pro-life' groups believe that abortion limits the life choices of the growing foetus. They believe that the foetus has a right to be born and a right to life.
- 'Right to Abortion' groups support women's rights. They believe that women have a choice; that a planned abortion is an appropriate medical intervention in an unwanted pregnancy, or in a pregnancy where the unborn child may have a genetic **disability**.

Because of the issues involved regarding the rights and choices of the individual, abortion is a controversial subject.

Abortion Act 1967: an Act of Parliament which enables a woman to terminate an unwanted and unplanned pregnancy. Under this Act, two doctors must agree to the abortion on the grounds of:

- 'risk' to the life of the pregnant woman
- 'risk' to the lives of her existing children
- 'risk' of abnormality in the **foetus**.

Under the Act the woman's emotional, psychological, social and physical **well-being** are taken into account by the doctors. (See **Human Fertilisation and Embryology Act 2008**.)

abuse: the deliberate act of injuring or intending to injure another person in order to cause them harm or discomfort. Acts of abuse can be:

- emotional – this involves ill treatment which causes damage to the emotional development of a child or adult. Examples include verbal threats, shouting, screaming and telling the child or vulnerable individual how stupid, hopeless or ugly they are. This may have a damaging and long-lasting effect on the **self-esteem** of the individual
- neglect – this involves persistently choosing to ignore a child or adult by not providing them with the care to meet their **basic needs** of safety, warmth, protection, food and affection. Examples of this include not feeding an elderly service user, leaving a child consistently unsupervised, with an inadequate diet and lack of parental care which could result in failure to thrive
- physical – this involves causing deliberate physical injury to a child or adult. Examples of this include hitting with a belt, smacking in anger and burning with a cigarette
- sexual – this involves the sexual exploitation of a child or vulnerable person. Examples include having intercourse with a person against their will, subjecting an individual or child

to sexual activities such as fondling, masturbation, oral sex and violating an individual or child's intimate and personal privacy

- self-harm – this involves the individual or child directing the injury or harm at themselves. Examples include pulling their hair out, scratching or cutting their wrists or other parts of the body
- financial – this involves the theft of money or the misuse of a service user's benefits
- institutional – this involves poor work practices where the needs of the service user are not considered
- domestic – this involves acts of violence in the family.

Groups of people who are the most vulnerable to abuse are children (see **child abuse**), women (see **domestic violence**), older people (see **older people – abuse**) and people with disabilities. There are strategies that organisations put in place to minimise abuse such as **Criminal Record Bureau** checks, **codes of practice** and legislation, policies and procedures, **advocacy**, **confidentiality** and staff training. The indicators of abuse include multiple bruising and unexplained injuries (see **models of abuse**).

access to information: the right that clients, patients and service users have to all information concerning their personal lives (see **Data Protection Acts 1984 and 1998**). Health and social care providers have different methods of storing information. These can be manual and/or computerised records. For example, the records which individual GPs maintain with regard to their patients and their different visits may be hand written. The drugs and personal details of a patient would however be fed into a computer system. Some agencies may have a limit on the length of time that they maintain an individual's records.

access to services: clients and service users are entitled to treatment and therapy provided through the **NHS (National Health Service)** and **personal social services**. Patients have rights to:

- receive health care on the basis of their clinical need, not on their ability to pay, **lifestyle** or any other factor
- be registered with a GP and be able to change their GP easily and quickly if they want to
- have access to emergency medical treatment at any time through their GP, the **ambulance service** and hospital **accident and emergency** departments
- be referred to a consultant acceptable to them, when their GP thinks it necessary, and to be referred for a second opinion if they and their GP agree this is desirable. (See **referral to health care services**.)
- **assessment** of their individual needs for continuing treatment and care.

Patients can expect the NHS to make it easy for everyone to use its services, including children, older people and those with physical or mental **disabilities**. For example, if a child needs to be admitted to hospital, parents can expect the child to be cared for in a children's ward under the supervision of a consultant **paediatrician**. Exceptionally, when a child has to be admitted to a ward other than a children's ward, a parent can expect a named consultant paediatrician to be responsible for advising on their care. There are other aspects of access to services which include adaptation of premises to enable everyone to have the right of access including those with **physical disabilities**. Distribution of information and campaigns can raise awareness of services that are available. **Advocacy** and support should be promoted as part of the services provided including making resources available to meet the individual needs of service users, clients and patients. Service users, clients and patients are entitled to treatment and therapy provided by the National Health Service and Social Services. (See also *barriers to access to health and social care services, resourcing of services*.)

accident: an unpredictable injury which affects a person at any time and which may require medical treatment. There are groups of people who are more at risk from accidents. They are:

- young children – because they are less aware of danger
- disabled people – because different impairments lead to vulnerability
- older people – because of diminishing *mobility*, or mental awareness.

Any individual can be at risk at certain times, for instance, a preoccupied adult may leave a toddler to wander out into a garden with a fish pond. The toddler does not have a sense of danger but is full of curiosity about the goldfish in the pond. She/he may lean over and fall in and within a matter of moments be in danger of drowning. All accidents in care settings should be recorded in an *accident book*. Accidents are identified in the *national health targets*. (See *Royal Society for the Prevention of Accidents*.)

accident and emergency: a special department at a hospital, which deals with accidents and acute illness; sometimes known as the 'A and E Department' or 'casualty'.

accident book: a method of recording *accidents* which occur in all organisations including those in health and social care. Information recorded should include:

- the name and address of the injured person
- the date and time of the accident
- details of the accident
- the type of injury
- the treatment given or action taken
- details of who was informed
- a signature of the person in charge at the time of the accident.

The accident book is often a requirement of the *health and safety* policy of a health and social care provision. This book should be accessible to all the members of staff (see *Regulations for Reporting of Injuries, Diseases and Dangerous Occurrences (RIDDOR) 1995*).

accommodation – in health and social care provision is a type of care which can be offered to clients in *residential homes*. It can be statutory, voluntary, private or informal care provision for:

- *children in care* – e.g. *children's homes* or in families through *foster care* and *adoption*
- clients with a disability – e.g. *hostels, sheltered housing*
- older people – e.g. *residential homes, nursing homes, sheltered housing*, family homes.

accommodation – of the eye: the ability of the *eye* to change focus so that both near and distant objects can be seen clearly. When a person looks at a distant object the rays of the light are bent (refracted) by the *cornea* and the lens and are focused on the retina. If the object is brought closer, the light rays have to be refracted more if they are to remain focused. This is done by contraction of the ciliary muscles which change the shape of the lens so that it becomes more convex.

accountability: responsibilities to meet the professional standards which are set by the appropriate government department or agency. This process reviews the ways in which primary care trusts work within the *health improvement programmes*. This term also applies to individual **health and social care workers** as they work with service users and employers within the **care value base** and with the different **codes of ethics** laid down by the professional bodies.

Acheson Report 1998: an independent study into **inequalities in health** in the United Kingdom. This was commissioned by the Labour Government in 1997 under the chairmanship of Sir Donald Acheson. The report findings mirrored those of the **Black Report 1980**, that the root cause of health inequalities was **poverty**. It concluded that, in order to improve the health of millions, the gap between the richest and poorest in UK society had to be reduced.

acquired disorder: a **disease** or **disability** which is contracted after **birth**. It is not **inherited disorder** or a **congenital disorder**. An example of an acquired disease would be an **infection** such as **meningitis** which is the inflammation of the meninges of the **brain** caused by a viral or bacterial infection.

acquired immune deficiency syndrome (AIDS): a **disease** which is caused by **HIV (human immunodeficiency virus)**. This virus attacks the immune system and therefore alters the body's response to infection. HIV is transmitted:
- through sexual contact via infected body fluids such as semen and vaginal fluid
- by injecting **drugs** – using previously infected needles
- through **blood transfusion** – using blood which is infected with HIV
- from a mother who is HIV-positive to her unborn child – the HIV virus can pass from the mother through the placenta to the **foetus**; the HIV virus is also present in the breast milk of an HIV-positive mother.

It is important to remember that *not* every person who is infected with HIV will go on to develop AIDS. The full onset of AIDS usually occurs after the following four stages have been completed. There is no set period of time for each stage.
- Stage 1 – symptomless stage, the person is infected with the HIV virus, but is producing antibodies to combat the infection and appears quite healthy. They can still infect others so health and safety precautions should continue to be taken, e.g. protected sex using a condom.
- Stage 2 – persistent generalised lymphadenopathy (swollen glands). This is the first sign that the immune system is breaking down, highlighted by swollen lymph glands in the neck, groin and axillae.
- Stage 3 – AIDS-related conditions such as weight loss, night sweats, fever, lack of resistance to disease, a general feeling of tiredness or fatigue and feeling unwell.
- Stage 4 – the immune system shows signs of failing and the lack of resistance can lead to different infections affecting the body. These include chest infections, brain infections causing blindness, loss of speech and tremors, skin diseases causing ulceration, boils, ringworm, **cancer** of the tongue and genital areas. This stage leads to death.

There are **health and safety** precautions which should be applied when working with people with HIV such as wearing gloves when attending to wounds.

active immunity: a type of resistance to **disease** in which individuals manufacture their own **antibodies**. This may or may not be the result of a natural **infection**. It is possible for the body to produce antibodies without suffering from the illness. This kind of *immunity* can be induced by the process of *vaccination*.

active listening skills: *listening skills* which are used during *interaction* between the client and the carer. There are two types of active listening:

- Paraphrasing – this is a way of summarising what the client has said and feeding back to the client for confirmation that what they have said has been understood. For example a carer could say to a client 'what you have just told me has raised these points, is that right?' Paraphrasing is an important way of checking for accuracy that what has been said has been understood by the carer. It also gives the client the feeling that the carer has been listening and is making an effort to understand their conversation. It is a means by which the carer can communicate that they want to care for the client. Often, this is the first step in building up an effective client–carer relationship.
- Reflective listening – concentrates on what is being said. The carer will either repeat what a client has said or use non-verbal messages and positive body language with space and silence for the client to respond further.

activities of daily living: daily tasks and activities associated with the process of living. They include washing, going to the toilet and dressing. Activities for daily living can be categorised into:

- self-care skills – personal care such as eating, drinking, washing, bathing, dressing, hair and skin care
- home care skills – caring for the home environment such as cooking and kitchen skills, gardening, washing, ironing, cleaning, budgeting and shopping skills
- employment skills – identifying skills which would be suitable for employment such as communication and computer skills
- *mobility* skills – using the body for daily tasks such as washing, dressing, shopping, housework
- social skills – making relationships such as friendships.

Understanding the activities of daily living is a vital part of assessing a client and the way in which they are able to cope with life. Development of these skills can be written into a client's individual *care plan*. Supporting clients with their daily living activities can be:

- short term – clients need support because they have had an *accident* or a surgical operation or are suffering from a temporary debilitating *disease* or *disorder*
- long term – clients need continuing support because the disorder, *dysfunction* or disease suffered restricts their *mobility*.

In some cases specialist aids or equipment are necessary in order to maintain the *health and safety* of both the client and the carer. (See *aids and adaptations, Disabled Living Foundation, occupational therapy, daily living task, independent living*.)

activities for health and well-being: tasks and activities which are based on meeting needs within the different aspects of an individual's development. Activities can be planned for different service user groups or individuals. Examples of activities to meet developmental needs are:

- physical needs of movement and mobility can be met through *exercise* classes, music and movement and dancing
- intellectual needs of thinking, *memory* and *language* can be met through crosswords, sudoku, *reminiscence*, jigsaw puzzles, *storytelling* and reading

- social needs of *interaction*, *communication* and building social relationships can be met through book clubs, leisure and special interest groups, *games*, *play*, *storytelling*, *music and singing*
- emotional needs of expressing feelings and building positive *self-esteem* and *self-confidence* can be met through creative activities such as art, drawing and play. Positive relationships can be developed through these different activities. (See *creative play*.)

Planning activities involves identifying an appropriate activity which meets the particular needs of the individual service user or group, i.e. children, teenagers, adults or older people. Timing and resources should be taken into account as well as the need for collaborating with others who may be involved. Activities should be evaluated following implementation. *Feedback* should also be in place to consider how the activity can be modified for future use.

activity-based interaction comprises the different activities which clients and carers can carry out together. These activities are designed to develop and promote their *communication skills* and *interpersonal skills*. Activities which can be provided to develop these skills include:

- 'one to one', e.g. discussion, practical tasks
- small group activities, e.g. discussion, debate, practical tasks
- large group activities, e.g. oral presentations, discussions, practical tasks.

(See also *interaction* and *activities for health and well-being*.)

acupuncture: a *complementary therapy* which originated in China. It is a relatively painless treatment which involves the insertion of fine needles at specific points on the skin. Acupuncture has been found to enhance *health* and the *immune system* as well as addressing specific symptoms. To qualify as an acupuncturist may involve full-time training lasting three to four years, or three to five years part-time.

acute: a disease or condition which is of quick onset. It is often short and severe. An example is appendicitis which involves inflammation of the *appendix*. The signs and symptoms are severe right-sided abdominal pain, sickness and high temperature. The treatment is immediate surgical removal of the appendix.

acute services: medical and surgical treatment and care mainly provided in hospitals.

acute trusts are trusts which manage hospitals. Their role is to ensure that hospitals provide high-quality health care.

addiction: the way in which an individual can become dependent physically, intellectually, emotionally and psychologically on a substance or activity, e.g. nicotine addiction, *heroin* or *alcohol* addiction.

additional needs: a term which applies to those service users who have requirements in addition to their existing disabilities. This includes physical disability, sensory impairment, *mental health disorder* or a combination of all of these. For example a child or adult with *Down's syndrome* will have educational and learning needs as well as supervision needs for any underlying medical conditions. (See *barriers to access to health and social care services*.) Positive working practice for service users with additional needs includes:

- assessment of individual needs and planning for *person-centred care*
- anti-discriminatory practice and empowerment

- supporting enablement and normalisation
- assisting coping mechanisms and using **strategies for effective communication** with the service user
- building positive relationships and building confidence in the service user.

However, there are barriers to the support that service users with additional needs receive. These are:

- environmental barriers which relate to limited physical access
- attitudes which promote discriminatory practice and social isolation
- economic barriers which lead to limited employment opportunities.

adenosine diphosphate (ADP) is a high *energy* compound found in cells. Its function is energy storage and transfer. When extra energy and phosphate are added it forms *adenosine triphosphate (ATP)*.

adenosine triphosphate (ATP) is a compound with a high level of *energy* found in cells. Its function is energy storage and transfer. It can be broken down so that ADP and phosphoric acid are formed. Energy is released in this process. Some of the energy is lost as heat, but a proportion of it can be used for biological activities. (See *glycolysis*.)

adipose tissue consists of cells containing fat which group together to form a protective layer under the skin. Extra layers of fat surround the organs of the body in order to provide protection and insulation.

administration consists of the procedures involved in managing services or organisations. These procedures usually relate to business management. They may be applied to health and social care organisations in the following ways:

- human resourcing, which includes staffing and personnel issues, e.g. employment of carers and client/staff ratios
- accounting and finance; budget issues such as costing of care packages and necessary resources to support the caring process
- marketing and product sales, for example advertising different caring services especially in the private or *independent sector*
- operations management; this includes reviewing the product and its production, for example *care management* which may involve setting up *care plans*, monitoring and evaluating the process.

Admiral Nurse Service is an example of a *voluntary sector organisation* which supports carers of people with a *dementia* illness. It aims to:

- provide information about the nature of dementia and the progress of the *disease*
- assist the carers in organising practical help
- enhance, increase and support the skills of carers in caring for a person with a dementia illness
- enhance the skills needed to deal with the *stress* and *anxiety* that may arise during the care process
- provide the carer with emotional *support* to reduce the sense of isolation and feeling of loss associated with the experience of bereavement and to continue to provide ongoing support after *bereavement*
- provide advice to other agencies and individuals in contact with people with a dementia illness and their care-givers, and to support efforts to meet their needs
- act as a training resource for informal carers such as family members.

admission: entry into hospital or residential care. The admission may be planned from a *waiting list*, or be an emergency via the hospital *accident and emergency* department. Admissions can also be arranged via the hospital outpatient department. Individuals may also be admitted to hospital under the *Mental Health Act 1983*. This procedure is called sectioning.

adolescence: the period of development starting with *puberty* and ending in *adulthood*. The age range is 11 to 18 years.

adoption: the legal transfer of an *infant* or child from their birth family to another family. Adoption was introduced under the Adoption of Children Act in 1926. A recent update in legislation is the Children and Adoption Act 2006 (England and Wales). This introduced a number of provisions with regard to arranging contact with children following parental separation and with regard to adoptions that have a foreign element.

adrenal glands are situated on the top of each *kidney*. These glands are divided into two parts:
- cortex – the outer part of the gland which produces steroid hormones, cortisol and *aldosterone*. Aldosterone helps to regulate the amounts of *sodium* and potassium found in the body. One of the functions of cortisol is to accelerate the conversion of proteins to glucose
- medulla – the inner part of the gland which produces the hormone *adrenaline*. Adrenaline prepares the body for the 'fight, fright and flight' response. This is the way in which the body responds during times of crisis, fear and danger. (See *endocrine system*.)

adrenaline (epinephrine) is the hormone which is produced in the medulla of the adrenal gland. It causes the body to respond physiologically to the effects of stress and sets up the 'fight, fright and flight' response. When adrenaline is produced in large amounts during times of crisis it has the following effects on the body:
- the skin becomes pale, because the blood vessels under the surface of the skin constrict and blood is diverted from the surface; this enables more *blood* to be supplied to the *muscles*
- *blood pressure* increases, the *heart* beats faster and more blood is pumped round the body
- the *liver* releases some of its stored *carbohydrate* to supply energy
- the pupils dilate.

adrenocorticotrophic hormone (ACTH): a *hormone* which controls the secretion of corticosteroid hormones from the *adrenal glands*. It is synthesised and stored in the anterior *pituitary gland*.

adulthood is a stage of life. It occurs when a person is fully developed and matured and has reached the full legal age, i.e. 18 years of age. It can be broken down into different stages such as:
- early adulthood (18–45 years)
- middle adulthood (46–64 years)
- later adulthood (65+ years).

advice: information which supports clients, service users and their carers. Advice may be given through advice centres. Such centres can be established by *statutory*, private and voluntary organisations which may also include friends, family or an informal caring network.

Advice can be offered through libraries, hospitals, town halls or other agencies such as the *Citizens Advice Bureau*. Advice centres have major roles in ensuring that information and advice is available to the general public.

advocacy: a procedure whereby a health and social care worker can speak or act on a client's, service user's or patient's behalf. The role of an advocate is to ensure that a person's rights and interests are represented. There are different types of advocate:

- citizen advocate – an unpaid member of the community, i.e. a member of a support group, a neighbour or volunteer
- volunteer advocate – an unpaid person who may receive expenses. Voluntary advocacy involves partnership with the person, focusing on specific tasks
- legal advocate – a legally qualified professional such as a solicitor
- professional casework advocate – a social care worker with a caseload of people that he or she supports. The person is usually a team-based paid worker. Each case is a partnership which is task-based with targets
- self-advocate – a person represents themselves
- formal advocate – an advocacy scheme set up by a volunteer or support group which is not user-led. It is usually managed by a voluntary service provider such as *SCOPE*
- peer advocate – may be a citizen advocate or active user of a service.

aerobic capacity: the capacity of the cardiopulmonary system, i.e. a measure of the way in which the *heart* and *lungs* function to supply oxygen to the tissues.

aerobic exercises: activities which result in physical exertion. These exercises are aimed at increasing oxygen consumption to benefit the *lungs* and *cardiovascular system*. Activities such as running, swimming and skipping are aerobic exercises.

aerobic respiration: respiration in which oxygen is used to oxidise food to carbon dioxide and water. There is a high yield of energy. The process is in two stages:

- *Glycolysis* – which does not require oxygen and takes place in the cell cytoplasm. It involves the conversion of glucose into pyruvic acid.
- *Krebs cycle* – which occurs only in aerobic respiration and takes place in the cell *mitochondria*. It is a complex cycle of enzyme-catalysed reactions in which pyruvic acid is oxidised to *carbon dioxide* and water, with the production of large amounts of energy.

aetiology is the science which investigates the causes of *disease*. For example, the aetiology of *typhoid fever* involves studying the causative agent, an organism called *Salmonella typhi*, which is found in contaminated water supplies containing sewage.

affection: the feeling of love, goodwill and kindness which a person shows to another. It is an important aspect of caring for others. For example, children need affection and love to promote their emotional growth and build their *self-esteem*. (See *emotional development*.)

after-school club: a place for children to go after the school day has finished but adult work hours haven't, usually from around 3.30pm to 6pm. The club may be in a child's school, another local school or different premises altogether. Sometimes *play workers* will escort children from the school to the club. The children are cared for by care workers who provide activities such as *creative play* with art and crafts, *games* and sports. A breakfast club can also be provided so that children can be dropped off before school and enjoy breakfast together. In the school holidays a holiday play scheme would operate, offering groups of children a range of organised activities as well as outings. They are usually open from 8.30am to 6pm. The clubs are registered and inspected by **OFSTED**. (See **out-of-school care**.)

age: stage of development in the life of a human being. This involves a number of processes and changes which take place in the body as it ages. (See also **ageing**.)

Age Concern – the National Council on Ageing: a voluntary organisation which works to improve the **quality of life** for the country's 12 million older people. It provides opportunities for the active and the able, as well as the frail and vulnerable. It is the centre of a network of 1100 local organisations and 180,000 **volunteers** offering a wide range of community-based services, including **day centres**, lunch clubs, home visiting and transport. Nationally, Age Concern supports this work through the provision of information and advice, policy analysis, publications, and grants towards training for the improvement of the quality of services for older people. It works closely with partner organisations in the UK, Europe and internationally, and is committed to teaching and research through the Age Concern Institute of Gerontology at King's College London. Age Concern is an organisation which campaigns actively on behalf of older people. (See **Employment Equality (Age) Regulations 2006**.)

age of consent: the age at which an individual can give their permission for any activity, treatment or therapy. Some examples which are covered by legislation include:
- 16 years of age – age of consent for heterosexual intercourse – 17 years in Northern Ireland
- 16 years of age – age of consent for **homosexual** intercourse – 17 years in Northern Ireland
- 16 years of age – age of consent for treatment.

Under the **Children Act 1989**, young people have the right to consent or to refuse consent to medical treatment (e.g. **immunisations**) provided such young people are deemed to be of an age or ability to make their own informed choice.

age profile: a method of looking at the structure of the population and predicting future trends. For example, increasing **life expectancy** is likely to lead to more people needing long-term care. (See **demography**.)

age structure and population: the way in which the ages of individuals are distributed in the national, international or global population. In the United Kingdom the age structure in the population has changed in the last 30 years. These changes include:
- an increase in the proportion of older people, particularly those over 75 years of age
- a decrease in the proportion of young people under 16 years old. (See **demography**.)

ageing: changes which occur in the body through the different stages of **human growth and development**. This process begins at **fertilisation** and continues throughout the life span to the end of a person's life which is **death**. Following conception the **foetus** grows and develops. After **birth** the changes occurring are part of the ageing process. The ageing process includes:
- rapid growth and development which take place in the early years of childhood
- physical changes which occur during **puberty**. The secretion of hormones leads to the development of secondary sexual characteristics in boys and girls
- changes in the chemical reactions in the body, e.g. the **basal metabolic rate (BMR)** which is affected by age. For instance, young people are able to take far more strenuous exercise and cope with a higher metabolic rate than most people in their seventies

- a decline in biological functioning, e.g. in females between the ages of 45 and 55 the reproductive system is affected by a reduction in **hormone** levels. This is called the **menopause**. For men at this age there are also some changes in the *reproductive system*. Other changes include loss of muscle elasticity, stiffness in bones and joints, slowing down of different functions such as those relating to the gastrointestinal system, e.g. constipation.

Effects of ageing include:

- increased isolation as a result of mobility problems, decreased income, decreasing motivation and loss of self-esteem
- increased dependency on others as a result of ill health and lack of self-confidence
- inability to cope as a result of confusion, dementia and mental health disorders which can lead to a breakdown in communication
- changes in role and lifestyle due to retirement and reduced income
- changes in health care needs and an increased need for formal and informal care. (See **caring**.)

There are a range of other factors which may be affected by the ageing process such as **education, employment, leisure**, recreation, **social class** and **status**.

Effects of ageing

Systems	Effects of ageing	Results
Digestive system including stomach, large and small intestines, liver, pancreas and rectum	Muscles become less efficient, so it becomes more difficult to push food along the alimentary canal	Constipation, bowel cancer, loss of appetite, weight loss
Eyes and ears	Vision and hearing impairment, i.e. affects the ability to see without glasses, and to hear	Long-sightedness, short-sightedness, formation of cataracts. Deafness which can affect communication as the older person cannot hear what is being said
Hair	Loses colour and hair loss	Grey hair and baldness especially in men
Heart and cardiovascular system	The function of the heart becomes less efficient in pumping the blood around the body	Less blood being circulated which can result in the organs of the body being less efficient. This can affect circulation and lead to hardening of the arteries, it can also affect walking and breathing
Heat regulating system	Body becomes less efficient at maintaining its body temperature	Can feel the cold and when atmospheric temperature drops can be prone to hypothermia

Systems	Effects of ageing	Results
Immune system	Body is less able to fight infection	Vulnerable to infection. Healing of cuts and wounds take longer
Lungs and air passages	An older person breathes in less air	Leads to breathlessness on exertion
Metabolism	Chemical reactions and the rate at which the body uses food slows down	Loss of energy, tiredness and lethargy
Musculoskeletal system	Muscles become less flexible and mobile and bones become brittle	Falls, fractures, arthritis, osteoporosis, changes in posture
Reproductive system	Menopause in women and decreased sperm count in men	Loss of sex drive and in men loss of fertility
Skin	Skin loses elasticity	Wrinkles
Urinary system	Less efficient kidneys and loss of elasticity in the bladder	Bladder capacity reduces with the need to pass urine more frequently
Mental and psychological health	Short-term memory affected, finds change difficult, changes in social role, amount of income, lifestyle and health status	Forgetfulness, confusion, finds it harder to cope with problems. Can lead to a decrease in social contact and social isolation

ageing theories: theories which describe the processes and patterns of development which affect older people. These are:

- disengagement – promotes the idea that as elderly people grow older, they withdraw from society and decrease their involvement in social activities. This can lead to a greater preoccupation with themselves as they feel less inclined to form new relationships and to interact with those they do not know
- activity – promotes the idea that older people who can adapt their activities to their age and who maintain their leisure pursuits and hobbies are more able to establish new roles and social relationships, and grow older with more positive *self-esteem*
- social creation of dependency – promotes the idea that, as people grow older, they become more dependent. When people retire their incomes decrease and there is a notion that they are more reliant on the state benefit system for support. This develops the view that social change in old age creates poverty, social isolation and dependency.

ageism: *discrimination* against or unfair treatment of individuals on the basis of their *age*. For instance when a person applies for a job they may not be considered as suitable for that post because they are over 50 years of age. Any language which is used to discriminate against people on the basis of age can be viewed as ageist, for example language which characterises older people as being inactive, sick and dependent. (See *Employment Equality (Age) Regulations 2006*.)

agnosia: a disorder occurring when the information from the sensory nerves is not properly interpreted in the sensory cortex of the *brain*. Auditory agnosia affects the ears and tactile agnosia affects the skin.

agranulocytosis: the reduction of *white blood cells* or granulocytes due to *disease*, an adverse reaction to medication, or as a result of *radiotherapy*. This condition may be evident during *chemotherapy* for cancer. Chemotherapy kills off the cancer cells but also destroys white cells in the process.

AIDS: see *acquired immune deficiency syndrome (AIDS)*.

aids and adaptations are used by individuals to enable them to increase, regain or retrain their ability to carry out the necessary tasks to support their daily lives, improve their *independence* and enable them to care for themselves. An example is special equipment used to help a person with severe rheumatoid *arthritis* to cook, clean, dress and undress. Stairs can be adapted to fit a chair lift. (See *activities of daily living, occupational therapists, Zimmer frame, callipers.*)

air: the mixture of gases which makes up the atmosphere. It consists of approximately:
- 78% nitrogen
- 21% oxygen
- 1% carbon dioxide and the five rare gases – argon, xenon, neon, krypton and helium.

air passages: the passages found in the nose and nasal cavities, the mouth, trachea, the bronchi and bronchioles. The bronchioles end in the *alveoli* of the *lungs*. These passages carry air which is breathed into the lungs and carry air, which is breathed out, back to the atmosphere. The trachea has a lining of ciliated *epithelial* cells. Mucus-secreting cells trap any particles of dust or dirt and the cilia sweep the mucus with the trapped dust to the back of the throat where it is swallowed, thus preventing dust entering the *lungs*.

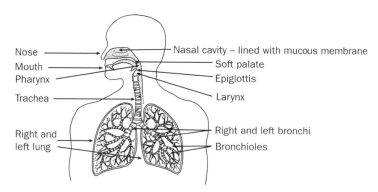

Air passages

air pollution: contamination of the air by potentially harmful substances; for example, the fumes from oil and petrol given off by motor vehicles can be harmful to humans. (See *environment*.)

alcohol (ethanol) is a depressant drug that is taken as a drink. It may be viewed by individuals in society as a means whereby they can:

- enjoy a 'better social life'; after a few drinks they feel more confident as alcohol depresses the nervous system and produces a sense of relaxation and calm
- enjoy a 'better sex life'; it is believed to be an aphrodisiac; however, it has been proved to have the opposite effect, increasing the desire but dulling sexual performance.

There are widely publicised safe drinking limits for men and women. These advise no more than 14 units of alcohol per week for women and up to 21 units per week for men, where one unit represents a half pint of beer, a small glass of wine, or one measure of sherry or whisky. Drinking above such limits could seriously affect a person's health. It can cause:

- psychological and physical *dependence* – people become 'problem drinkers'
- increase in violence – there are links between violence and alcohol
- dangerous driving – people who drink and drive are more likely to have accidents
- serious effects on a person's health – on damage to the heart, brain, liver, kidneys and digestive system.

Alcoholics Anonymous was set up in 1935 in New York. It is a voluntary fellowship of men and women who are/were alcoholic who help each other to achieve and maintain sobriety by sharing experiences and giving mutual *support*.

aldosterone: a hormone secreted by the *adrenal glands* which functions in the *kidney* and is responsible for maintaining sodium and potassium levels in the blood. It aids water balance in the body.

Alexander technique: a complementary therapy which enables the individual to become more aware of balance (see *ears*), *posture* and movement. Individuals are taught to use their muscles more efficiently. It is based on the theory that *ill health*, injury and pain can be due to the physical aspects of the body being out of balance. (See *complementary and alternative medicine*.)

alimentary canal: a long tube which runs from the mouth at one end of the body to the anus at the other. The alimentary canal has a number of different functions. These are:

- ingestion – taking food into the mouth
- *digestion* – breaking large insoluble molecules like starch and *protein* into smaller soluble ones like glucose and *amino acids*
- absorption – the process by which the soluble molecules resulting from digestion pass through the wall of the alimentary canal into the body
- assimilation – the process whereby simple soluble food materials are incorporated into the *cells* and are either built up into complex materials or broken down for *energy* release
- egestion – the removal of waste material from the gut in the form of faeces.

The main regions of the alimentary canal are the oesophagus, stomach, duodenum, ileum, colon and rectum (see diagram overleaf).

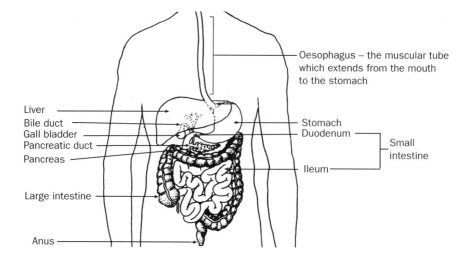

Alimentary canal

allergies are reactions by the *immune system* to different substances. These can be:
- airborne, e.g. pollen, dust mites, mould spores, feathers and animal hair
- food, e.g. eggs, fish, nuts and fruit.

During an allergic reaction, the body releases a chemical called histamine in response to the allergen. Skin tests can be carried out to check for whatever is causing the allergy.

alveolus: (plural alveoli) one of the many air sacs in the lungs where *gaseous exchange* takes place. The alveoli are lined with very thin, flat cells known as squamous epithelial cells. A number of adaptations make the alveoli efficient gas exchange surfaces:
- the walls of the alveoli are very thin so that there is minimum resistance to the diffusion of gases from one side to the other
- there is a very large number of alveoli and these provide considerable surface area over which *diffusion* can take place
- the alveoli are in close association with an extensive system of blood capilliaries; there is a difference in the concentration of respiratory gases either side of the alveolar wall. This difference is kept as high as possible so oxygen is continually being removed by combining with haemoglobin in the blood in the capillaries to form oxyhaemoglobin. (See *gaseous exchange*.)

The air in the alveoli is regularly replaced by the ventilation mechanisms of breathing.

Alzheimer's disease: a neurological disorder which has serious *degenerative* effects on an individual. These effects include:
- difficulty in remembering recent events – leading to confusion and forgetfulness
- developing disorientation – leading to increasing confusion, an inability to recognise people or places
- episodes of hallucinations – leading to the seeing of objects or individual people that are not there
- paranoia, leading to feelings of anger, or feelings that they are being watched
- violent mood swings.

Alzheimer's disease results in patients losing the ability to care for themselves and to carry out daily activities such as washing, dressing, eating meals, reading and writing. Possible causes include *genetic* inheritance, abnormal deposits of protein in the brain or the inhalation of environmental toxins. (See also *dementia, Admiral Nurse Service*.)

ambulance service: a service which deals with emergency (999) calls to road traffic collisions, general accidents, major disasters and to people who become suddenly ill or injured. The service also deals with non-urgent cases such as taking patients and clients to and from hospitals and *day centres*.

ambulance trusts: provide emergency access to health care and in some areas they also provide transport to enable patients to get to hospital for treatment. There are 11 ambulance trusts covering England.

amino acids: the basic components of *protein* molecules. Hundreds of amino acids are linked together by peptide bonds to form long chains of peptides, polypeptides and proteins. Of the hundred amino acids that occur in nature, twenty-three are the building blocks of human proteins. The arrangement of amino acids determines the type of protein molecule.

Proteins are broken down into amino acids as part of the process of *digestion*. Amino acids then enter cells where they are built back up into the types of protein which the body requires, for example muscle fibres or plasma proteins. Any excess amino acids are broken down by a process of deamination in the *liver*. During deamination the amino groups are broken off, one at a time and ammonia is formed. Ammonia enters the ornithine cycle, in which it reacts with carbon dioxide to form urea. This urea is taken to the *kidneys* and excreted.

Amnesty International: an organisation which investigates reports of *abuse* and torture suffered by individuals in different parts of the world. It is a *pressure group* which works on behalf of global *human rights* including the rights of political prisoners. It is also a charity which depends on voluntary contributions to maintain its activities.

amniocentesis: a technique carried out on a pregnant woman to enable genetic screening of a *foetus* inside the womb. *Ultrasound* is used to determine the precise position of the foetus and the *placenta* within the *uterus*. A fine needle is then inserted through the abdominal wall into the amniotic cavity. A sample of amniotic fluid is removed. This will contain some foetal cells which can be examined for any defect in the chromosomes. Amniocentesis is used to detect a range of diseases, disorders or dysfunctions which may be affecting the foetus (e.g. *Down's syndrome*).

amnion: one of the membranes that surrounds a developing *foetus* in the *uterus* of its mother. The cells making up the amnion secrete amniotic fluid which fills the space between the membrane and the foetus. This fluid provides protection and support for the delicate foetal tissues. (See *foetal growth and development*.)

amphetamines: (street names: pep pills, speed) *drugs* which act as stimulants to the *central nervous system*. These drugs are used to treat different medical conditions and sometimes to reduce weight as part of a slimming programme. Tolerance to amphetamines can develop rapidly, leading to *dependence*.

amylase: an *enzyme* which digests starch. Amylase breaks down starch into soluble sugars by means of hydrolysis (a chemical process which involves the addition of water).

Salivary amylase is found in saliva and pancreatic amylase is found in pancreatic juices. (See also *digestion*.)

anaemia: a condition in which there is a reduced amount of *haemoglobin* in the blood. People suffering from anaemia tire easily. They have pale skin and get out of breath if they exert themselves. Causes of anaemia include:

● a shortage of iron in the diet – iron is an important part of haemoglobin molecules

● conditions which lead to a loss of blood – these may be due to accidents or the development of disorders such as ulcers which bleed over a period of time

● conditions which result in the destruction of *red blood cells* – an example is *sickle-cell disorder*, an inherited disease in which the affected person has a type of haemoglobin which is less efficient at transporting oxygen than normal haemoglobin; the red blood cells of someone with this condition also have a shorter lifespan than normal red blood cells.

anaerobic respiration is a form of respiration which takes place in the absence of oxygen.

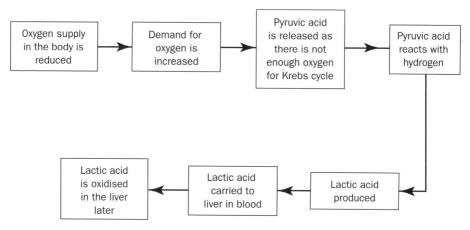

Anaerobic respiration

anatomy: the study of different parts of the body and the structural relationships between them. This is linked to *physiology*.

angiogram: an *X-ray examination* of *blood* vessels using a dye that is opaque to X-rays. An example is cardiac catheterisation which is an examination of the blood vessels surrounding the *heart*.

anorexia nervosa: an *eating disorder* which is characterised by severe weight loss. It is particularly common in young adolescent girls who have a fear of becoming fat. Signs and symptoms include:

● obsession with food and eating, not eating large amounts, feeling very uncomfortable about eating anything which might be fattening (fussy eaters)

● over-activity and an obsession with *exercise*

● continuing weight loss to a dramatic and life-threatening degree

● excessive tiredness and weakness

● cessation of *menstruation* due to *hormone* imbalance

● fine hair covering the body (called lanugo); the hair on the head thins.

About 50% of all patients need hospital treatment, and 5–10% die from starvation. (See also *bulimia nervosa, eating disorders*.)

antagonistic muscles are *muscles* which produce opposing effects to enable movement to take place. An example of antagonistic muscle action is that of the biceps and triceps muscles of the arm. When the biceps contracts to bend the arm the triceps muscle relaxes. When the triceps muscle contracts to straighten the arm the biceps muscle relaxes.

Muscles are called either flexor or extensor muscles depending on their function.

- Flexor muscles pull two parts of a limb towards each other, e.g. contraction of the biceps muscles causes the arm to bend.
- Extensor muscles pull two parts of a limb away from each other, e.g. contraction of the triceps muscle straightens the arm.

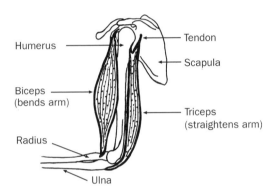

Antagonistic muscles

antenatal: the period of time when the *foetus* is growing in the *uterus* of the mother. Developments are closely monitored by a medical team which includes the GP, the obstetrician, the *midwife* and the health visitor.

antibody: a *blood* protein produced in lymphoid *tissue*. Antibody production is a response to the presence of foreign substances, for example bacteria, viruses or other antigenic substances. Antibodies circulate in the *plasma* and attack the *antigen* making it harmless to the body. Every antibody produced is specific to a particular antigen. (See *immunity*.)

anti-discrimination policies: policies which are put together as part of a framework for good practice in organisations. They serve as a deterrent to *discrimination* against individuals on the basis of age, class, culture, gender, health status, HIV status, marital status, cognitive ability, mental health, offending background, physical ability, place of origin, political beliefs, race, religion, sensory ability and sexual orientation. Gender, race and disability policies are supported by legislation.

(See also *Sex Discrimination Acts 1975 and 1986, Race Relations Acts 1976 and 2000, Disability Discrimination Act 1995 and 2005, Employment Equality (Age) Regulations 2006, Civil Partnership Act 2004.*)

anti-discriminatory practice: action which is taken to prevent discrimination against people on the grounds of race, class, gender, disability, sexual orientation, etc. It promotes equality as a result of the introduction of **anti-discrimination policies** in the workplace (e.g. **care settings**). It is also known as anti-oppressive practice. It promotes the principles of anti-discrimination by:

- applying the **care value base** in all practice
- balancing the individual rights of an individual service user with the rights of others
- dealing sensitively with conflicts if and when they arise
- identifying when discrimination is present and challenging that discrimination
- putting the service user at the centre of service provision and ensuring that their care supports their culture, individual rights and choices, personal preferences and beliefs
- supporting diversity and tolerating differences
- working within legal policies and guidelines.

anti-diuretic hormone (ADH): a hormone which is produced in the posterior lobe of the **pituitary** gland. It increases the reabsorption of water in the renal tubules of the **kidneys** leading to less water being lost in the **urine**.

anti-social behaviour: behaviour that does not conform to that which is considered normal or the 'norm' by certain groups of people in society. An example of this is a person shouting obscenities at people walking past them in the street oblivious to the effect that they are having, and the fear and uncertainty that they are promoting. Anti-social behaviour has increased in society with more violence on the streets and more drunkenness in public places.

Anti-Social Behaviour Act 2003: an Act of Parliament which addresses **anti-social behaviour**. It deals with different issues which have been causes for concern in local communities. These include:

- gang activity amongst young people leading to increasing violence on the streets
- public drunkenness, which is on the increase, especially at weekends in city centres
- making false reports of an emergency which causes disruption to emergency services
- graffiti has been identified with anti-social behaviour because of the damage caused to properties. As a result, councils have been given authority to ban the sale of spray paint.

antigen: a foreign substance, chemical, bacteria or virus which enters the body and provokes an immune response. (See **antibody**.)

antitoxin: a type of **antibody** produced by the body to counteract a toxin or poison formed by a bacterium or **virus** which has entered the body.

anxiety: a normal reaction to **stress** or to a situation which poses a threat or uncertainty. Anxiety can also occur in discrete panic attacks when the person is feeling nervous and helpless. However, anxiety can become a focus of a person's life when they worry and feel fearful about everyday situations. The anxiety in these cases can lead to a psychological disorder called neurosis. Anxiety also produces physical symptoms such as dizziness, headaches, tremors, lack of concentration, diarrhoea and breathlessness.

aorta: the main **artery** in the body. Other arteries branch off from it to supply **blood** to all the organs in the body. The walls of the aorta contain baroreceptors which monitor the **blood pressure** and chemoreceptors which monitor the amount of chemical compounds in the blood.

aortography: an *X-ray examination* of the aorta. This procedure involves the injection of a radio-opaque dye into the aorta. X-rays are taken and any defect, *disease* or degeneration is shown up.

Apgar score: a scoring system which is used to assess the general health of a baby immediately after birth. A maximum of two points is given for each of the following signs measured at one minute and five minutes after delivery. The features recorded are:

- breathing and type of breathing
- heart rate
- colour, the healthy appearance of the baby's skin
- muscle tone
- response to stimuli such as light.

aphagia: the inability to swallow. This can be life threatening in situations such as choking. However, the loss of the ability to swallow can also be a symptom of severe anxiety.

aphasia: the loss of the power of speech due to a defect or disorder affecting the speech centre which is situated in the cerebrum of the *brain*.

aphonia: the loss of the power of speech due to a localised problem of the throat or mouth. Such problems can include any disease of the nerves and muscles which affects the production or articulation of speech.

appendix: a small tubular organ which is attached to the end of the caecum. It is composed of lymphoid tissue and does not have any known function. It can become infected and inflamed (appendicitis). The treatment for appendicitis is the surgical removal of the appendix under general anaesthetic. Appendicitis requires immediate treatment as it can cause an abscess or generalised peritonitis (inflammation of the lining of the *abdomen*).

approved social worker: a *social worker* who has been specially trained in the area of *mental health*. An approved social worker is one of the professionals who is required to carry out an *assessment* of a client, taking into account all the circumstances of the individual. They are required to consider the least restrictive options for care and treatment of clients, while retaining the decision for compulsory admission to hospital under the *Mental Health Act 2007*.

aromatherapy: a *complementary therapy* which uses essential oils and hydrosols (the water-soluble part of a plant or flower) to promote personal health. Essential oils are concentrated essences extracted from plants and flowers. The healing and therapeutic uses of such oils are achieved either by inhalation or by direct application on to the body using *massage*. Examples of essential oils used in aromatherapy are:

- rosemary – a decongestant oil
- rose – a calming oil
- peppermint – an oil to relieve nausea
- lavender – an oil to relieve insomnia.

arrhythmia: a deviation from the normal rhythm of the *heart*. The normal rhythm is called sinus rhythm. Arrhythmia can include extra or ectopic beats and rapid heart rate (tachycardia). However, it is important to remember that there is a normal variation to the heart beat which speeds up slightly on breathing in (inspiration) and slows down on breathing out (expiration).

art therapy: the use of art as a means whereby individuals learn to express themselves through drawing, painting and modelling. It helps people to release their tensions and stress and promotes positive *self-esteem*.

arteries: blood vessels which carry *blood* away from the *heart*. Arteries have a lining composed of *epithelial cells* (endothelial layer). The walls of the arteries are very thick and contain a large amount of elastic tissue and muscle. When the ventricles of the heart contract, blood at high pressure is forced into the arteries. This causes the walls to stretch. When *ventricular* contraction stops, the pressure of the blood falls and the elastic tissue contracts. This stretching and contraction of the elastic tissue in the artery walls helps to even out *blood flow* throughout the body. (See *cardiac cycle*.)

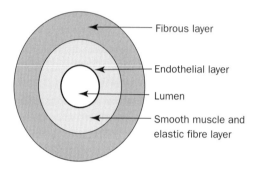

Fibrous layer

Endothelial layer

Lumen

Smooth muscle and elastic fibre layer

A section of an artery

arteriole: a vessel which takes *blood* from the smaller *arteries* to the *capillaries*. Arterioles are very small in diameter and, like all blood vessels, have a lining of epithelial cells. Their walls contain large numbers of muscle fibres. Many arterioles also have rings of muscle called sphincter muscles where they join with the capillaries. By contraction of the muscle fibres in the walls and the sphincter muscles, the blood supply to particular capillary networks can be regulated to meet the needs of each part of the body.

arthritis: a disease which attacks the *joints* of the body causing damage and discomfort. It is closely associated with rheumatism which is a general term used to cover aches and pains in the body. There are two main types of arthritis:

- Rheumatoid arthritis is a condition characterised by inflammation of the joints especially of the hands and feet. It can also affect the knees, elbows, hips and other joints in the body. The patient or client complains of pain and lack of movement in the joints. As the disease progresses the joints become more enlarged and disfigured due to the formation of granulation tissue which limits movement and attacks the *cartilage* at the end of the bones. This causes deterioration of the muscles.
- Osteoarthritis is a degenerative disease affecting the cartilage in the joints causing deterioration. As the cartilage is destroyed new bone grows in its place leading to increasing pain and stiffness. The hips, knees and spine are mostly affected causing lack of mobility.

arthrography: a procedure using X-rays to examine the *joints*. This involves injecting a radio-opaque dye into the joint space. It shows up the outline and contents of the joint and any disease or dysfunction which may be affecting this part of the body.

artificial respiration: an emergency procedure which maintains a flow of oxygen into and out of a person's lungs when the normal and natural breathing reflexes are insufficient. The best-known method of artificial respiration is mouth-to-mouth ventilation or resuscitation. (See *ABC of resuscitation*.)

artificial resuscitation: procedures which are used to revive a person from an unconscious state or possible death. In hospitals, artificial resuscitation may take the form of cardiac massage, manually giving heart resuscitation and or the use of electric shock treatment or defibrillation to restore the heart beat. The heart muscle must be revived within three to five minutes or permanent brain damage can occur. (See *ABC of resuscitation*.)

Asperger syndrome: a disorder which shares many of the same characteristics as *autism*. Certain traits such as clumsiness are typical in those suffering with Asperger syndrome. The key characteristics are:
- difficulty with social relationships – unlike those affected by autism, some who suffer with Asperger syndrome try hard to be sociable. They find it difficult, however, to understand non-verbal signals, including facial expressions
- clumsiness – difficulty with co-ordination skills
- difficulty with *communication* – those with Asperger syndrome may speak very fluently but may not take much notice of the listener's reaction; they may talk on regardless of the listener's interest and may appear insensitive to their feelings.

Despite having competent language skills, sufferers may sound over-precise and take words too literally. They can learn facts and figures but find it difficult to think in abstract ways. They may develop obsessive interests in hobbies or collections. Sufferers may feel secure with their routines and prefer to order their day in a set pattern. (See *autism*.)

asphyxia or suffocation: a life-threatening condition in which oxygen is prevented from reaching tissues in the body due to obstruction or damage to parts of the *respiratory system*.

assertive skills are developed to deal with and cope with certain social situations. They are based on the ability to control emotions and confront difficult circumstances in a calm and reasonable way. Health and social care workers often train in assertiveness to help them in their work with different client groups. (See *communication, strategies for effective communication*.)

assessment: a method used to determine the different needs of a client, patient or service user. It is an important part of setting up a *care plan* as part of the *care management* process. The types of assessment which can be applied to different client groups and care settings are as follows:
- initial assessment – at the beginning of a period of care such as within a care plan or in the case of a child with *safeguarding* issues
- medical assessment – a specific examination by a doctor for a definite purpose, e.g. a court request or as part of a *child health surveillance programme*. Medical assessment of a client may include recommendations for a client's ongoing care
- development assessment – an objective assessment of a client, often to some agreed protocol or method of treatment to be carried out by a doctor, *health visitor* or *psychologist*, for the purpose of determining a child's developmental progress, or a client's *daily living skills*

- *special education needs* assessment – a requirement when a child is in need of support for their learning
- health assessment – an examination undertaken by a health visitor or school nurse to ascertain a child's health status. The health assessment will include information on height and weight, *immunisation*, vision and hearing
- comprehensive assessment – a structured time-limited exercise to collect and evaluate information about clients and their families on which to base long-term decisions, for example assessment of an older person with regard to their long-term care
- family assessment – a report prepared over a period of time to assess the functioning of a particular family in relation to the needs of a child. The assessment is usually undertaken by a *social worker* but may be undertaken by a psychologist or *family support worker*.

assessment of need: assessment to determine the specific needs of the service user as part of their *care plan* or as part of their ongoing treatment and support within the *care management* process.

assessment tools: materials or resources used to gather information as part of the *assessment* process. These include *observation* records, forms, checklists, diaries recorded by the *health and social care worker* and the service user, questioning, personal history flow chart and discussions.

assist describes the role of carers when they support clients or someone else in a particular activity.

association area: a part or area of the cerebral cortex in the *brain*, which is responsible for receiving sensory impulses and for starting the motor impulses. The *neurones* which link these impulses are called association fibres.

Association for Real Change: (formerly the Association of Residential Care) an organisation which exists to promote the quality of life, maintenance of standards and diversity of residential and day care provision for people with *learning disabilities*. It is a *pressure group* which provides support including:
- a national voice for all members
- a code of good practice to promote professional standards
- access to expertise and support on a local and national level.

Association of Workers for Children with Emotional and Behavioural Difficulties: a voluntary group which was set up to support children with behaviour difficulties and their families. The aims of the group are to:
- voice their concern on behalf of children and young people with emotional and behavioural difficulties and those who work with them
- offer support to the parents and workers involved with children suffering from attention deficit hyperactivity disorder
- promote publicly the belief that the needs of children and adolescents with emotional and behavioural difficulties should be identified and supported.

(See also *attention deficit hyperactivity disorder*.)

assumption: a pre-judgement about a person or situation. It relates to *attitude* formation. In health and social care, it should be part of *anti-discriminatory practice* not to make pre-judgements or assumptions about service users, clients, patients and colleagues. (See also *stereotyping*.)

asthma: an obstructive disease of the bronchial airways. This may be caused by a trigger response in the airways leading to constriction of the muscles, inflammation and oedema (collection of fluid) in the bronchioles and an increased production of mucus. The asthmatic person begins to cough, starts wheezing and complains of a tight chest and breathlessness. There are a number of triggers or irritants which can cause asthma:

- *allergies*, e.g. dust, animals, food
- *environment*, e.g. changing weather condition/smoky atmosphere
- *infections*, e.g. colds, sore throats
- *stress*, e.g. *anxiety* about exams
- *hormones*, e.g. during the pre-menstrual period
- air temperature, e.g. weather, either cold or hot and dry
- medicines, e.g. aspirin.

astigmatism: a defect in the function of the eye. An abnormal curvature of the cornea and lens causes astigmatism. As a result the visual image is distorted because not all the light rays can focus on the retina. Astigmatism can be corrected by using cylindrical lenses in spectacles. These lenses effectively refract the light in one plane only.

ataxia: abnormal or unsteady movements in the limbs of the body. This is the result of damage or injury to the cerebellum, the part of the brain responsible for balance. There are different causes of ataxia such as alcoholism, brain tumours, *multiple sclerosis* and thyroid disease. (See also *Friedreich's ataxia*.)

atheroma: the formation of fatty deposits or plaques on the inner lining of the *arteries*. This causes degeneration and thickening of the artery. When the atheroma is extensive the inner lining of the artery may become rough and the *blood flow* in the artery turbulent. A clot or thrombosis may form and the whole vessel then becomes blocked so that blood flow is cut off. Atheroma occurring in the heart or brain is likely to result in death. Factors which contribute to atheroma and atherosclerosis include smoking, high *blood pressure* and high *cholesterol* levels.

atrioventricular bundle: (bundle of His) collection of modified cardiac muscle fibres called Purkinje tissue situated in the septum of the heart between the right and left ventricle. It maintains the rhythm of the heart and the contraction of the heart or cardiac muscle.

atrioventricular node: a small area of specialised muscle in the wall of the *heart* between the atria and the ventricles. The atrio-ventricular node co-ordinates the heart beat. At the start of each beat, a wave of electrical activity spreads from the sino-atrial node or pacemaker over the walls of the atria. This brings about contraction of the atria. The muscle fibres in the atria are completely separate from those in the ventricle, except in one small area, the atrio-ventricular node. Through this node electrical activity can pass from the atria to the ventricles. There is then a short delay before the electrical activity spreads to the base of the ventricles. This delay allows emptying of the atria to be completed before the ventricles start to contract.

atrioventricular valve: this is situated between the atrium and the ventricle. There is one valve on either side of the *heart*. These valves are made of fibrous tissue and are opened and closed by *blood pressure*. During the *cardiac cycle*, when the pressure in the atrium is higher than that in the ventricle, the valve is open and blood is able to flow through into the ventricle. During ventricular systole, the muscle in the wall of the ventricle starts to contract and the pressure of the blood in the ventricle rises. As a result, the valve shuts so that blood is pumped out leaving the heart through the arteries, preventing any backflow of blood into the atria. Heart sounds can be heard when a stethoscope is placed against the chest wall. The first of these in each cycle is due to the atrioventricular valves closing. The valve on the left side of the heart has two flaps of fibrous tissue and is known as the bicuspid valve; that on the right side has three flaps and is called the tricuspid valve.

atrium: one of the two upper chambers of the *heart*. The right and left atria are relatively thin-walled and receive blood from the veins. The right atrium receives deoxygenated blood from the body, while the left atrium receives oxygenated blood from the lungs. The deoxygenated blood from the body enters the right atrium from the venae cavae; oxygenated blood from the lungs enters the left atrium via the pulmonary veins.

attachment: the early relationship which develops between an *infant* and his or her mother or primary care giver. Another term for attachment is *bonding.* (See *Bowlby.*)

attention deficit hyperactivity disorder: (ADHD) a behavioural disorder in children. The child's behaviour may be characterised in different ways such as:
- hyper- or over-activity leading to disruptive behaviour, such as fidgeting and restlessness
- an inability to concentrate
- easy distraction in play and learning tasks
- forgetful and disorganised behaviour
- short memory span
- low self-esteem leading to negative behaviour patterns.

Children with this disorder and their parents may need multidisciplinary support. Agencies may work together to produce a co-ordinated procedure so that the individual needs of the child are considered and met. (See *Association of Workers for Children with Emotional and Behavioural Difficulties*.)

attitudes: the way in which an individual organises their thoughts, *beliefs*, feelings and reactions towards themselves and others in society. Attitudes are developed through the process of *socialisation*. Fixed and inflexible attitudes can lead to categorising people and events so that individuality is not recognised. (See *stereotyping*.)

audiogram: a method of measuring an individual's hearing. Hearing is measured at different sound frequencies and results are recorded on a graph. This shows up any defects such as 'glue ear' in children. The machine used for hearing tests is called an audiometer.

Audit Commission: a public spending watchdog, a central government agency which audits the activities of local authorities and the *NHS (National Health Service)*. The Audit Commission's methods are based on the policies of *economy, efficiency and effectiveness*. Each organisation is required to conduct an annual audit and examination of their accounts. This annual audit is open to scrutiny. Such precautions are extremely important where public sector organisations are using public money. The reports by the Audit Commission relate to many issues in health and social care. Examples include:
- Are We Choosing Health? (2008) – a joint report with the Health Care Commission reviewing how well the NHS and local government are tackling issues of health improvement and health inequalities at local and national level
- Sports and Leisure, Anti-social Behaviour and Young People (2008) – a report which identifies how councils, public and private sector partners are working together through sport, leisure and developing activities to combat anti-social behaviour.

auditory impairment: see *deafness or hearing impairment*.

auditory nerve: the nerve leading from the inner ear to the brain.

auriscope: an instrument which is used by doctors or nurses to examine the eardrum and the ear canal. An auriscope enables any inflammation or infection of the eardrum to be detected and treated.

autism: a disorder which disrupts the development of social and ***communication*** skills. There is no known cause for autism. Up to 75% of those with autism have accompanying learning difficulties, but whatever their general level of ability, they share a common problem in trying to make sense of the world. The degree to which autism sufferers are affected varies but there are common characteristics:

- difficulty with social relationships – autistic children and adults often seem indifferent to other people, even to their parents. The ability to develop friendships is impaired, as is the capacity to understand other people's feelings
- difficulty with communication – autistic individuals lack the ability and understanding necessary to engage in meaningful communication. Language is slow to develop and speech patterns are affected
- those with autism find it hard to recognise or interpret messages and signals that others take for granted
- difficulty in the development of play and imagination – children with autism do not develop creative 'let's pretend' play in the way that other children do
- difficulty with change – individuals with autism often become obsessed with particular objects or behaviour, focusing on them to the exclusion of everything else. In marked contrast to these are the 'islets of ability', which some autistic individuals display; for example, some autism sufferers who may be severely disabled in most ways will display a special talent for music, art, mathematics or mechanics.

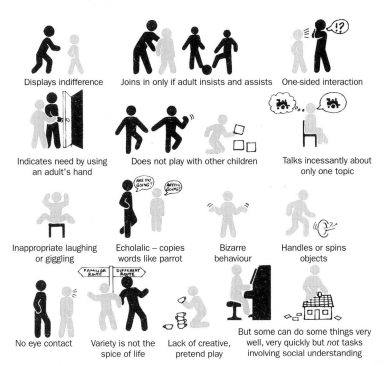

The aspects of autism

Early intervention and specialist education are vital if children with autism are to develop to their full potential. The National Autistic Society was established by parents in 1962 to encourage a better understanding of autism and to pioneer a range of appropriate services for those with autism and for those who care for them. (See also *Asperger syndrome*.)

autoimmune diseases are caused by the body when it produces antibodies which destroy normal body cells. An example of an autoimmune disease is rheumatoid arthritis. Autoimmune diseases are more common in older people.

autonomic nervous system: the part of the nervous system which controls muscles and glands but is not under conscious control. It co-ordinates mainly involuntary body activities such as digestion, blood pressure, heartbeat or pulse and peristalsis. (See *autonomic response*.)

autonomic response: a response evoked by the *autonomic nervous system*. There are two sub-divisions of the autonomic nervous system. The effect of one system counteracts and balances the effect of the other. The sympathetic system prepares for action. The parasympathetic system prepares for rest.

The *sympathetic nervous system*:
- accelerates the heart
- constricts the arterioles
- dilates bronchioles
- dilates the iris
- slows gut movements
- contracts bladder and anal sphincters
- causes contraction of the bladder
- increases sweat secretion.

The *parasympathetic nervous system*:
- slows the heart
- dilates arterioles
- constricts bronchioles
- constricts the iris
- stimulates the tear glands
- speeds up gut movement
- relaxes the bladder and anal sphincters
- inhibits sweat secretion.

autonomy: personal freedom to act and make choices in a way that a service user thinks is right for them. Individual clients should have their different rights and choices respected. This is a major factor in caring. Carers should encourage clients to be independent and to be involved in all decisions related to their care.

axon: one of the components of a *nerve cell*. The axon conducts impulses away from the nerve cell body. It is enclosed within a fatty, myelin sheath which protects the nerve fibre and speeds up the transmission of impulses.

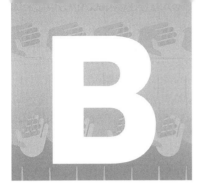

baby: see *infant*.

bacillus: a rod-shaped bacterial cell. Examples of bacilli include *Lactobacillus bulgaricus* which is found in yoghurt and **salmonella**, many species of which cause **food poisoning**.

bacteria: an important group of micro-organisms. Bacteria are small and do not have nuclei or other organelles. Some bacteria can be harmful and cause diseases such as cholera. There are different types of bacteria and they can be classified according to their different shapes. These are:
- bacilli or rod-shaped bacteria, e.g. *Salmonella typhi* which causes typhoid fever
- cocci or round bacteria, e.g. *Staphylococcus aureus* which causes boils
- spirilla or spiral shaped bacteria, e.g. *Treponema pallidum* which causes syphilis
- vibrio or curved shaped bacteria, e.g. *Vibrio cholerae* which causes cholera.

Another approach to classification which helps to identify bacteria is a technique called **Gram staining**.

Bacilli – rod-shaped   Cocci – spherical   Spirilla – corkscrew-shaped   Vibrio – curved

Types of bacteria

balance and the ear: see *ear*.

balanced diet: a diet which contains all the essential **nutrients** in the appropriate quantities for the body to grow and function efficiently. There are seven components to a healthy diet. (See **carbohydrates**, **fats**, **proteins**, **minerals** and **vitamins**.)

A balanced diet

Food component	Function	Examples of sources
Carbohydrate	Provides energy	Bread, sugar
Fat	Provides energy and insulation	Dairy products, milk, meat
Fibre	Healthy functioning of the digestive system	Vegetables, potatoes, cereals
Minerals	Maintain body metabolism	Vegetables, milk
Protein	Used for body growth and repair	Chicken, cheese, nuts, eggs
Vitamins	Maintain body metabolism	Green vegetables, fruit
Water	Supports chemical reactions in the body	Water supply

Bandura, Albert (1925–): a psychologist who claimed that the *environment* is a major force and influence in the way in which people think and behave. In experiments he was able to show that children learn from observing others. He suggested that individuals imitate and copy each other's actions and so adopt *social roles* and *behaviour*.

banning or time out: a procedure which is a form of *behaviour management* involving the exclusion of a child or young person from a play or care setting for reasons of unacceptable *behaviour*. A child should always be warned of banning in advance and the banning should always be for a fixed period of time. (See *ABC of behaviour*.)

bar chart: a chart or graph which shows a comparison between variables. It is a method used to present information and is widely used in health and social care research. An example of a bar chart used in such a research project would be one showing the number of children who attend nursery school over a period of three years. (See *histogram*.)

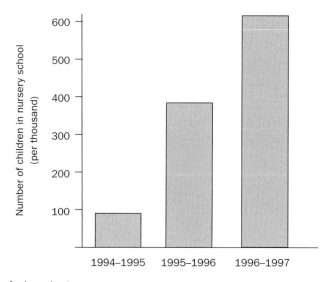

An example of a bar chart

Barnardos: a charity set up in 1866 by Dr Thomas Barnardo in response to the growing needs of young children mistreated, abused or exploited in the workplace. For many years Barnardos was associated with children's homes and orphanages, but over the last 25 years the long-stay homes have closed down. Most of the children in Barnardos were not orphans, but were placed with Barnardos either because their families were too poor to care for them, or because social attitudes at the time did not approve of mixed race, disabled and illegitimate children. Modern-day Barnardos is an organisation which tackles issues such as:

- *unemployment* and *poverty* – offering support with welfare and advice, community shops and credit unions, providing holidays for poor families
- *disability* – offering support in the form of advice and counselling, advocacy, short-term breaks, residential care, befriending clubs and supporting families with disabled children
- *foster care* and *adoption* – Barnardos is one of the UK's leading fostering and adoption agencies
- families – providing parent support, child protection, counselling and advice, parent and toddler groups, toy and book libraries and after-school and holiday activities

- *homelessness* – providing emergency accommodation, support and advice, drop-in centres which offer a service to refugees and travelling families
- advising and helping young people to develop the skills to be independent
- *HIV/AIDS* – supporting families and young people affected with HIV and AIDS through counselling, education and advice
- sexual *abuse* – offering support and counselling for abused parents, children and young abusers, helping them cope with their difficulties
- lobbying – working towards influencing public policy to highlight disadvantage and inequality.

barriers: difficulties experienced by service users in a variety of situations related to health and social care organisations.

barriers to access to health and social care services: difficulties which are experienced by clients and service users in terms of access to the health and social care services which they need. These can be due to a number of factors:
- physical access, e.g. stairs with no lift, narrow doorways limiting access for wheelchairs
- financial access, e.g. services are expensive and the client is unable to pay
- location, e.g. the service is in a geographical area which clients without transport will have difficulty in reaching
- psychological factors, e.g. clients may lack confidence and may be anxious about visiting a service
- *culture*, e.g. a client may be self-conscious because they cannot speak English very well and there is no provision in the service to accommodate this
- non-provision of services, e.g. the client may live in a rural area, where the services may be limited
- lack of knowledge/information – client may be unaware of the existence of the service.

(See also *access to services*.)

barriers to communication: difficulties which can occur when a careworker is working with clients. Barriers are put up when misunderstandings occur and individuals feel that their rights and abilities are not respected. Factors may include *attitudes* with regard to *culture, learning disabilities* and *physical disabilities*. There are common problems which arise within care practice, such as:
- lack of awareness of the needs of the client – this includes not listening to the client, not giving the client time to express themselves, no eye contact with the client, no rapport or other evidence of the carer trying to make conversation with the client. In addition to this there are no devices in place to enhance communication for those service users with sensory impairments
- lack of sensitivity during the practical care of the client – this could include carers rushing the client during bathing, not cutting their fingernails, not washing their hair, or not attending to their personal needs with gentleness. These tasks are reinforced by the carer working in silence
- the carer may use their position to control the client. An example of this is when the carer makes all the decisions for the client, decides what they should wear, where they should sit, who they should see and talks to them without waiting for a reply
- negative verbal communication towards the client – this is where the carer shouts at the client, calls them names such as stupid, silly or dirty or any term which makes the client

feel embarrassed. Such abuse may cause the client to become silent and withdrawn. This can also include using unexplained slang and medical jargon which the service user does not understand

- negative body language – this may involve the carer using non-verbal signals to communicate. This might include gestures such as rolling the eyes, not engaging in eye contact, shrugging the shoulders or wearing a worried and anxious expression
- lack of resources – which includes various communication systems for clients who have hearing and visual impairments, those who are unable to speak, those with learning disabilities, and clients where English is a second language
- physical factors – which relate to room size, furniture arrangements, decoration and number of people (see **personal space**).

The relationship between client and carer is a very important one and is a focus for all the aspects of care given to clients. Barriers to communication which are apparent and affect the health and well-being of a client should be recognised and handled by the appropriate manager. (See also **care relationship, team, care management, building confidence, strategies for effective communication**.)

barriers to effective caring: difficulties which arise within care relationships such as:
- inappropriate **attitudes** such as discrimination and **stereotyping**
- lack of motivation demonstrated by the carer in the caring process
- preoccupation with the carer's own needs, lack of caring skills.

This also includes service user barriers such as lack of status and influence, loss of **self-confidence** and **self-esteem.** (See **barriers to communication, discriminatory practice.**)

barriers to organisational culture: difficulties experienced by workers within health and social care organisations. These include:
- having to meet unrealistic deadlines and targets
- having to work within restricted resources, i.e. budgets.

basal metabolic rate (BMR): the measurement of the energy given off by the body while it is at rest. It is an indication of the way in which oxygen is taken up by the body. Before the BMR is measured, the person concerned undergoes a standardised rest period of 12–18 hours of physical and mental relaxation. No meal is eaten during this time. This ensures that the **alimentary canal** is empty before measurements are taken. 'Basal' refers to the energy required to maintain the continuing activities of the body (i.e. heart beat, respiration, kidney function). The oxygen consumed by the individual is measured for at least ten minutes and this value is converted into oxygen consumption per hour. The BMR is measured either in calories per second or joules per second.

A number of factors affect BMR, such as:
- age – the basal metabolic rate has a maximum value at about one year old. It then falls more or less continuously for the rest of a person's life
- sex – at all ages, females have a slightly lower basal metabolic rate than males
- state of nutrition – people who are undernourished tend to have a lower basal metabolic rate
- health – a fever raises the BMR
- environment – a cold environment raises the BMR
- thyroid activity – a high metabolic rate can indicate an excess of thyroid hormone; a low metabolic rate can indicate too little thyroid hormone. (See **metabolism**.)

baseline observations: the recording of certain measurements such as *temperature*, *pulse*, respiration rate and *blood pressure*. These measurements are taken by a GP, nurse or carer and recorded on a chart. They are the patient's own 'norms', against which any subsequent changes can be compared.

bases of discrimination: terms which apply to the different aspects of discrimination such as age, gender, ethnicity, disability, sexual orientation and religious belief.

basic needs: basic requirements which should be met. These include food and clean water, shelter and protection from harm, rest and sleep, stimulation, warmth and appropriate clothing, fresh air and exercise, love and affection, friendship and support. (See *Maslow*.)

behaviour: the way in which people are observed to act and conduct themselves. Behaviour often reflects *attitudes* towards certain issues and events. There are influences which affect behaviour such as low self-esteem in early years, negative self-concept, stress and an inability to cope with situations, labelling, stereotyping, discrimination, depression, relationship breakdown, addiction, bereavement, ethnicity, violence, bullying, poverty and social influences such as social class, social exclusion, and biological influences such as genetic inheritance.

behaviour management: methods and strategies used by health and social care providers to control undesirable and *challenging behaviour*. Guidelines in *behaviour* are often designed to meet the needs of clients in different health and social care provisions. They may involve *discipline* codes for clients; for example, clients learn to cope with their own negative behaviour and begin to appreciate what is acceptable. (See *behaviour modification, banning*.)

behaviour modification: a method used to teach individuals to change their negative *behaviour* by using reinforcers to produce positive behaviour. It is a way of removing the unwanted behaviour and increasing that which is socially appropriate. For instance, a child who is constantly misbehaving and distracting others in class may be given a star for the first ten minutes that they are able to work on their own without causing a distraction. This is a method of positive reinforcement to encourage acceptable behaviour in the classroom. Behaviour modification can be reinforced through a knowledge of behaviour and *learning theories*. (See *ABC of behaviour*.)

behaviour theories: theories which give an understanding of how individuals behave and therefore can provide a practitioner with different strategies on how to modify that behaviour. Behaviour theories are those which can be applied to the ability to learn behaviour and therefore provide a framework which practitioners can use in order to help an individual:
- gain more control over their feelings and behaviour and therefore give them more autonomy
- try to control their behaviour and feelings towards individuals
- look for strategies to influence their feelings and behaviour
- understand and predict their behaviour patterns (See *development theories*, *learning theories*, *ABC of behaviour*.)

Behaviour theories include:
- behaviourist theories – which are about learned behaviour and use techniques such as token systems, i.e. giving tokens for positive behaviour and using behaviour modification (see *Pavlov* and *Skinner*)
- cognitive theories – which are about how individuals think and use information in their mind and use techniques such as information processing, i.e. using the information

from the service user to help them understand the processes involved in their own thinking and to learn strategies of control over negative thought (see *Bruner*)

- humanistic theories – which are about the individual person and can be described as the person-centred approach. It uses techniques such as helping the individual to find inner resources to help them learn to come to a place of *self-actualisation* (see *Rogers*)
- psychodynamic theories – which are about the instincts that individuals are born with, and which exist in the unconscious mind. As an individual grows, they have to learn to control their instincts. Techniques used are methods of therapy or *counselling* which explore the difficulties that the individual is experiencing from the perspective of subconscious thought (see *Freud*).

behaviour therapy: any technique of *behaviour* change that is based on the procedures of *classical conditioning*. Other methods of behaviour therapy include modelling, token economics and shaping. (See *behaviour modification*.)

beliefs: thoughts, feelings, *attitudes* and *values* which enable a person to identify with the world in which they live. Beliefs may or may not have religious significance, but they are an expression of a person's *identity* and how they live their lives. In health and social care, the personal beliefs of the client should always be respected even if they conflict with the beliefs of the carer. Ethical dilemmas may be experienced when religious beliefs prohibit necessary medical intervention e.g. a blood transfusion. (See *religion*.)

benefit trap: a situation that arises from the *welfare state* concentrating on directly supporting people rather than helping people to support themselves. (See *poverty trap*.)

benefits: the *statutory* amounts of money which are issued and distributed to those members of society who need this form of support.

benign: a condition or illness which is not malignant, for example, if a tumour or growth is benign then it is not cancerous.

bereavement: the loss of a loved one through death. Bereavement affects individuals in different ways and they suffer from *grief*. In the United Kingdom every year over 600,000 people die, leaving at least 1.5 million friends and family members who suffer a major bereavement. CRUSE Bereavement Care is an organisation which was set up in 1959 to offer personal and confidential help to bereaved people and to those who care for them through counselling, information and social support groups.

Best Value is a statutory approach to service delivery which emphasises improvement. *Local authorities* have a duty to provide Best Value especially where the role of local people is a key factor in influencing service delivery. In addition to this, importance is attached to making the best use of partnerships with the private and voluntary sectors and with other public sector bodies to deliver services jointly. It requires that social care workers should:

- adopt new approaches in which they challenge accepted procedures and identify new ways of doing things
- listen to service users, and take what they say into account
- understand the links and connections that there are with other services.

Each local authority should produce an annual Best Value Performance Plan and services are reviewed every five years. Service users are expected to take part in satisfaction surveys in all areas of work including social services, and councils are expected to report on these.

Better Home Life 1996: (update of *Home Life 1984*) a *code of practice* for nursing and residential care homes. It sets out a model of good practice and describes the principles that underpin good quality care. It applies to residential *care homes*, nursing homes and, where appropriate, long-stay hospital wards and units, sheltered housing and *sheltered housing* with extra care. (See *older people*, *residential homes*.)

Beveridge Report 1942: a government report which led to the creation of the *welfare state*. The Beveridge Report identified five major problems which were affecting life in Britain. These were poverty, ignorance, disease, squalor and idleness. The report made recommendations which included the introduction of:

- a social insurance scheme to which employees paid a small sum out of their wages; they could then claim benefits through periods of unemployment, sickness and retirement (this is known as *National Insurance*)
- *benefits* paid at a flat rate regardless of any other forms of income and to be funded by a flat rate national insurance scheme
- maternity grants and benefits for widows
- a 'safety net' which was a means whereby those people not covered by an insurance scheme could have their needs met through unemployment benefit ('the dole')
- an information system to provide individuals with a knowledge of employment opportunities.

bias: the tendency to treat one group or individual in a different way to others. Bias can be either positive or negative. In positive bias, favourable treatment is shown to a group or individual. In negative bias, unfavourable behaviour is shown. Bias can reflect attitudes and prejudices towards a group or individual and in some cases leads to *discrimination*. Within health and social care, bias is actively discouraged as it does not meet the requirements of the *care value base* underpinning care practice.

biased sampling: the over-representation of one category of participants in a survey. For instance the proportion of males, females, students or people of a certain age in a sample may fail to adequately represent the population from which it is taken. There are many ways in which a researcher may unwittingly introduce *sampling* bias. These include:

- giving insufficient thought to the sampling technique being used (e.g. only choosing people who happen to be in the college canteen during a psychology or sociology or health and social care course)
- only using people who volunteer – people who volunteer to take part in a research project may not be typical
- only using students – the sample will not represent the population as a whole. (See *research, data collection*.)

bibliography: a list of books or articles that have been used in researching a subject for assignments, essays, reports or projects. It is usually included at the end of a report, essay or project. (See *referencing*.)

bile: a solution produced by the *liver* and stored in the *gall bladder*. It is a mixture of substances not all of which are involved in digestion. It aids the digestion of fats by bringing about their emulsification. Bile neutralises the acid from the stomach to help the pancreatic enzymes to work. It also contains two bile pigments, bilirubin and biliverdin, products which are a result of the breakdown of **haemoglobin**.

bile pigments: chemicals formed by the breakdown of **haemoglobin**. *Red blood cells* die after about 120 days in circulation. When this happens the haemoglobin which is contained in the cells is broken down and the waste products of this process are converted into bile pigment and excreted in *bile*.

bile salts: components of *bile* which are involved in the *digestion* and absorption of fat. Although bile does not contain any digestive *enzymes*, it does contain bile salts which aid the breakdown of fats in food. Without the presence of bile, the digestion of fats would be less efficient and there would be an increased amount of undigested fat passed out of the body in the faeces. Most of the bile salts are reabsorbed in the small intestine and transported back to the *liver* for re-use.

bilingualism: the fluent use of two languages. (See *English as a second language*.)

biochemistry: the study of the chemical processes which occur in living things.

biofeedback: a process which has been developed to control physiological responses such as heart rate, blood pressure and muscle tension. In certain situations, these responses can have negative effects on the body. For instance when a person is under *stress*, the heart beats faster, the blood pressure increases and there are generalised aches and pains. In biofeedback, the person looks at ways in which these responses can be controlled by using relaxation techniques, deep breathing exercises and massage. This technique has been used on individuals who suffer from anxiety attacks. Such attacks cause the heart to beat faster, the breathing to be more rapid and shallow, the skin to break out in a cold sweat and the mouth to become dry. When clients feel these symptoms approaching, they are encouraged to undertake deep breathing exercises to alleviate *anxiety*.

biographical and health data: information which is collected at the initial *assessment* of a patient or client. This is the first part of the admission procedure when they enter hospital or community care. The details collected include:

- name, address, telephone number, family members, next of kin, date of birth and religion
- health history – any diseases or inherited conditions, previous treatments which include operations, drug treatment or any other therapy/previous admissions
- allergies to certain foods, materials or drugs
- different terms for daily items or tasks. With children it is important to find out their likes, dislikes, their favourite toy, if they have a special name for anyone or anything which is important to them. For example, some children have a special name for going to the toilet
- disabilities – the patient's daily living skills, how they cope with everyday activities, what is the level of their dependence/independence (see *activities of daily living*).

biological determinism: a psychological theory by which it is believed that an individual's growth and development are determined by their inherited characteristics. The opposite view is social determinism where an individual's growth and development are said to be affected by social influences on their lives such as their social status and the *social class* to which they belong.

biology: the science of life which examines the structure, function and organisation of living things.

biopsy: the removal of a sample of tissue for examination, often by microscopy. It is done to observe any evidence of disease or degeneration, so assisting diagnosis and treatment. (See *pathology*.)

birth: contraction of the muscles of the mother's *womb* in order to expel the *foetus*. When the baby is ready to be born and the birth is about to start the mother will have some of the following signs:

- 'a show'; a plug of blood-stained mucus discharged through her *vagina*
- her waters will break; the membranes which contain water and surround the baby rupture
- contractions of the muscles in the wall of the *uterus*; these become regular and strong and the intervals between contractions shorten (labour pains).

There are three stages involved in birth:

- Stage 1 – the cervix widens or dilates so that the baby's head can pass through. The length of time for this stage can be anything from two to twenty-four hours. Most babies are born head first but in some cases the baby may come feet first in what is called a *breech presentation*.
- Stage 2 – the baby is pushed out by the mother. At this stage every time the uterus contracts the mother pushes very hard so that the baby can be born.
- Stage 3 – the placenta and membranes are pushed out. These are examined and checked. Pieces of placenta left in the womb can cause further blood loss.

Stage 1

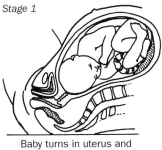

Baby turns in uterus and is in a position for birth

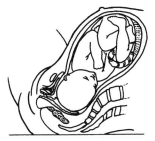

The baby's head pushes the cervix; a plug of mucus is released and 'waters break'

Stage 2

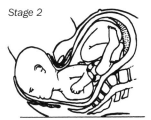

The uterus contracts and the baby is pushed out through the vagina

Stage 3

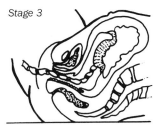

The placenta becomes detached from the wall of the uterus

Stages of labour

birth injuries or trauma: injuries to a baby during delivery and at the end of labour. These may result in damage to bones, nerves or skin and can cause infection or brain damage.

- *bones* – during difficult births, breech deliveries and the birth of big babies, bones may fracture. Fracture to the legs and arms are recognised immediately as the baby may not be able to move the damaged limb. Fractures of the skull are usually associated with the use of forceps during a difficult delivery
- *nerves* – nerves to the neck may be stretched during delivery and the nerve known as the brachial nerve may be damaged. This will affect the nerve supply to the upper arm muscles and the arm will hang down at the baby's side and turn inwards. Nerves supplying the face may be damaged by a forceps delivery
- *skin* – minor scratches and abrasions may appear on a baby's face after a forceps delivery. When a baby has been born as a result of a *breech* delivery the baby's bottom and genital area may be bruised
- *infection* may be contracted during birth
- brain damage can be caused by a lack of oxygen in the baby's bloodstream.

birth statistics/birth rate: the number of children who are born each year. This is recorded as children born per 1000 people within the population. (See *demography*.)

Black Report 1980: a government report, 'Inequalities in health', produced by Sir Douglas Black in 1980. The report was based on research carried out in the late 1970s. The report highlighted different aspects of material deprivation, poverty and social class. There were clearly defined areas of *inequalities in health* and status between the different social and economic groups. In the Green Paper *Our Healthier Nation – A Contract for Health*, the social case indicated that income, class and health are connected. (See *Acheson Report 1998*.)

bladder: a muscular sac situated in the lower *abdomen.* The bladder acts as a container for *urine*. Urine is passed into it from the *kidneys* for temporary storage. Urine is held in the bladder by a small muscle called a sphincter muscle which closes the exit from the bladder. When the bladder is full the pressure on the nerves in the bladder causes a message to be sent to the brain and the person feels the need to pass urine. Understanding this process is an important part of working with clients. Children are trained to use their bladders through toilet training. In the elderly, the sphincter muscles of the bladder often lose their elasticity and the older person may dribble urine frequently. In both cases regular toileting is an essential part of the caring process.

blind and partially sighted: see *visual impairments*.

Bliss system: an electronic board which shows up different words and phrases. It is used specifically for people with a speech impairment. A person touches the words or phrases that they want to use to convey a message.

blood: a vital body fluid which consists of *plasma, platelets*, *red blood cells* and *white blood cells*. An adult has about 5.5 litres (9.5 pints) of blood circulating in their body. Blood is a type of *connective tissue*.

The functions of blood are:

- to carry different substances such as oxygen, carbon dioxide, dissolved food materials, hormones and urea around the body
- to produce antibodies, to engulf bacteria and to produce histamine
- to aid the blood clotting process using platelets.

blood cells: cells which are found in blood. There are two main types of cells:

- *red blood cells* or erythrocytes. Their main function is to carry oxygen from the respiratory organs to the tissues
- *white blood cells* or leucocytes. Their main function is to provide the body with a defence against disease.

blood clotting: the way in which blood forms a solid mass where there has been damage to the tissues and bleeding. When the body is wounded, soluble fibrinogen which is present in *blood plasma* is converted to insoluble fibrin. This forms a mesh over the surface of the wound where red blood cells are trapped and form a clot. Clots stop further blood from escaping and also help to prevent the entry of pathogenic bacteria. A complex mechanism controls the process of blood clotting. Fibrinogen can only be converted into fibrin in the presence of prothrombin which is converted into thrombin by the enzyme thrombokinase.

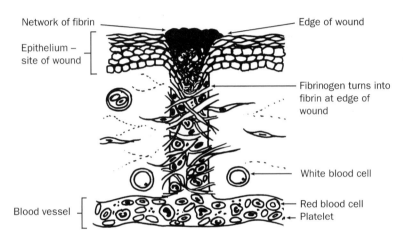

Blood clotting

blood count: a term used to describe the number of each of the different types of blood cells in a given volume of *blood* (e.g. per cubic millimetre of blood).

blood culture: a method of testing for micro-organisms in blood. A sample is taken from an individual and is tested for evidence of *bacteria*. The sample is also examined under a microscope. Blood cultures are taken if septicaemia (infection of the blood) is suspected.

blood flow: the way in which *blood* is pumped around the body via the *heart*. The speed of blood flow is measured by recording the *pulse*. This indicates the frequency at which the blood pulsates through the body. The flow of blood is maintained by the pumping action of the heart, by muscle contraction and by the *breathing mechanism*. (See *cardiac cycle*.)

blood groups: a system used to categorise blood types. *Red blood cells* have protein molecules on their cell surface membranes. Some of these proteins act as *antigens* and it is the presence or absence of specific types of these antigens which determines blood group. There are many different systems of grouping blood but the ABO system is probably the best known. There are four blood groups in this system; A, B, AB and O. These are determined by the presence of the antigens A and B. Individuals with blood group A have antigen A in their red blood cell membranes; those who are group B have antigen B; group AB individuals have both antigen A and antigen B while group O have neither A nor B. It is the presence of these and other antigens which determines whether or not one person's blood may be safely given to another during **blood transfusion**.

blood plasma: the liquid part of blood. A pale straw-coloured liquid composed mainly of water containing a variety of dissolved substances; it is transported from one part of the body to another. Plasma carries food substances from the small intestine to the liver, hormones from the ductless glands to their target organs, urea from the liver to the kidneys, and carbon dioxide from the cells to the lungs. Plasma is the medium through which continual exchange takes place. Plasma also contains proteins including albumin, globulin, fibrinogen and the antibodies. Other important constituents of plasma are the ions of sodium, potassium, calcium, chloride, phosphate and hydrogen carbonate. Blood plasma from which the fibrinogen has been removed is called serum.

blood pressure: the pressure of **blood** against the walls of the main arteries. Blood pressure is highest during systole, when the ventricles are contracting (systolic pressure) and lowest during diastole when the ventricles are relaxing and refilling (diastolic pressure). Blood pressure is measured in millimetres of mercury using an instrument called a sphygmomanometer placed on the brachial artery of the arm. To measure blood pressure, an inflatable cuff is placed around a person's upper arm and the pressure in the cuff is increased until it is above the pressure in the artery. As the pressure is released, the blood begins to flow in the artery and can be felt at the pulse or heard with a stethoscope. The procedure is not painful but creates a sensation of pressure. It is important to explain the procedure to the client since distress or even mild anxiety can raise the blood pressure. Blood pressure should be taken with the person in a lying or sitting position in order to obtain an accurate reading. The expected systolic pressure should be approximately 120 mm and the diastolic pressure 80 mm. High blood pressure is called hypertension and low blood pressure is called hypotension. Another method is to use an electronic machine with an inflatable cuff which is either battery or mains operated. It produces the reading electronically.

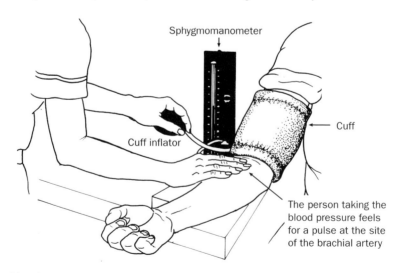

Taking blood pressure

blood sugar level: the amount of *sugar* or glucose which is contained in the blood. The blood glucose level is controlled by the secretion of insulin from the **pancreas**. The normal blood glucose level is 4–6 mmol per dm^3 of blood.

blood system: the human body's transport system. Its functions include:

- the transport of nutrients, blood gases, hormones and waste products from one part of the body to another
- the distribution of heat from respiring tissues (e.g. the liver and muscles) to other parts of the body.

blood tests: examination of blood samples to detect disorders or disease. For example, a test for **haemoglobin** detects how much iron is in the blood and therefore detects anaemia, i.e. lack of iron in the body. The presence of certain cancers such as ovarian **cancer** can be detected through blood tests.

blood transfusion: the transfer of **blood** from one person to another. The ability to do this safely depends on the **blood groups** of the individuals concerned. **Red blood cells** have **protein** molecules in their cell surface membranes. Some of these proteins act as **antigens** and it is the presence of these which determines blood group. For example, the red blood cells belonging to group A individuals have antigen A on their surface while those belonging to people with group B blood have antigen B. In addition to this, these individuals also have antibodies present in their plasma. Someone with group A will have a specific antibody against antigen B. It is convenient to call this antibody b. Similarly, a person with group B blood will have antibody a.

body language: see *communication*.

body mass index: (BMI) a way of calculating a person's desirable weight. It is calculated by dividing the weight in kilograms by the height in metres squared. BMI measures and assesses whether an individual is obese, overweight, average weight or underweight.

BMI measurements:

- Less than 18.5 = underweight for height
- 18.5–24.9 = normal weight for height
- 25–29.9 = overweight for height
- 30+ = obesity.

body temperature: the amount of heat produced in the body is balanced by the amount of heat which is lost. This is the way in which a healthy body maintains a stable temperature of 37 degrees Celsius (98.4 degrees Fahrenheit). Body temperature is regulated by the heat-regulating centre in the hypothalamus of the **brain**. Body temperature may be measured using:

- disposable oral probe thermometers which are placed under the tongue and thrown away after use
- tympanic thermometers which are placed in the ear. A disposable cover is placed over the nozzle and a bleeper sounds when the temperature is ready to be read. The disposable cover is thrown away
- LCD or liquid crystal display thermometers which involve placing a strip across the forehead. They are thrown away after use.

bolus: the mass formed as a result of chewing food in the mouth through movement of the jaw and the muscles of the mouth. The tongue rolls the food into a ball or bolus which is then pushed to the back of the throat for swallowing.

bonding: the development of a close relationship between two individuals. This is the first relationship in the life of a **newborn baby** when an **attachment** is formed between the baby and its mother or primary care giver. The bonding process is reinforced by:
- eye contact with the baby
- holding the baby closely and securely
- skin contact – holding hands, breast feeding
- talking – cooing at the baby and making sounds.

In the early months of a baby's life these actions from their carer help to promote a sense of love, security and well-being. This gives the baby a positive view of itself and the world it lives in. As the baby grows into a child this sense of security will help the development of relationships with others. (See also **Bowlby.**)

bone: a **connective tissue** which is impregnated with large deposits of calcium salts, mainly calcium phosphate. The salts make the bone extremely hard. Bone is formed by the process of ossification which is the formation of bone tissue from cartilage or membrane. This involves the laying down of bone by bone cells or osteoblasts. The osteoblasts arrange themselves in rings around nerves and blood vessels. Eventually the osteoblasts surround themselves with bone and at this stage they are called osteocytes. This type of bone is called compact Haversian bone. Spongy bone is less compact and not as hard as compact bone. Compact bone is found in the shafts of the limb bones, while spongy bone is found at the ends of these bones. Covering the bone is a dense layer of connective tissue called the periosteum.

Bones have a variety of functions including:
- movement and stability – bones form a supporting body framework and provide attachments for muscles, ligaments and tendons which reinforce the support and movement of the body
- protection – bones form a framework which protects the organs of the body
- storage – bones store minerals such as calcium, phosphorus and magnesium
- cell production – **red blood cells** are manufactured in the **bone marrow**.

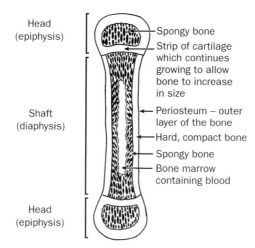

The structure of a long bone

bone marrow: a substance which fills the cavity in certain bones. There are two types of bone marrow. They are:

- red bone marrow – where all the *red blood cells* and some white cells are made
- yellow bone marrow – which stores fat.

boundaries: see *discipline*.

boundaries of service user's rights within health and social care contexts: boundaries of behaviour which are reinforced by policies and procedures. These are applied when a service user is:

- at risk of being harmed or injured by another service user or of causing harm to themselves
- intending to harm others
- intending to or is breaking the law.

bowel disorders are diseases or dysfunctions of the bowel. Examples include irritable bowel syndrome, Crohn's disease, constipation and bowel *cancer.*

Bowlby, John (1907–1990): famous for his views on the importance of *attachment* or *bonding*. He investigated the bond that forms between the primary care giver and the infant or young child. Deprivation of this bond may have consequences for the infant or young child, on both their short- and long-term development.

Bowlby believed that an infant should experience a warm, intimate and continuous relationship with his or her mother. Drawing upon evidence gathered from a variety of sources, including studies of hospitalised children, institutionalised children and evacuees, as well as experimental work with motherless monkeys, Bowlby suggested that prolonged *separation* from the primary care giver (usually the mother) or the failure to form an attachment bond (privation) leads to adverse effects in later life. This may include the development of difficulties in forming intimate relationships with others. Bowlby claimed that children who were deprived of maternal love would always be disadvantaged in some way, either physically, socially or emotionally.

Braille: a type of writing and printing using raised dots to represent letters, which allows blind and *visually impaired* people to read and communicate by touch.

brain: the most highly developed part of the *nervous system*. It is contained in the cranial cavity of the skull and is surrounded by three membranes called meninges. The brain is made up of the:

- cerebrum – this is the most highly developed part of the brain consisting of two cerebral hemispheres. It is the site of functions such as vision, smell, hearing, touch, speech and memory
- midbrain – which is an area which joins the diencephalon to the pons. It carries impulses in towards the thalamus and out from the cerebrum towards the spinal cord
- medulla or medulla oblongata – the area of the brain which is responsible for many involuntary actions such as breathing. (See *hypothalamus*.)

Brain stem is a term used to describe the area comprising the midbrain, pons and medulla. See the diagrams below.

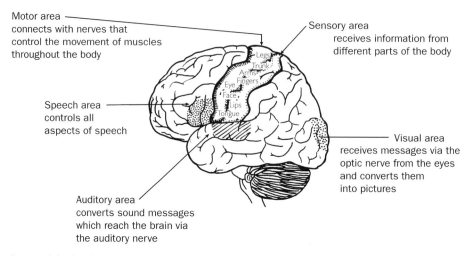

Areas of the brain

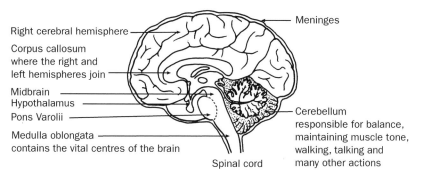

A section through the brain

breast self-examination: a method which women use to examine their *breasts* to check for abnormalities. It is recommended that in the first part of the examination of her breasts a woman should sit in front of a mirror and look carefully at each breast. She should note the normal size, shape and position of the nipple, checking that there has not been any change in size, texture of skin, swellings, discolouration, rash or very prominent veins. In addition to this she should check the nipple to see if it has become retracted or turned in. Self-examination and palpation of the breasts should never be rushed. The woman should give herself sufficient time for this process. Having completed the self-examination she should decide whether her breasts have undergone any changes or if any unusual swellings or other features have appeared. If she is worried she should contact her doctor or visit her family planning clinic which can offer help and advice. It may be that she should have a test or special X-ray of her breasts (called a mammogram, see *mammography*). These procedures can be viewed as a method of breast screening, to check a woman's breast for any lumps or tumours which could result in breast *cancer*. (See *screening programmes*.)

breasts: mammary glands which are situated in the upper part of the chest. They are important parts of a woman's anatomy because:

- they are stimulated by hormones to produce milk following the birth of a baby
- they are significant in terms of sexuality; they contain sensory areas which are sensitive to touching and stroking, they are erogenous and the nipple responds when the woman becomes sexually excited
- they are an essential part of early contact between the mother and baby; this includes breast feeding and skin-to-skin contact between mother and child.

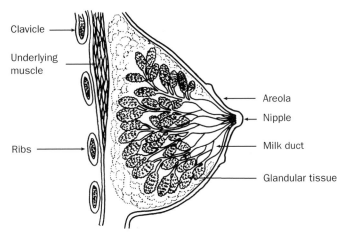

A section through the breast

breathing mechanism: the way in which the body:

- takes in air by inspiration; this enables oxygen to be taken to all parts of the body via the *lungs* and the *heart*
- lets out air through expiration which enables carbon dioxide to be excreted from the body via the heart and the lungs. (See *respiratory system, gaseous exchange*.)

breech presentation: the position of the baby in the uterus before birth which suggests that the bottom or buttocks of the baby will be born first. The normal position is head first.

British crime survey: a survey which involves interviewing a *sample* of 10,000 adults about their experiences as victims of crime. These surveys are carried out by Home Office researchers.

British Heart Foundation: a voluntary organisation which aims to highlight the issues relating to heart disease. Heart surgeons, hospital doctors, nurses and GPs rely on funding from the British Heart Foundation to support their research, education and training. The Foundation is a charity which receives no government funding.

British Red Cross is an international organisation which helps to meet the needs of *vulnerable people* in times of emergency, both in the UK and in countries across the world. The British Red Cross espouses a policy that they:

- are neutral in conflict – impartial to race and creed. Because of their neutrality they can work in a battle zone, bringing food and medical supplies
- care for people in the local community – there are over 90,000 volunteer workers offering a range of services in the community, including *first aid* training
- have staff who are trained and skilled to respond to emergencies.

The principles of the Red Cross stand for humanity, impartiality, neutrality, independence, voluntary service, unity and universality.

British Sign Language: one of the languages used by those with a hearing *impairment*. Language users make *gestures* involving movements of hands, arms, eyes, face, head and body, to conduct a conversation. The development of British Sign Language has been an amazing breakthrough and it is much used by those with severe hearing loss. (See *sign language, Makaton*.)

bronchitis: inflammation of the *air passages*, that is the bronchii/bronchioles of the lungs. This causes coughing, shortness of breath and a general feeling of being unwell (malaise). Treatment involves rest and the taking of fluids. In some cases, when bacterial infection is evident, antibiotics are given.

bruise: a discolouration of the skin due to any impact or injury. A bruise is formed when the tiny blood vessels in the skin bleed and there is swelling and discolouration under the surface of the skin.

Bruner, Jerome (1915–): a cognitive psychologist. He believed that intellectual development in a child depends very much on the way in which the mind uses the information that it receives. Bruner believed that children develop different ways of representing the environment around them. These ways of using information include:

- enactive – children represent the world through their sensor-motor actions for example, trying to describe a spiral staircase without using physical actions is a means of making an individual aware of the nature of this type of representation
- iconic – thinking based on the use of mental images
- semantic – the representation of the environment through language; this enables the child to access much of the knowledge available in their surroundings and to go beyond the information given.

Bruner believed that *language* is the vital component which opens up new horizons of *intellectual development* for the young child.

buddies: those individuals who become friends, partners or counsellors. They usually help a person cope through a particular health condition and treatment, psychological problem, period of study or any life stage change when support is valuable. Examples include:

- buddies who are recruited to support people with cancer, AIDS or any other serious illness
- study buddies, where two students will support each other through a course or programme of study
- birth buddies, when a friend will support a woman through the antenatal phase and through the labour and birth of her baby. (See *coping*.)

budgets: see *funding*.

building a positive relationship is about strategies or methods used by the health and social care worker to develop a positive relationship with individual service users. (See *care relationship, building confidence, effective communication, strategies for effective communication, interaction, active listening, interpersonal skills*.)

building confidence: a method by which the carer can help a client to feel more positive about themselves. This can take the form of:

- attention – the client feels that a carer is taking time to be with them
- praise – when a carer says 'well done' for a task achieved
- listening – the client feels a sense of self-worth when a carer takes time to listen
- seeking client opinions – the client feels that their opinion is valued
- decision making – the client gains a sense of independence when they are able to make decisions for themselves
- creating a positive environment, enabling the client to feel at home, safe, happy and positive about themselves.

(See *care value base, interpersonal skills, strategies for effective communication*.)

bulimia nervosa: a compulsive *eating disorder*, characterised by episodes of compulsive overeating, usually followed by self-induced *vomiting*.

bullying: the way in which a person may intimidate, threaten or harass another person. Bullying is closely linked to *abuse* as it often involves name calling, aggression and in some cases acts of violence. In schools, a group of children may single out one child because they think he or she is different. For example a child may wear glasses and the group will constantly threaten this child. The child becomes frightened and often does not want to go to school. The victim will be threatened to keep silent and will often find this a major stress in their life. In some cases bullying has led to the victimised child committing suicide. Schools have developed anti-bullying policies where children are encouraged to talk about bullying and the perpetrators are disciplined within the framework of a *code of practice*.

Bullying does not just take place amongst children, it can happen in the workplace. For instance, recent reports suggest that employers, managers, supervisors and work colleagues are just as liable to bully others in the workplace. This includes health and social care settings. Bullying in whatever form should be treated as dangerous behaviour particularly when it involves clients, service users and workers. Trade unions are now recognising the need to address bullying in the workplace. (See *harassment*.)

Bullying can also take the form of electronic or cyber bullying. This includes the use of text messages, mobile phone calls, internet sites and e-mails to embarrass, harass, intimidate and threaten individuals.

A–Z Online

Log on to A–Z Online to search the database of terms, print revision lists and much more. Go to **www.philipallan.co.uk/a-zonline** to get started.

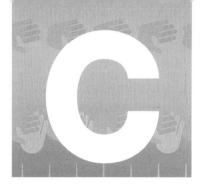

calliper: a metal frame which gives support to a weak limb (leg, ankle or foot). It provides an individual with the support needed for increased *mobility* or walking. Callipers can be full limb length or half limb length. (See *aids and adaptations*, *Zimmer frame*.)

campaign: an organised course of action which is carried out by a group in order to increase awareness of a particular issue in society. For example, the *Child Poverty Action Group* draws attention to the issues of *poverty* and the needs of children.

cancer is a disease of which there are over 200 types. Each cancer starts in the same way. It is linked to changes in the normal make-up of a *cell*, leading to the uncontrolled growth of abnormal cells. There are differing views as to why this occurs. For instance, *stress*, excessive *smoking* or intake of *alcohol* are viewed as predisposing factors. Cancer can affect many parts of the body including the bowel, lung, breast, prostate, testicles and skin. There are different methods of treatment which include *chemotherapy*, *radiotherapy* or surgery (operations) or a combination of two or three of these.

Cancer Relief Macmillan Fund: an organisation which provides care and support for cancer patients in hospitals, *hospices* and patients' homes. It was founded in 1911 by Douglas Macmillan. Macmillan nurses and doctors are skilled in the treatment and nursing care of cancer patients and are financed through the Macmillan Fund. The fund also provides financial support for patients and their families and for the development of *day care* and information centres.

Cancer Research UK: the largest *cancer* charity in the world, brought about by the merger of the Cancer Research Campaign and the Imperial Cancer Research fund in February 2002.

cannabis: an illegal *drug* derived from the plant *Cannabis sativa.* Cannabis may be used to relax the person and give them a sense of well-being. There has been some debate re the classification of cannabis and it was downgraded to a class C drug. Then it was upgraded back to a class B drug. Increasing research has made links between cannabis and *mental health disorders*. It is illegal to grow, produce, possess or supply cannabis. It is also an offence to allow any building or place to be used for growing, preparing, supplying or smoking cannabis. Cannabis can produce psychological dependency, making the person dependent upon smoking it in order to cope with life. Cannabis smoked regularly can have harmful effects on the body. Some of the organs affected are the:

- *brain* and *central nervous system* – cannabis causes short-term memory loss, poor concentration, anxiety and panic attacks
- *heart* – cannabis speeds up the heart beat and therefore increases blood pressure

- reproductive system – cannabis causes a decrease in the sperm count, causes egg damage and alters hormone levels; newborn babies of habitual cannabis users may have a lower birth weight
- *lungs* – cannabis causes damage to lungs; this is increased when cannabis is smoked together with tobacco
- *immune system* – cannabis affects the way in which the body protects itself against infection.

The use of cannabis for therapeutic purposes is on the increase. There is a growing debate with regard to the possible medicinal benefits of cannabis, e.g. in the treatment of *multiple sclerosis* or for individuals who suffer from disorders which cause acute pain such as severe *arthritis.*

capillaries: small blood vessels which connect *arteries* and *veins* and form a network in the tissues. The walls of capillaries are one cell thick. Arteries and veins carry blood but the important exchange between the blood and the tissues takes place in the capillaries. High pressure in the arterial end of the capillaries forces water and small soluble molecules out through the walls forming the tissue fluid which surrounds the cells of the body. Much of this water flows back into the capillary at its venous end since the water pressure of the tissue fluid is higher than that of the blood plasma at this point. There is, therefore, a continuous circulation of fluid out of the capillaries and back into them. This takes useful substances to the cells and returns waste products to the *blood* and then to the *kidneys* and the *respiratory system*. *Blood flows* into capillaries from arterioles. Arteriole walls contain muscle fibres which can contract to reduce the diameter of the vessel. In this way the blood supply to the capillary system in a particular organ is always being adjusted to meet its needs.

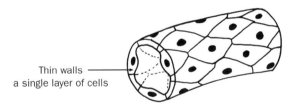

Thin walls — a single layer of cells

A section through a capillary

carbohydrates are made up of carbon, hydrogen and oxygen. The simplest carbohydrates are monosaccharides. These can be built up into disaccharides and polysaccharides through the process of condensation involving the removal of water. The function of carbohydrates in the body is the production and storage of *energy*. They are a main energy source for the different chemical reactions in the body and an integral part of a healthy *diet*. (See *balanced diet, sugar.*)

carbon is a non-metallic element which occurs in all living matter. It combines with other elements as a result of chemical reactions. Examples of the compounds formed include:
- *carbon dioxide* – a waste product of metabolism in the body
- *carbon monoxide* – a poisonous gas which is released through *smoking* or pollution
- *carbohydrates* which are composed of carbon, hydrogen and oxygen.

carbon dioxide: chemical formula CO_2. A colourless gas produced as a result of chemical processes in the body. It is a **waste product** which is carried in the **blood** from the different parts of the body via the **veins**, through the venae cavae to the right atrium of the **heart** and to the pulmonary arteries from the right ventricle, where it is pumped to the **lungs** and breathed out into the general atmosphere.

carbon monoxide: chemical formula CO. A poisonous gas found in smoke. It is either drawn into the body or released into the atmosphere through tobacco **smoking** and exhaust fumes from motorised vehicles. Carbon monoxide once in the system combines with **haemoglobin** in the **blood** to form carboxyhaemoglobin. This reduces the blood's ability to carry oxygen to all parts of the body. Oxygen is vital to the different chemical reactions and functions in the body. A lack of oxygen and an increase in carbon monoxide can lead to:
- increased risk of blood clots or thrombosis
- the formation of **atheroma** – which leads to atherosclerosis, fatty deposits which occur in artery walls; this in turn can lead to the narrowing of the arteries.

cardiac catheterisation: a test on the **heart** used to diagnose a heart disorder. It involves inserting a long thin plastic tube or catheter into a vein in the arm or groin so that it passes into the right **atrium**, **ventricle** and pulmonary artery for the purpose of recording pressure in these parts of the heart. A contrast medium or dye, sometimes also taken before the test, is monitored by **X-ray examination** and photography.

cardiac cycle: the events which take place to produce a **heart** beat. It is a continuous cycle which is controlled by the sino-atrial node (the pacemaker) situated in the wall of the right **atrium**.

The cardiac cycle:
- The walls of the atria contract and blood is forced into the ventricles. This is called the atrial systole.
- The walls of the ventricles contract and blood is forced out of the heart into the pulmonary artery and the aorta. This is called the ventricular systole.
- The walls of the atria relax and **blood flows** into the atria from the venae cavae and pulmonary veins.
- The walls of the ventricles relax and blood flows into the atria. This is called the ventricular diastole.

cardiac muscle tissue: **muscle** tissue which is found only in the **heart** walls. It consists of many branching fibres which contain nuclei and striations. The cardiac muscle contracts and relaxes causing the heart to beat and pump **blood** around the body. It works under involuntary control and produces its own electrical impulses. These nervous impulses increase or decrease the heartbeat.

cardiograph: an instrument used to record the force and form of the heartbeat. The results are recorded graphically. (See **electrocardiograph**.)

cardiology is the study of the structure and function of the **heart**. This includes any heart disease, degeneration or functional disorders. A cardiologist is a fully trained doctor who specialises in the diagnosis and treatment of heart disease.

cardiorespiratory system includes the **heart** and **lungs** and the blood vessels associated with them. The cardiorespiratory system can be monitored by a carer by measuring and recording **pulse, blood pressure**, and the efficiency of breathing (i.e. respiration rate and **lung** volume) which relate to the supply of oxygen and the removal of **carbon dioxide**.

cardiovascular system: the heart and its associated blood vessels, i.e. *arteries*, *veins* and *capillaries*.

care: an umbrella term for the different types of caring which take place under the auspices of health and social care. (See *health care*, *nursing care*, *personal care, caring*.)

care assistants or clinical support workers provide practical help, support and care. They give *direct care* to a range of client groups in different settings which may be residential, day care or in the client's own home. A *residential care* assistant helps residents with their daily *routine*, including getting up, bathing, dressing and any toileting which may be necessary. The care assistant also serves food and helps with feeding residents as necessary. National Vocational Qualifications are a means whereby care assistants can be trained in the workplace.

care environment and care context: the setting, time and surroundings in which caring takes place. *Health and social care workers* are expected to be able to optimise or make as effective as possible the caring process which takes place within a care context. This includes:

- communicating with colleagues – sharing experience and knowledge through discussion, *reflective practice* and *feedback*
- communicating with service users in a positive manner (see *effective communication*, *interaction*, *interpersonal skill*, *strategies for effective communication*, *active listening* and *building confidence*)
- making a service user comfortable by ensuring that they are warm, happy and secure and have sufficient personal space (see *basic needs* and *Maslow*)
- providing a safe *environment* – ensuring premises and equipment are made safe for service users, monitoring that there are adequate numbers of staff on duty to care for them (see *safety*, *risk assessment*, *positive care environment*)
- providing stimulating activities to build up positive personal relationships (see *activities for health and well-being*)
- working with a number of clients at the same time, but prioritising the *individual needs* of each service user and supporting *anti-discriminatory practice*.

(See also *positive care environment*, *health and safety*, *care value base*, *codes of practice*, *life quality factors*, *physical life quality factors*, *psychological life quality factors*.)

Care Homes for Old People National Minimum Standards 2003 set out the key standards that apply to all care homes that provide accommodation and nursing or personal care for older people. These standards are of primary importance to the service users and include:

- choice of residential home
- complaints procedures and protection
- daily life and social activities
- environment
- health and personal care
- management and administration
- staffing.

(See *care value base*, *life quality factors*, *care environment and care context*, *national minimum standards*.)

care management: co-ordination by a named care manager appointed to supervise the *assessment* and purchasing of appropriate care for clients. The process involved in care management of a service user is:

- referral to the appropriate care manager from relevant agencies
- assessment of the service user using the types of assessment identified in the Fair Access to Care Service produced by the Department of Health. It will take into consideration the holistic needs as well as the life quality factors of the service user
- care planning, taking into account the requirements and priorities of the service user. The resulting care plan is agreed
- identifying the resources necessary for the care plan to be implemented
- monitoring and review of the care plan as it is being implemented
- recognition of any need which is developing through the care plan which may result in the care plan being changed or modified or re-assessed
- evaluating the care plan. Is it working? Is it meeting the service user's needs?

There are a number of issues which relate to the care management process. These are:

- meeting the needs of the service user ensuring that they are realistically assessed following referral. This includes meeting the criteria of the Fair Access to Care Services in terms of eligibility criteria. These criteria are determined by the seriousness of risk to the service user if their presenting needs are not met. These criteria are Critical – is it life threatening? Has serious abuse or neglect occurred? Substantial – less critical but is the service user still at some substantial risk? Moderate and low which indicates that the service user is at a lower level of risk
- following assessment, do they meet the eligibility criteria?
- resourcing and cost of the care plan in terms of implementation
- reviewing and timetabling service provision and use of equipment by the service user.

care order: an order made by the court under the *Children Act 1989*. It relates to placing a child in the care of a designated *local authority*.

care organisations are *statutory, voluntary, private, independent, self-help* and support agencies which provide care for different client groups in a number of different ways. These include:

- *day care* – luncheon clubs and day centres for older people, *parent and toddler groups* for parents with young children, day nurseries and playgroups
- *health centres* – GP surgeries
- *residential care* – for those clients who will benefit from full-time caring, e.g. children, vulnerable adults, older people and people with disabilities
- information centres – offering information and advice in a number of areas, e.g. *Citizens Advice Bureau*
- voluntary groups such as parent and toddler groups, clubs for children and older people
- *counselling* and *support* – offering opportunities for people to talk about the different issues affecting them
- *respite care* – offering carers a break from the heavy responsibility and the often exhausting burden that long-term caring for a family member can bring
- hospitals
- transport – Dial-a-Ride provides transport for disabled and older people to go shopping or to the theatre

- *support groups*, e.g. those organised by *charities* such as *Age Concern*
- *pressure groups* – to highlight the needs of clients and their carers, e.g. *MIND.*

care plan: a procedure set up to outline a course of care, treatment or therapy between professional carers and their clients, service users or patients. Setting up care plans is an important aspect of a professional carer's work. There are stages of development in the care plan:

- assessing the client's needs
- identifying their current provision
- deciding the type of care needed and how the services will be provided
- setting aims and goals for the client and writing these into the care plan
- implementing the care plan
- monitoring the care plan
- reviewing the care plan
- evaluating the care plan.

Care plans may be:

- developed by one professional, for example a care manager, nurse or social worker
- jointly devised by a multi-professional or *multi-disciplinary team*, e.g. a team of people who may be responsible for developing a care plan for a client with *physical disabilities*
- developed by the client themselves, working with the appropriate health and social care professionals. This is an important aspect of setting up a care plan as it enables the client to take control of their own care. The role of clients in their care planning is recognised in legislation such as the *Children Act 1989, NHS and Community Care Act 1990* and the *Carers (Recognition and Services) Act 1995*. This plan is set up as a continuous cycle of events.

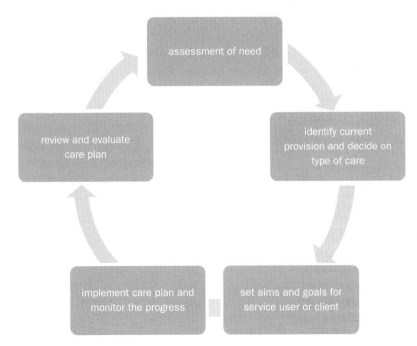

Care planning cycle

care practice: the care and support which is given to service users in their different care settings. This practice must be underpinned with the care value base and equal opportunities legislation, policies and procedures. Person-centred care should be the focus of all care practice and care management. Effective care practice is dependent on:

- building positive professional relationships with service users, colleagues and managers
- dealing with issues which relate to labelling and stereotyping in a sensitive way
- implementing the care value base, policies and procedures
- promoting strategies which empower service users and build their self-esteem and self-confidence. (See *anti-discriminatory practice*, *care relationship*, *building confidence*, *effective communication*, *strategies for effective communication*.)

care practitioner: a term to describe the carer or carers who offer a range of health and social care support to service users.

Care Quality Commission: the independent regulator of health and social care in England. Its aim is to make sure better care is provided for everyone, whether in hospital, in care homes, in people's own homes, or elsewhere. It is responsible for regulating health and adult social care services, whether provided by the NHS, local authorities, private companies or by voluntary organisations. It protects the rights of people detained under the *Mental Health Act 2007*.

care rationing: the way in which care is prioritised with regard to the allocation of health and social care services. It is linked to the distribution of resources in a geographical area and the decision-making process involved. For example, as these areas are split into the responsibility of primary care trusts, some trusts will refuse drugs and treatment in their area because they are too expensive whilst other trusts will be prepared to pay.

care relationship: the rapport, respect and the professional relationship which is developed between clients and their carers. This involves:

- assessing and monitoring a client's individual needs
- maintaining rights and choices, creating autonomy and independence, enabling the client to feel that they are in control of decisions affecting their lives
- respecting the client's sense of dignity with regard to personal and cultural lifestyle and beliefs
- retaining professionalism within the caring relationship; this is based on both the client and carer setting boundaries for the relationship which involves partnership and working together.

(See also *codes of practice*, *care value base*, *equal opportunities policies*, *positive care environment*, *building confidence*, *strategies for effective communication*, *interpersonal skills*, *care environment and care context*.)

care settings: places where health and social care practice is carried out. These are *residential*, hospital, *domiciliary*, and *day care*. Each of these settings is regarded as important in supporting client care. They include:

- residential care – carried out in different nursing and residential homes, hostels, sheltered housing and warden-controlled accommodation
- hospitals
- *domiciliary services* – carried out in the client's home
- *day care* provision – carried out to offer *direct care* and provide assistance whenever necessary including support with the development of daily living skills (see *activities of daily living, enablement*)

- social services carried out by *social workers* working with different client groups
- education provision carried out by nurseries, schools, colleges and universities.

Care Standards Act 2000: an Act of Parliament which was introduced to:
- make provision for the registration of children's homes, residential homes, independent clinics and hospitals, different care groups including fostering and voluntary adoption agencies
- establish the *General Social Care Council* and the Care Council for Wales
- establish a *Children's Commissioner for Wales*
- make provision for registration, regulation and training for those providing childminding or day care
- make provision for the protection of children and vulnerable people
- amend the law for children looked after in schools and colleges.

care strategies: methods or ways of working within health and social care provisions to minimise risk to service users and their carers. For example, *legislation*, *policies* and procedures are put in place to protect vulnerable people. (See *Protection of Vulnerable Adults*.)

care system: the arrangement of care and support which is set up by *health and social care organisations*. These organisations can be voluntary, statutory, independent or informal caring networks.

care team: a group of carers who have the formal or informal responsibility of caring for the service user. They may be paid or unpaid. The care team will include the service user.

care trusts: organisations that work in both the health and social care sectors. They carry out a range of different services related to social care, mental health services or primary care.

care value base: a theoretical framework which promotes good practice within health and social care. It provides carers with a common set of values and principles within which to work. The care value base addresses the following:
- to foster people's *rights and responsibilities*. These include rights such as that to be different, freedom from discrimination, confidentiality, choice, dignity, effective communication, safety and security
- to foster equality and diversity of people. This includes understanding common assumptions such as those which surround gender, race, age, sexual orientation, disability and social class, and understanding prejudice, stereotyping and labelling and their effects. It is important to understand one's own beliefs, assumptions and prejudices and, in addition to this, the benefits of diversity
- to maintain the *confidentiality* of information. This involves using the legal framework included in the *Data Protection Acts 1984 and 1998*. Policies and procedures relating to confidentiality are implemented to value and protect the rights of a client.

care values in early years: a theoretical framework which promotes practice within early years work with children and describes a common set of values and principles within which to work. Care values address the following:
- ensuring that the welfare of the child is paramount, i.e. first and foremost, within the early years setting
- keeping the child safe and maintaining a safe environment

- making sure that children are offered a range of experiences and activities to support every aspect of their development
- maintaining confidentiality
- promoting equality of opportunity and anti-discriminatory practice
- valuing diversity
- working in partnership with parents
- working with others in a positive and professional way
- working with practitioners who implement reflective practice.

(See *paramountcy principle*.)

care workers: see *care assistants or clinical support workers*.

care workers' responsibilities: see *health and social care workers*.

carer: the individual who takes responsibility for the care and support of a person who cannot care for themselves, such as a child, a disabled person or an older person. Carers can either be formal or informal carers. (See also *caring, Carers National Association*.)

Carers and Disabled Children Act 2000: this Act places new responsibilities on *local authorities* to help support carers. It provides:

- *assessment* of carers' needs
- services to help carers
- payments to carers and disabled children.

Carers (Equal Opportunities) Act 2004: an Act of Parliament which requires carers to be offered an assessment of their needs in relation to gaining fair access to work, training and leisure.

Carers National Association: an organisation set up to represent the interests of all carers. It has four aims which are to:

- encourage carers to recognise their own needs
- develop appropriate advice for carers
- provide information and advice for carers
- bring the needs of carers to the attention of government and those responsible for making care policies.

Carers (Recognition and Services) Act 1995: an Act of Parliament which sought to provide an assessment of the ability of carers to provide care. It includes:

- the assessment of carers who provide care in England and Wales. It will take into account the service which the carer provides or intends to provide on a regular basis. This includes provision for a disabled child under Part III of the *Children Act 1989* or person under Section 2 of the Chronically Sick and Disabled Persons Act 1970
- the assessment of carers who provide care in Scotland. This includes Section 12A of the Social Work (Scotland) Act 1968 which was amended with regard to the local authority's duty to assess the needs of a person and their carer. It addresses similar issues as for England and Wales.

The Act does not apply to Northern Ireland. (See *caring for the carer*.)

caring is supporting and looking after another person. This can be formal or informal caring:

- formal care is provided on an organised and paid basis through health and social services

- *informal care* is provided on an unpaid basis, usually because the person being cared for is a family member, close friend or partner.

People who work in health, social care and the early years service may be involved in direct care or indirect care:

- direct care is caring and working with clients, patients and service users providing the appropriate health or social care support (e.g. nurses, **nursery nurses, physiotherapists**)
- indirect care is providing the support services which are necessary for care (e.g. hospital laboratory staff, catering or security staff).

caring for older people involves using *care strategies* which meet the *holistic* needs of the older person. These strategies include:

- being able to make a realistic assessment of their individual needs, i.e. physical, intellectual, social, emotional, spiritual and cultural needs
- being aware of the problems that arise in old age such as ill health and decreasing mobility, retirement and decreased income and isolation
- ensuring that an older person's right to choice, respect and dignity is met by a caring carer who is sensitive to their needs
- helping them with adapting to change and maintaining their independence
- promoting a healthy and balanced diet and helping them to choose suitable exercises or an exercise programme
- providing the relevant support through a care plan when appropriate.

Disorders affecting older people include:

- circulatory system, e.g. cardiovascular disease
- digestive system, e.g. constipation
- nervous system, e.g. cerebrovascular accident or stroke, dementia
- respiratory system, e.g. lung cancer, breathing difficulties
- musculoskeletal system, e.g. arthritis
- sensory impairment, e.g. vision and hearing loss.

(See *older people* and *ageing*.)

caring for the carer: a term indicating an awareness of the needs of carers who care for others in a variety of settings. In the last 20 years there has been a growing awareness of the needs of those who care for relatives long term. Such issues have been at the centre of the **Carers Recognition and Services Act 1995** and the philosophy of the **Carers National Association**. (See *young carers*.)

caring skills: skills developed in the care and support of service users, clients and patients. They include:

- using strategies for effective communication
- being able to assess individual needs
- building confidence amongst service users and maintaining positive care relationships
- modelling the positive behaviour of colleagues and managers
- having a positive attitude and good interpersonal skills.

cartilage: a hard, flexible supporting tissue important to the skeletal system. Cartilage has various functions. It is more compressible than bone so cartilage is found at the ends of *bones* and between the *vertebrae*. It enables the body to withstand the shocks and jarring which accompany movement. Its flexibility is ideally suited to supporting such structures as the nose, the larynx and the trachea.

case conference: a formal meeting. It consists of different professional representatives who get together to exchange information and to decide on a course of action in relation to a particular client (or family) with whom they have been working.

case control study is a method used to combat epidemic *disease*. It involves finding the cause of the disease and the means of control for future prevention.

case history: an historical account of a person and their family. This may include any significant *life events* which might explain any of the problems that the person or family may be experiencing. These events are recorded in chronological order and are kept up to date by the relevant health or social care professional. Some agencies may use the term 'social history' and in the health service the term 'medical case records' is used. (See *diagnosing disease*.)

case study: a *research method* which explores the in-depth behaviour and experiences of an individual, small group, organisation, community, nation or of an event. Case studies enable researchers to explore wider issues surrounding their chosen subject. Health and social care students may find this method useful if they wish to study a particular area of health and social care, such as the roles and responsibilities of *social workers*.

cell: a living structure, millions of which make up the human body. Cells vary in size and shape. In all cases, they are bound by a plasma membrane which encloses the cytoplasm. The cytoplasm contains the following cell organelles:

- nucleus – containing nucleoplasm bounded by a nuclear membrane. The nucleoplasm contains *chromosomes* made mostly of *deoxyribonucleic acid (DNA)*. DNA provides the information which determines the characteristics of the organism and transmits hereditary characteristics to the next generation
- centrioles – found outside the nucleus and necessary for cell division
- ribosomes – responsible for protein synthesis
- endoplasmic reticulum – canals in the cytoplasm which form a connecting network and are responsible for transporting nutrients and substances around the cell
- mitochondria – oval structures in the cytoplasm which produce energy and are sometimes called the 'powerhouses' of the cell. The more energy a cell requires, the greater the number of mitochondria it contains. These are the sites for the *Krebs cycle*
- lysosomes – membrane-bound organelles which contain enzymes. These enzymes digest bacteria and any damaged or worn-out part of a cell. Lysosomes may be thought of as disposal units.

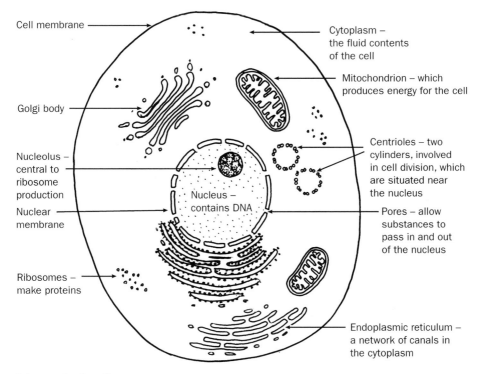

Cell membrane

Cytoplasm – the fluid contents of the cell

Mitochondrion – which produces energy for the cell

Golgi body

Nucleolus – central to ribosome production

Centrioles – two cylinders, involved in cell division, which are situated near the nucleus

Nucleus – contains DNA

Nuclear membrane

Pores – allow substances to pass in and out of the nucleus

Ribosomes – make proteins

Endoplasmic reticulum – a network of canals in the cytoplasm

A human body cell

cell cycle: the sequence of events between one **cell** division and the next. The cell cycle consists of three main stages.

- Stage 1 interphase – the cell grows and increases in size and prepares for the next division. New proteins are synthesised and new cell organelles are made.
- Stage 2 **mitosis** – the genetic material (DNA) divides.
- Stage 3 cytokinesis – the cytoplasm of the cell and its organelles divide more or less equally between two daughter cells.

The length of an individual cell cycle, even in the same organism, is very variable. Many factors combine to determine its precise length. It depends, for example, on temperature and the supply of nutrients.

The cells of many organisms are generally only able to go through a limited number of cell cycles. Once they have become specialised, they are unable to divide any more. Cancer cells, however, can carry on dividing indefinitely. Greater understanding of the mechanism which controls the cell cycle may lead to the discovery of ways in which tumour growth may be limited.

Celsius: a scale of **temperature**. The scale is divided into small divisions called degrees Celsius (°C), with the freezing point for water being 0°C and the boiling point for water at 100°C. Temperatures in degrees Celsius are for practical purposes the same as those in degrees centigrade, which may still be encountered.

census: a national social survey. It has been instigated by the government every 10 years since 1801 (except 1941). Every household in the United Kingdom is required to take part. The information gathered is used to provide statistics which relate to all aspects of national life (e.g. *family structures*).

centile charts: charts which are used to record a child's body measurements such as height and weight. The measurements can be taken in the following ways:

- standing height measurements are taken from age two years onwards. The measurement is taken without shoes, standing with heels, buttocks and shoulders in contact with an upright wall. The child is encouraged to look straight ahead
- supine height measurements are taken with the child lying down on his or her back
- weight measurements are taken with the baby or young child lying, sitting or standing on the scales. Children under one year should be weighed without clothes or nappy for an accurate reading.

The child's measurements are carefully recorded at each age and stage. The distribution of the measurements is expressed in *percentiles*. A percentile refers to the position which a measurement would hold in a recording series of 100 children. The 50th percentile represents the middle measurement or median. Such a percentile chart shows the normal growth curve. A number of measurements are taken over a period of time so that the growth curve can be plotted.

central government: see *government.*

central nervous system (CNS) consists of the *brain* and *spinal cord*. It is composed of:

- types of matter – consisting of grey matter, which contains *blood* vessels and *nerve* cells, and white matter, which contains nerve fibres and a few blood vessels
- meninges – consisting of three membranes with a tough outer layer and a middle layer with spaces filled with cerebrospinal fluid which acts as a shock absorber. A lining membrane containing blood vessels supplies the nervous tissue. *Meningitis* is inflammation of the meninges due to infection.

The central nervous system is the body's control centre. It co-ordinates both mechanical and chemical actions. The millions of nerves in the body carry 'messages' or nervous impulses to and from the following central areas:

- brain – the organ which controls most of the body's activities. It is made up of millions of neurones (nerve cells) arranged into sensory, association and motor areas. The sensory areas receive information via nerve impulses from various parts of the body. Association areas in the brain analyse the impulses and make decisions. The motor areas send impulses or information back to muscles or glands. The impulses are carried by the fibres of 43 pairs of nerves – 12 pairs of cranial nerves serving the head and 31 pairs of spinal nerves (see *cerebrum*)
- spinal cord – a long string of nervous tissue running down from the brain inside the vertebral column. *Nerve impulses* from all parts of the body pass through it to the brain and back again. Some are carried into or away from the brain, some are dealt with in the cord (i.e. involuntary actions). Thirty-one pairs of spinal nerves branch out from the cord through the gaps between the vertebrae. Each spinal nerve is made up of two

groups of fibres called the dorsal root and the sensory root. They comprise fibres of sensory neurones (bringing impulses in) and a ventral or motor root, made up of the fibres of motor neurones (taking impulses out)

- neuroglia – special cells which support and protect the nerve cells (neurones) of the central nervous system.

Dysfunctions of the central nervous system include *multiple sclerosis* and *Parkinson's disease.*

Centre for Policy on Ageing is an independent organisation. It was established in 1947 following the publication of the Rowntree Report, 'Old People'. It aims to raise issues of public importance on matters connected with *ageing* and old age. It raises awareness, promotes debate and influences policies which further the interests of older people. The Centre for Policy on Ageing provides:

- a policy and research department
- a library and information service
- the publication of policy and research papers highlighting issues associated with ageing and the ageing process.

cerebral palsy: a medical condition caused by damage or injury to the developing brain. This may occur during pregnancy, birth or in the early post-natal stages. There may be minor disabilities such as late walking and clumsiness or more severe disorders of *posture*, movement and co-ordination. There are different types of cerebral palsy depending on the part of the body affected. Children with cerebral palsy may suffer from movement which is jerky and uncontrolled. Often one movement will start off a series of other movements, which can be distressing to the child. Children with cerebral palsy may need continuous medical treatment and social support throughout their lives.

cerebrospinal fluid: a colourless fluid which is found in the *ventricles* of the *brain* and the central canal of the *spinal cord*.

cerebrovascular accident (CVA) or stroke: the effect of a serious interruption of the *blood* supply to the *brain*. It may be caused by a blood clot or by the rupture of an *artery* wall. The actual effects vary according to the part of the brain involved. Damage to the right side of the cerebellum, for example, may produce loss of feeling or *paralysis* of the left side of the body.

cerebrum: part of the forebrain, made up of the two cerebral hemispheres. These hemispheres are responsible for the control of voluntary behaviour. This part of the *brain* is very large and covers most of the midbrain and hindbrain. Different parts of the cerebrum have different functions:

- sensory areas – these receive sensory information. They include areas such as vision and hearing, as well as those concerned with sensory information from the general body surface. The size of the area is related to the number of receptors involved
- association areas – those parts responsible for interpreting sensory information in the light of experience. They are principally associated with memory and learning
- motor areas – the areas from which originate the impulses which go to voluntary muscles.

cervical smear: a test which involves removing some *cells* from the neck of the cervix as part of an investigation for degenerative disease. It is integrated into the cervical *screening programme* which was set up in 1987. This offers cervical smears to women over the age of 25 years and under the age 65 years, at least every five years. Some GPs recommend a smear every three years. Cervical smears are an important procedure in detecting early signs of cervical *cancer*.

challenging behaviour: displays of difficult or problem *behaviour* which affect the safety of the person, their carer and others. This includes verbal *abuse,* physical abuse, self-destructive behaviour and destruction of property. Triggers for this behaviour can be discomfort, the influence of alcohol or drugs, disability, noise, stress, difficulty in *communication*, a difficult environment such as too hot or too cold or too noisy.

Challenging behaviour may be displayed by people with learning difficulties, children or any individual client, care manager or carer who is under stress. It may take the form of:

- shouting, screaming, biting and kicking (e.g. child's *tantrum*)
- uncontrolled outbursts of temper leading to violence, which can be dangerous to the instigator and to others (e.g. a schizophrenic client who is suffering from delusions and may be hearing voices)
- periods of disorientation and confusion (e.g. a client with learning difficulties who may also suffer from *epilepsy*)
- excessive mood swings and periods of frustration if a person's routine is interrupted (e.g. an older client who finds moving into residential care a difficult transition).

Working with clients with negative or challenging behaviour may involve *behaviour management* to help the clients manage their behaviour. Carers under *stress* can develop difficulties in their behaviour which may take the form of shouting and *bullying* clients and colleagues or physically hitting out at helpless clients. Carers should be supported with strategies on *stress management* such as *relaxation techniques*. It is important to carry out a *risk assessment* and identify the appropriate *behaviour therapy* which would be an effective means to modify challenging behaviour. Other strategies could be using methods of intervention such as diversion, i.e. showing them something to divert their attention, rewards for good behaviour, medication and possible appropriate physical restraint. (See *anti-social behaviour*.)

challenging discriminatory behaviour: see *anti-discriminatory practice*.

change: experiences which occur during the life stages can be predictable or unpredictable, negative or positive. Predicted change is that which may be controlled or managed by an individual. For instance, if a person feels that their life has become routine and that they are in a rut, then change could be a relief and could present them with a fresh challenge and cause for excitement, for example falling in love, changing jobs, planning a foreign holiday. However, unpredicted change could be another matter. For instance, there are those incidents which happen 'out of the blue' (e.g. an unexpected and distressing phone call with news that the return of a daughter from abroad has been delayed due to a road traffic accident). Other situations may include redundancy, sudden illness or a breakdown in a long-term relationship. It is inevitable that many changes do occur in a person's lifetime. However, it is the methods of *coping* with these changes that are the most relevant to health and social care workers.

Predictable events	Unpredictable events
Giving birth	Miscarriage, stillbirth
Starting school	Child death/terminal illness
Leaving school	Lack of education opportunities due to family illness or family problems
Further education/employment	Unemployment/redundancy
Partnership/marriage	Divorce/separation
Permanent housing	Homelessness
Financial security	Sudden loss of income

charities are non-profit-making organisations. Charities were first set up during the eighteenth and nineteenth centuries as a response to the nation's *poverty*, failing education and poor health and living standards. They were organised by wealthy people who believed in 'doing good'. In recent years some charities have developed into large voluntary organisations which play an important part in community life. There are now approximately 175,000 charities registered under the Charities Act 1993. Information about different charities can be found in the Charity Commissioners Central Register. In order to qualify as a charity, an organisation must be set up with the aim of developing initiatives which will benefit the community. They are funded from various sources including:
- central government grants to finance specific projects
- local authority grants – usually to provide non-statutory services
- grants from organisations and business
- contracts with health authorities and social services departments, who employ voluntary organisations to provide statutory or non-statutory services
- fundraising
- individual donations
- benefit from charitable status, related to taxation (e.g. covenant schemes).

(See also *Barnados, National Society for Prevention of Cruelty to Children, funding.*)

Charter Mark: a mark of quality service or excellence in public sector organisations. The Charter Mark is issued to organisations who have been assessed with regard to the service they offer. The views of the service users are taken into account during this process. The Charter Mark is seen as a recognised achievement for achieving *quality* standards.

charters: documents which tell clients, patients and service users what they can expect from a service. They set out the rights and responsibilities of an organisation. Examples include:
- The NHS Charter 1998 which informs clients, patients and service users of the treatment and care they can expect from the NHS
- The Better Care, Higher Standards, a national charter which informs clients, patients and service users who need support and care what they can expect from health and social care services and local housing. The national charter requires local authorities and health services to publish local charters which set out key standards such as: finding out about services, helping people remain independent, finding a suitable place to live and caring for carers.

charts: a way of documenting relevant information. Charts are used by health and social care workers to:

- record the results of *research* (e.g. used by health and social care students in the production of their assignments)
- record the readings of *temperature, pulse,* respiration and *blood pressure*, and fluid balance, for example in hospital by doctors and nurses
- record the administration of *drugs* in the form of medication charts
- record the observation of growth in the form of *centile* charts.

chemical poisoning is one of the harmful effects of chemicals. Chemical substances can be dangerous to work with as they can be corrosive, explosive, toxic or highly inflammable. Any chemical which can be hazardous should carry a symbol enabling it to be identified. All chemical experiments require a risk assessment before they are undertaken. Factors such as the chemicals, techniques and apparatus used are considered and recorded. The *Health and Safety at Work Act 1974* reviews safe practice and is reinforced by the *Control of Substances Hazardous to Health (COSHH) Regulations 1993*. The Health and Safety at Work (Offences) Act 2008 imposed stricter penalties for breach of safety.

Chemical poisoning can occur due to:

- uncontrolled experiments in the laboratory
- over-dosage of *chemotherapy* in the treatment of *cancer*
- explosions where poisonous gases are released into the atmosphere
- high toxic levels in the atmosphere as a result of *pollution*.

chemicals are used to:

- conduct experiments to produce substances required in many areas such as industry, manufacturing, the treatment of sewage, the manufacture of fuels and disinfectants and in agriculture
- combat disease in the treatment of cancer.

(See also *chemotherapy*.)

chemotherapy is the use of specific drugs and chemicals to treat cancer. *Cytotoxic drugs* are used to either kill or prevent cancer cells from reproducing. However, in the act of working on the cancer cells, these drugs can also kill the body's healthy cells, such as the *white blood cells*. Other side effects of this treatment can include hair loss and baldness, nausea, sickness and vomiting.

child abuse: deliberate ill-treatment of a child. It can take the form of:

- abandonment – a child is left alone with no adult care
- educational neglect – a child does not attend school and has no parental guidance
- emotional *abuse* – a child may be subject to name calling, negative reinforcement, lack of love or building of *self-esteem*
- emotional neglect – a child is ignored and isolated
- medical neglect – the general health of a child is not considered, no medical supervision is encouraged, or there are no *immunisation* or *child health surveillance* checks
- physical abuse – a child may be hit or hurt in some way, such as smacking or suffering cigarette burns
- physical neglect – a child is not given an adequate diet or physical care

- sexual abuse – a child is subjected to sexual acts
- multiple maltreatment – a combination of different forms of *abuse*. (See *safeguarding.*)

In November 1998, government changes redesigned child abuse procedures to include:

- a *Criminal Record Bureau* – keeping track of people with criminal records who want to work with children (see *Vetting and Barring Scheme – Every Child Matters*)
- the age for duty of care by each local authority being extended from 16 to 18 years.

Child Accident Prevention Trust: a voluntary organisation which works closely with health, social and childcare professionals to draw attention to issues relating to child *safety*.

Child Care (NI): a charity which promotes the rights of the child in Northern Ireland. The aims of Child Care (NI) are:

- to promote in Northern Ireland the preservation and protection of health and personal development of children without distinction of sex, race or political, religious or other opinions
- to advance public education in child care by associating the appropriate voluntary agencies with the object of improving life for children.

The charity offers training and information services. It provides an overview of the child care issues in Northern Ireland. (See also *Children in Wales, Children in Scotland, National Children's Bureau.*)

child development: see *growth and development, P.I.E.S.*

child health clinics are run by *health visitors* and doctors as part of a community service for families. Health visitors and GPs offer routine *child health surveillance*, programmes of *immunisation* as well as general information and advice.

child health surveillance programme: designed to ensure that the developmental progress of a child is reviewed at certain times during their first eight years of life.

Child Poverty Action Group is a *pressure group*. The CPAG is committed to raising awareness and working towards eliminating poverty for children and their families. It offers an information service with publications available which provide advice on benefits, etc.

child protection involves a series of guidelines which promote and safeguard the welfare of children. Child protection was supported by the *Children Act 1989*. This Act sought to protect children from harm arising from failures within the family and as a result of unwarranted intervention in family life. It enables *social workers* to investigate children's circumstances and to make decisions about them. *Working Together to Safeguard Children 1999* provided the necessary guidance with regard to child protection. This was updated in 2007. The protection of children is at the heart of all work with children. Since the Children Act 1989 legislation has been updated with the emphasis being on *safeguarding children*. This is enshrined in the *Children Act 2004*. It places a statutory requirement on those involved in caring for children to make arrangements to safeguard and promote their welfare.

Child Support Act 1991: an Act of Parliament passed in 1991 and implemented in April 1993. It created a new child benefit system designed to replace existing procedures. Child maintenance was assessed using a formula with set rules and amounts, instead of being left to a negotiable formula followed by the Department of Social Security, by reliable relatives, or at the discretion of the courts. Maintenance henceforth would be assessed, collected and enforced by the *Child Support Agency*. The Child Support Act was amended in 1995 to make provision for child support maintenance and other maintenance and to provide for a child maintenance bonus, i.e. provision for payment by the Secretary of State in certain circumstances. In 2000 the Child Support Pensions and Social Security Act made changes to the child support scheme in order to make the process easier both for parents and for those working within the Child Support Agency.

Child Support Agency: a government agency set up in 1993 following the implementation of the *Child Support Act 1991*. It has responsibility for the assessment, review, collection and enforcement of child maintenance payments from estranged parents. The law also requires that absent parents should make regular payments for child maintenance.

childcare: the care of children in a variety of settings which include their family homes, *day nurseries*, homes of *childminders, pre-school groups* and *family centres*. Childcare involves caring for the different physical, intellectual, emotional, cultural and social needs of children and young people. The Secretaries of State for Scotland, Wales and Northern Ireland are responsible for policy relating to the development of childcare in those parts of the UK and each of the Secretaries of State plan to issue their own documents on childcare. In England, the care of children is the responsibility of the *Department for Children, Schools and Families.*

Childcare Act 2006: an Act of Parliament with a focus on early years and childcare. The Act takes into account some of the key commitments from the Ten Year Childcare Strategy (2004). It requires that all work with pre-school children is based upon the five *Every Child Matters* outcomes. *Local authorities* are held accountable in ensuring that this happens within their *early years provisions*. It also stipulates that there are sufficient childcare places for working parents.

child-centred: policy and practice that starts with a child's needs being the principal consideration in the health and well-being of the child.

childhood is the period in a child's life which extends from *infancy* to *puberty*. There are different stages of childhood:
- infant (less than 2 years)
- toddler (2–3 years)
- pre-school (3–5 years)
- school age (5 years +).

Childline: a free, confidential, 24-hour helpline for children and young people in trouble or danger. Childline was set up in Spring 1986 after the BBC consumer programme 'That's Life' (presented by Esther Rantzen) appealed to viewers for their help in conducting a survey on *child abuse*. The response was overwhelming and, following the programme, a special childwatch team was set up. The childwatch team met with childcare professionals from both the voluntary and statutory sectors and it was decided to establish a permanent free telephone helpline, which would provide a way of comforting and advising those who could not be reached in any other way. Children phone about many problems, including sexual and physical abuse, bullying, problems with families, friends and worries about schoolwork. Each of the phone calls is followed up by the Childline team at the request of the child.

childminders offer day care for young children in their own homes. Childminders are registered and the home is inspected according to criteria which include the number and size of rooms, toilets and washing facilities. There are standard ratios for minders/children: one minder to one baby under one year, one minder to three children under five years of age, one minder to five children between five and seven years of age, one minder to six children under eight years of whom no more than three should be under five years of age. The childminder's own children are taken into account when the number of places are allocated to a childminder by a local authority. Monitoring and inspection of childminders is the ongoing responsibility of *OFSTED* which inspect each childminder every three years.

Children Act 1989: an Act of Parliament which was introduced to bring about radical changes and improvements in the law with regard to children especially with regard to *child protection*. The Act deals with issues such as:

- children, families and parental responsibility
- court proceedings with the welfare of the child being viewed as paramount
- children in the care of local authorities and adoption.

(See *United Nations Convention – The rights of the child*.)

Children Act 2004: an Act of Parliament which lays out the legal framework for change to the different services provided for children from birth to 19 years of age. The Act implements aspects of the *Every Child Matters* framework.

children in care or looked-after children: children who are being cared for by a *local authority* following the imposition of a *care order* with the agreement of the parents due to:

- family-related difficulties such as ill health, abuse, bereavement, substance misuse, or mental health disorders
- a child or young person with difficulties such as ill health, challenging behaviour, learning disabilities or who has committed an offence.

Care for these children can be temporary or permanent through a number of care settings such as *foster care*, *respite care*, residential child care, or through other relevant agencies such as *Barnardos*. Care is arranged through the local authority, i.e. by the Director of Social Services and his or her staff. Although looked-after children can be cared for successfully, there are some children who can be at *risk* from exploitation and *abuse* even within such arrangements. (See *children's homes*.)

There should be strategies in place to minimise the risk for looked-after children, such as:

- making children aware of the possibility of abuse, no secrets
- working closely with the children and their families
- ensuring that relevant procedures are in place when abuse is suspected or confirmed. (See *child protection* and *safeguarding*.)

Children in Scotland is the national agency for organisations and individuals working with children and their families in Scotland. It exists to identify and promote the interests of children and their families and to ensure that relevant policies, services and other provisions are of the highest possible quality and are able to meet the needs of a diverse society. The framework for Scotland's children, young people and families includes:

- supporting families
- recognising diversity and promoting equal opportunities

- supporting children and families in the early years
- preparing young people for adult life.

Children in Scotland works in partnership with the **National Children's Bureau** and **Children in Wales**. (See also **Child Care (NI)**.)

Children in Wales is an organisation which offers advice and support with regard to children and their families in Wales. It was established as a charity in 1993. Its purpose is to identify and promote the interests of young people in Wales and to improve their status in a diverse society. It publicises good practice in children's services through research, policy development, publications, seminars, conferences and training and through links with influential opinion and the media. The service includes:

- the early childhood unit – offering support and advice to staff involved with young children in early years groups
- library and information service – providing a reference library of books, journals, reports, statistics, news cuttings, booklists and lists of organisations; there is access to the **National Children's Bureau** library database, which is the largest in the country concerned with children
- membership – providing regular updates of information relevant to children, young people and their families.

children with disabilities: children with different disabilities such as physical disabilities, sensory impairments and learning disabilities and difficulties. In the **Children Act 1989** a framework was set up to support such children. This was updated in the **Special Education Needs and Disability Act 2001**. There is legislation and **codes of practice** in place to support the needs of these children. Integrating children with disabilities into mainstream service provision is viewed as a way of meeting their individual and holistic needs. In addition to this, the process of integration involves:

- different agencies such as teachers, speech therapists and physiotherapists working together
- physical health and safety and access being made available within the learning environment
- sufficient staffing in terms of regulated staff/child ratios being in place, and specialised training being given to staff, e.g. **portage**, **sign language**, **Braille**, **Makaton**.

Some children's disabilities may be so severe that they require separate services. In such cases, where possible, this provision is attached to a service used by other children so that joint activities can be arranged from time to time. (See **special needs**.)

Children's Commissioner in Wales Act 2001: an Act of Parliament which extends powers to a Children's Commissioner. The role of the Commissioner is to safeguard and promote children's rights and welfare. This involves representing the rights and welfare of children in Wales at the Welsh Assembly. (See **Children in Wales**.)

children's homes: 24-hour **residential care** for children and young people. There are four different types of residential care:

- community homes maintained, staffed and controlled by local authorities
- homes maintained, staffed and controlled by the voluntary sector
- registered children's homes run by private companies
- independent homes accommodating between 4 and 50 pupils.

children's rights are protected by the *Children Act 1989* in terms of their treatment and welfare. Children's rights require that the wishes and feelings of the child should be taken into account at all times. (See also *United Nations Convention – the Rights of the Child, Children Act 1989, child protection, safeguarding*.)

children's trusts: organisations set up under the *Children Act 2004* to bring together health, education and social services for children, young people and their families. This will involve workers such as family support workers, health visitors, school nurses, social workers, speech therapists and teachers. In some areas, the Trust may also include the *Sure Start* programme.

chiropody is the theory and practice relating to the maintenance of healthy feet. It involves the treatment of feet and their associated disabilities and diseases.

chiropractic: a *complementary therapy* which uses a technique involving the manipulation of the spine. It is based on the belief that disorders of the body are due to the incorrect alignment of *bones* causing abnormal functioning of *nerves* and *muscles*. Chiropractic treatment is performed by trained chiropractors. Training as a chiropractor involves four years' study at the British College of Chiropractic.

choice: the option for the service user to make a decision. This should be an integral part of their daily life. Choice gives an individual a sense of freedom and *empowerment*. Being offered a choice builds positive self-esteem and self-confidence. (See *rights and choices, building confidence*.)

cholesterol: a lipid (fatty substance) which plays an important part in living organisms. Some of the cholesterol required by the body is taken in the *diet* and some is formed in the *liver*. Cholesterol is an important component of cell membranes and is a precursor of *bile* salts and steroid hormones such as testosterone and progesterone. High levels of cholesterol in the blood are associated with *atheroma*. Its level is often monitored in older people or people with high cholesterol levels in the blood. Drugs may be given to reduce blood cholesterol.

Christmas disease: a disease which is due to a defective gene in the *X chromosome*. It is a sex-linked recessive disease which means it affects only males. It is similar to *haemophilia* and inhibits the blood clotting process. This is due to a deficiency in factor IX in the *plasma*.

chromosomal defects are the abnormal structure of *chromosomes*. These can cause medical conditions and disabilities of varying severity. Examples of conditions caused by chromosomal defects are *Down's syndrome* and Turner's syndrome.

chromosome: one of the thread-like structures found in the nucleus, in which the genetic material of the *cell* is organised. Chromosomes consist of DNA and protein. There are 23 pairs (46) of chromosomes in all human body cells. The gametes (eggs and sperm) have 23 unpaired chromosomes.

chronic conditions and illness: *diseases* or disorders which are long-term and lead to slow and progressive deterioration despite treatment. An example of such a disease is chronic myeloid leukaemia which occurs mainly in men and may be present for many years with few symptoms.

cilia: microscopic hair-like projections, drawn out from the cell membrane. Mucus-secreting cells are usually associated with ciliated cells. The cilia exhibit a continual flicking movement, keeping up a constant stream of mucus in the cells lining the *air passages* of the respiratory tract; *smoking* has a harmful affect on these cilia.

circulation: the passage of fluids around parts of the body. Examples of circulation in the body include:

- the passage of *blood* from the *heart* to the *arteries* to the *capillaries* and from the capillaries to the *veins* and back to the heart
- the passage of *bile* from the *liver* cells, where it is made, to the small intestine via the *gall bladder* and bile ducts (some constituents are reabsorbed into the bloodstream in the small intestine and returned to the liver).

(See *circulatory system*.)

circulatory disease: any disease which affects the *cardiovascular system*.

circulatory system: a network of *blood*-filled tubes (blood vessels) which circulate fluid to different parts of the body. There are three main types of blood vessels known as *arteries*, *veins* and *capillaries*. A thin *tissue* layer (endothelium) lines arteries and veins and is the only layer in capillary walls. Blood is kept flowing one way by the pumping of the heart, and by the muscular tissue in the walls of arteries and veins. In different parts of the body muscles contract and relax and these actions encourage blood flow.

cirrhosis of the liver: a disorder of the *liver* in which liver tissue becomes damaged and the healthy tissue is replaced by fibrous tissue. This scarred or fibrous tissue affects the normal working of the liver. The main cause of cirrhosis is 'heavy drinking' or excessive intake of *alcohol*. The best treatment is for the person concerned to stop drinking alcohol. This usually helps the liver to recover.

Citizens Advice Bureaux: (CAB) a service which provides valuable information to members of the public. The Citizens Advice Bureaux are situated in all parts of the United Kingdom. They offer general advice on a number of issues including *housing* and *benefits*. If more specialised or detailed advice is needed then the CAB will be able to tell a client where to go to receive further help. Some of the Bureaux provide a free appointment with a solicitor. At present, there are 700 Citizens Advice Bureaux with 1000 service outlets in England, Wales and Northern Ireland. Approximately 5.5 million people seek help from the Bureaux each year.

Civil Partnership Act 2004: an Act of Parliament which allows same sex couples to form a legal commitment to each other. Gay men and lesbian women have campaigned for this Act for several years in order to receive official recognition for their relationships. Civil ceremonies have followed this Act, where same sex couples have exchanged vows similar to a wedding ceremony and have become civil partners.

class: see *social class or socio-economic group*.

classical conditioning: see *learning theories*.

classification of care services is a method of dividing and grouping health and social care services with regard to *care settings*, client age and individual client need.

classroom assistants work in the classroom to give learning support to individuals or groups of children under the direction of a qualified teacher. Classroom assistants are also known as teaching assistants or learning support assistants.

client: an individual receiving support, treatment or therapy from a health or social care service. The individual is the focus of the health or social care activity.

client classification is a way in which clients can be grouped together. Clients may be grouped according to:
- age – child, adult or older person
- needs – mental health, learning disability or physical disability
- type of care – acute, chronic, social care or priority care
- level of care – primary, secondary or tertiary
- care setting – domiciliary, day care, clinics, residential or hospital care
- service being supplied – physiotherapy, chiropody, probation, hostels, psychiatric care, etc.

clinic: a department in a hospital, or at an established service provider, which specialises in a particular *disease*, *disorder* or *dysfunction*. Its services include:
- a follow-up appointment in the outpatient department of a hospital
- a group of medical professionals and students at a hospital ward specialising in a particular disease, providing examination and treatment of patients
- an established service in the community which advertises a specialist diagnosis and treatment of specific diseases or conditions
- a system for monitoring and maintaining health, such as child health, Well Man or Well Woman clinics.

clinical governance: a government initiative which assures and improves clinical standards at local level, throughout the NHS. This includes action to ensure that risks are avoided, adverse events are rapidly detected, openly investigated and lessons learned, good practice is rapidly disseminated and that systems are in place to ensure continuous improvements in clinical care. (See *The New NHS – Modern, Dependable, hospitals*.)

clinical medicine: the study of *disease* by *diagnosis* and treatment through direct contact with the patients/individuals suffering from the disease. This is different to diagnosis of a disease through the study of body or *blood* cells. Direct contact with the patient is an important part of this branch of medicine.

clinical nurse specialist: a qualified nurse who has developed skills and experience in treating a group of patients suffering from a certain condition or disease. Examples include nurses who work with cancer patients, nurses who work with patients who suffer from diabetes or from head injuries following a car accident.

clinical procedures: any clinical activity, treatment or care in which health care workers may be involved.

***Clostridium botulinum*:** a common type of bacterium frequently found in the faeces of humans, in animals, soil, dirt, flies, raw meats, poultry and dehydrated food. *Clostridium* spores can survive cooking and grow without oxygen. Infected meat or poultry left out on warm and unwashed surfaces or stored before it has fully cooled down can activate the organism. The toxins are released when infected food is eaten and cause abdominal pain and diarrhoea within 8–22 days. The disease lasts for 1–2 days and can be fatal in sick and older people.

Clostridium difficile: a bacteria which lives in the gut of some adults and children. It is the cause of infections mostly in a health care environment. *C. difficile* infections are usually evident when the antibiotics taken by the patient or service user upset the balance of good bacteria in the gut. The signs and symptoms are diarrhoea and a high temperature. It is infectious so it is essential when working with vulnerable groups such as sick children and older people that good *hygiene* practice and meticulous hand washing is maintained.

cluster sampling: a *sampling* method, used in research, which looks at the *survey* population and divides this into smaller groups or clusters. It is used when the survey population is unusually large. For example, a London Borough will have a large population, so it may be appropriate to break the sample down into groups by *race, class, gender, age*.

cocaine: a stimulant derived from the leaves of the coca shrub. It produces temporary euphoria and makes the user feel more alert. In its purified form it is taken intra-nasally ('snorted'). It is classed as an illegal *drug* because of the danger of *addiction*.

code of conduct: a statement which sets out a framework of professional *behaviour*. (See *code of practice*.)

code of ethics: a statement of *beliefs* held by a professional organisation or body. It would be expected that the professionals involved would adhere or stick to these beliefs in their professional practice, e.g. doctors who take an oath to preserve life.

code of ethics for social work: a framework of professional behaviour for social workers. It sets out the values, principles and ethics which underpin social work. This code was set up to ensure that the individual rights of service users are met.

code of practice: a theoretical framework which shapes how practitioners behave in a professional setting. These are designed to advise health and social care workers of their roles and rights and responsibilities. Each code of practice is underpinned by the care value base. They also provide guidance to patients, clients and service users on the support and behaviour they can expect from the worker caring for them. (See also *codes of practice for social care workers and social care employers, code of ethics for social work, code of standards of conduct, performance and ethics for nurses and midwives 2008*.)

codes of practice for social care workers and social care employers: standards of professional practice to which all social care employers and social care workers should adhere. The codes of practice for social care workers and social care employers are as follows:

Social care workers must:
- protect and promote the rights of service users and carers
- strive to establish and maintain the trust and confidence of service users and carers
- promote the independence of service users while protecting them as far as possible from danger or harm
- respect the rights of service users whilst seeking to ensure that their behaviour does not harm themselves or other people
- uphold public trust and confidence in social care services
- be accountable for the quality of their work and take responsibility for maintaining and improving their knowledge and skills.

The social care code of practice applies to qualified *social workers* and over a million other people working in a range of jobs in social care, most of whom do not have formal qualifications. All social care workers are expected to sign a general social care register.

Social care employers must:
- make sure that people are suitable to enter the social care work force and understand their roles and responsibilities
- have written policies and procedures to enable social workers to meet relevant codes of practice
- provide training and development opportunities to enable social care workers to strengthen and develop their skills and knowledge
- put in place and implement written policies and procedures to deal with dangerous, discriminatory or exploitative behaviour and practice
- promote codes of practice to social care workers, service users and carers and co-operate with care councils' proceedings.

code of standards of conduct, performance and ethics for nurses and midwives 2008 sets out the standards that are required of nurses and midwives. The standards state that nurses and midwives should:
- be trustworthy with the health and well-being of their patients
- treat patients as individuals and respect their dignity
- be able to work with others to protect and promote the health and well-being of those in their care, their families and carers, and the wider community
- provide a high standard of practice and care at all times
- be open and honest and able to act with integrity and uphold the reputation of their profession.

cognitive development: the development of an individual's thinking systems linked to problem solving and reasoning. This is particularly important to children as part of their *learning*, *intellectual development* and *language development*. Cognitive skills are acquired as children grow and develop their thinking and reasoning. Cognitive skills include:
- attention and concentration – the ability to give concentration and thought to a particular subject or object over a period of time
- classifying – the ability to sort, order and match according to size, shape and colour
- memory – the ability to remember and recall incidences.

colon: the part of the *alimentary canal* between the small intestine and the rectum. Its main function is the absorption of water. The colon contains many bacteria. Some of these are mutualistic (both human and bacteria gain a nutritional advantage). These bacteria receive a continuous supply of nutrients from the material in the intestine, in turn they synthesise a number of *vitamins* which may be absorbed by the body. The food passes from the colon to the rectum and is then evacuated from the body through the anus.

coma: a state of unconsciousness which can last for hours, days or longer. It is a state which indicates that the functioning of the *brain* has been affected. A person in a coma cannot be woken up or roused. There are different degrees of coma. In some patients there may be a pupil reaction to light, some restlessness, or some movement when touched. Other patients can be deeply unconscious and make no response to any stimulus such as light and touch. Causes of coma include severe injuries suffered due to a car accident, barbiturate poisoning or inflammation in the brain or encephalitis. (See *consciousness*.)

Commission for Social Care Inspection: an independent organisation established by the Health and Social Care (Community Health Standards) Act 2003. The role of the Commission was to inspect all care services and councils to ensure that a high standard of care is being given. It was replaced in 2009 by the *Care Quality Commission*.

commissioning is a process by which local authorities plan, organise and buy services that are required for care in the community.

Committee on Medical Aspects of Food Policy: (COMA) a committee of the Department of Health which produces important reports relating to nutrition and food. (See *National Advisory Committee on Nutrition Education*.)

Committee on Toxicology: (COT) a committee of the Department of Health which advises the government on the safety of food additives. (See *E numbers*.)

common assessment framework: a method and strategy of *assessment* used across all children's services to identify a child's need. It is a means whereby action can be taken to support a child before an issue reaches crisis point. The common assessment framework is used by different practitioners using the same method or common approach.

common health emergencies are those which occur most frequently in care settings. These include:

- *asthma* – supporting a client with breathing difficulties
- broken bones or *fractures* – supporting clients who have broken bones as the result of a fall, a heavy blow to a bone, or twisting and wrenching a bone; older people tend to be more vulnerable to broken bones because age and disease can weaken bones
- burns or scalds – supporting a client with a burn or scald which has damaged the skin; burns are caused by fire, dry heat, chemicals, friction, the sun's rays, or radiation while scalds are caused by the wet heat from boiling liquids and vapours
- choking – supporting a client with an obstruction in their *throat* which can block the passage of air and therefore requires quick action to remove it
- concussion – supporting a client who has had a blow to the head causing loss of *consciousness*
- cuts – supporting clients who have cut or scratched themselves on a sharp object
- electric shock – supporting a client who has suffered an electric current running through their bodies (in these circumstances it is crucial that the carer does not touch the body of the client, the source of electricity should be first identified and turned off using a broom handle or other non-conducting object)
- *heart attack* – supporting clients with chest pain.

Dealing with these health emergencies is an important aspect of a carer's work. Whenever an emergency arises a carer should:

- think 'danger' (check their own safety)
- determine the response of the casualty (levels of *consciousness*)
- check the casualty's airway, breathing and circulation and if necessary carry out the *ABC of resuscitation*
- place the casualty in the *recovery position* if this is appropriate
- get help – using the telephone, knowing what to say and giving the relevant information to the paramedics or *ambulance* crew.

(Source: *First Aid Manual.*)

Whenever possible carers should be trained as *first aiders* by appropriate agencies such as St John Ambulance.

communicable disease: a disease which is transmitted from one person to another, e.g. by *droplet infection* through coughing and sneezing. (See *infection*.)

communication: the exchange of information between individuals, groups and organisations. There are different methods of communicating such as:

- verbal/oral communication – which involves using voice including variation of the voice's tone and pitch. Use of *language* is also an important part of oral communication. Verbal communication is used in conversations, speaking on the telephone, in team and group meetings, conference speaking or giving a 'talk'. Interacting with clients using conversation enables the carer to offer encouragement and support and show interest. Asking questions and finding out how the client is feeling is an important aspect of care. There are some clients with disabilities which may make oral communication difficult. For example clients who are unable to speak may use a system called a *Bliss* board. Clients with visual impairments can use *Braille*. Clients with hearing difficulties can use *sign language* or special hearing aids. In other cases where clients do not speak English, information can be translated into their first language or an oral interpreter can be provided. (See *giving a talk* and *creating a PowerPoint presentation*)
- non-verbal communication – body language includes the use of the eyes and eye contact, facial expressions, body movement, posture which relates to how people sit or stand, proximity to others, touching and gestures and physical body movements such as the use of arms and legs. Non-verbal communication is a way in which messages can be conveyed to others. Positive non-verbal communication can involve maintaining eye contact, or leaning towards a person. Facial expressions, smiling, looking interested, with *gestures* such a putting a hand on the arm of another person, can convey support. However, sometimes these messages can be misunderstood; for instance in some cultures, maintaining eye contact can be viewed as being too confident, while looking away is seen as being 'sly'. Learning the different aspects of body language from a trans-cultural perspective is an important aspect of working in the caring profession
- visual communication includes writing, typing and illustrating information which is sent and received by individuals, groups and organisations. Every day millions of letters, memos, reports or lists are written and used to convey a message to others
- multi-media communication includes the use of television, video, computer, CD-ROM, telephone, fax, e-mail, texting using mobile phones and the internet. These methods support global, national and local communication networks
- using advocates when necessary to support a client, patient or service user
- communicating in groups.

Communication is viewed as an integral part of the caring process and developing such interpersonal skills can enhance this process. (See *active listening, interpersonal skills, barriers to communication, building confidence, care value base, culture, warmth, interaction, effective communication, strategies for effective communication, communication skills, conversational skills, communication of values in a care context*.)

communication cycle: the cycle of *interaction* which takes place between individuals within the communication process. It relates to the way that messages are received and understood by people who are communicating with each other.

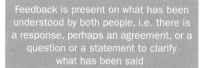

Feedback is present on what has been understood by both people, i.e. there is a response, perhaps an agreement, or a question or a statement to clarify what has been said

Ideas occur and the message is coded and sent to the other person, i.e. the person is expressing their ideas

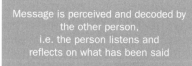

Message is perceived and decoded by the other person, i.e. the person listens and reflects on what has been said

The communication cycle

communication difficulties arise when there are blockages between people within the communication process. This can be the result of impaired hearing or vision or lack of equipment or a language difficulty when those people involved in the process are not speaking the same language. (See *barriers to communication*.)

communication of values in a care context describes the methods used by *care assistants or clinical support workers* to develop effective care practice. These are carried out by:

- considering the service user's rights, choices and personal preferences
- demonstrating the ability to show awareness of the individual needs of the service user
- establishing, building and maintaining positive relationships
- encouraging independence, giving support and empowerment
- protecting confidentiality of information in discussions
- showing respect for individual differences and maintaining a service user's dignity.

communication skills are the developed and proven ability to communicate and interact with others. This involves the ability to:

- apply positive body language using appropriate facial gestures, open or closed body positions, e.g. not sitting directly in front of the service user staring at her with arms folded across the chest, and not using eye contact to build rapport, because of an awareness of the cultural variations in the appropriateness of eye contact

- build positive relationships with service users by maintaining confidentiality, setting professional boundaries in the relationship, and building a rapport, i.e. a relaxed and friendly attitude between both carer and service user (see *effective communication, building confidence, strategies for effective communication, conversational skills*)
- communicate the care values by showing respect for individual differences, considering the service user's choices, encouraging independence and meeting the individual and different needs of each service user (see *communication of values in a care context*)
- listen with active listening skills which includes eye contact, being receptive, attentive and responsive, showing sincerity as well as being able to ensure the service user feels relaxed
- use appropriate language to carry out a number of tasks such as questioning, using different verbal prompts to develop an interaction between the carer and the service user. In addition to this the carer should be able to give out information in a way which is easy to understand and to be aware of any barriers to communication which might present themselves.

community: a group in society which may be determined by factors such as geographical boundaries, common values, *culture* and *religion*. The idea of 'community' implies shared *lifestyles*, relationships and individuals being in regular contact with each other.

community action is the process whereby locally based groups organise themselves to achieve objectives. They are usually associated with disadvantaged groups who seek redress for their grievances through *self-help* organisations. They organise themselves as *pressure groups* to draw attention to the different needs of their groups. In addition to this, they tend to look for funding from national and local government to help them achieve their objectives.

community care: a service which provides care in a person's home (*domiciliary services*). This can include a house which provides living accommodation for three or four people. *Sheltered housing*, offered to people with mental health disorders coming from long-stay institutions, is another example. Community care may enable a person to carry on their daily routine within the comfort of their own home. It can involve a number of the following services:

- family support services support family members who provide the vast bulk of caring. Probably over 80% of those being cared for receive little or no help from formal agencies, and are instead looked after by a wife, daughter or husband (see *informal care*)
- home carers support clients in a wide range of domestic tasks including cleaning, shopping, making beds. The extent of services offered depends on assessment by a home help organiser. In some areas, charges may be made through the process called *means-testing*
- community psychiatric nurses support clients with *mental health disorders* and there is a specialised branch for people with learning difficulties
- *district/community nurses* support patients across the entire range of physical illnesses and disabilities
- *health visitors* support specific client groups such as young children and their parents, and elderly clients
- *social workers* support and visit clients and assess their social needs. They then arrange appropriate services whenever possible
- *general practitioners (GPs)* support and treat patients in surgeries or *health centres* or at home, and will liaise with social and health services (particularly through district/community nurses) to address the needs of the client

- *day care* support takes place within a centre run by Social Services or by a health authority. The services vary, but usually there are meals, activities and other facilities such as bathing available. The health authority centres provide a range of medical services. Transport can also be arranged to these centres if necessary
- Meals on Wheels provides cooked meals for the elderly and disabled in their homes. All clients pay a standard charge which may differ from area to area
- Macmillan nurses support those who are suffering from *cancer* and wish to remain in their own homes. They are specially trained in cancer care
- *respite care* is offered in the form of a centre that takes elderly or ill people for a week or for a few days, so that the carer can have a break from his/her task
- *occupational therapists* provide support which includes assessment of the limitations of physical abilities, and organise appropriate aids, such as chair lifts, etc. They are also trained to help people work with their disabilities so that clients are able to become more independent. (See *aids and adaptations*.)

community care charters are documents which apply to key health, housing and social services. They form an essential part of effective community care which includes the assessment process. Such charters are developed locally to make sure services work well together to meet the needs of clients identified under community care legislation. Individual service providers have developed standards which are worked towards to ensure quality care. Working together is a means whereby the arrangements in caring for people can be linked to provide a co-ordinated service. (See *charters, Charter Mark*.)

Community Care (Direct Payments) Act 1996: an Act of Parliament which gives *local authorities* the power to give disabled people the relevant finance they need in order to buy their own health and social care services. The Act applies to England and Wales and there are corresponding procedures in Scotland and Northern Ireland. Local authorities have set up procedures under the Act which provide advice and information to clients with regard to their needs, requirements and appropriate care which they must have to support their daily living.

community health services are provided for people wherever they are, in homes, schools, clinics and on the streets. Examples are health visiting, school nursing, chiropody, speech and language therapy. Services such as community nursing, psychiatric nursing and physiotherapy can enable people with short- or long-term illness or disability to be cared for in their own homes.

community midwife: a qualified professional whose main role is to care for women through *pregnancy* and up to 28 days after the *birth*. They work closely with GPs and *health visitors* in providing *health promotion* advice to expectant mothers. (See *midwife*.)

community nurse: see *district nurse*.

community rehabilitation team: a specialist *multi-disciplinary team*. It assesses the needs of people at home or who have just returned home from hospital and organises packages of services to meet rehabilitation needs.

community work involves the tasks and activities which explore and review the needs of a local community. It includes:
- encouraging members of the community to act together to confront and deal with problems or difficulties as they arise
- stimulating neighbourhoods to form groups and provide *self-help*

- co-ordination and liaison between groups which can be *voluntary groups*, *support groups* for informal *carers*.

In addition to this, community work looks at improving the *quality of life* of those individuals who live in the local *community* or neighbourhood. (See *community action, pressure groups*.)

competence is the ability to apply knowledge learned in a practical situation or context with skill. Developing competence can involve learning through observation, problem solving, decision making with reflection of practice and evaluation.

complaints and complaints procedures: a complaints procedure is a formal way in which a service user can make a complaint, e.g. to voice a grievance or concern about medical treatment or social service. Within the procedure there are usually requirements for each health or social care provision to respond to that complaint. A complaints procedure requires the following:

- the complaint should be made in writing and each of the issues must be addressed
- a named member of staff is designated to deal with complaints
- a clear timescale is laid down for any complaint to be carefully examined
- a complaints committee is set up to hear the complaint; an independent member should be present at the hearing
- a method of responding to the complaint is formulated.

complementary and alternative medicine is used as an alternative or different method of treatment to that which is considered as conventional treatment. It can either be used as an independent alternative, or a complementary, treatment alongside the existing conventional approach. In 2000, a decision was made in the House of Lords Science and Technology Committee to combine complementary and alternative medicine so that it is now known as CAM and the treatment involved is known as therapies. Appropriate techniques may be selected which relate to the patient's physical, mental, spiritual and emotional needs. Complementary medicine adds another dimension to the healing and treatment of *disease* (see *holistic care*). Using CAM helps individuals recognise that they have a crucial part to play in their treatment. The therapies are divided into a range of methods, groups or categories such as:

- cognitive therapies, e.g. those which promote mind/body healing by using the power of positive thinking and promoting a sense of control in self
- expressive therapy, e.g. art therapy as individuals are encouraged to express their feelings to promote a sense of release and well-being
- medical systems, e.g. Chinese herbalism which uses different alternative or non-traditional therapies, such as acupuncture, to treat signs and symptoms and promote physical healing
- physical therapies, e.g. yoga which uses exercise to release thoughts and self-expression and promote a sense of well-being
- sensory therapies, e.g. aromatherapy. These are therapies that work in conjunction with the five senses and promote relaxation.

CAM looks at treating the whole person. There are some therapies which are professionally recognised such as chiropractic, osteopathy, acupuncture, herbal medicine, reflexology, massage and homoeopathy. (See *holistic care*, *holistic health*.)

complementary therapy: see *complementary and alternative medicine*.

compounds: two or more different *elements* chemically bonded together. Examples of compounds within the human body are water, *carbohydrates, lipids, proteins* and *vitamins*.

compulsory admission to hospital: legal procedures employed under the *Mental Health Act 1983* to admit a person to hospital. The person may be suffering from a *mental health disorder* and can be detained in hospital for up to 28 days for their own health and safety and/or the safety of others.

computed axial tomography: (CAT scanning) a method of diagnosing disease using radiology to examine the soft tissues of the body. *X-ray examinations* scan the body and view differences in tissue density. The computer then constructs on a screen cross-sectional images of what is being examined. *Tumours*, abscesses and other types of disease can be seen, diagnosed and treated with the aid of such visualisation. (See *magnetic resonance imaging*.)

conception is the biological process which involves an egg being fertilised by a sperm so that it then becomes implanted in the wall of the womb or *uterus*. (See *fertilisation*.)

conciliation: a service which is offered to couples who are considering separation or *divorce*. The Court Welfare Service gives assistance and support to this as a means whereby couples can discuss their problems either for the purpose of reconciliation or to form a working relationship which should prove a positive aspect of post-divorce care for their children.

confidence building: see *building confidence.*

confidentiality is a legal requirement to maintain the privacy of the personal details of a *service user*. These details must be restricted to carers on a need-to-know basis. It is accepted that *carers* in direct contact with the service user do need to know about the service user as part of the care process. However, information should not be shared without permission and then only to those identified people who also need to know, such as the appropriate manager, colleagues working with the same service user and other professionals who have co-ordinated the care of the service user. This is part of the *care value base* which underpins all care practice. (See *Data Protection Acts 1984 and 1998*.)

conflict of interest relates to decisions being made for a service user by professionals involved who have their own reasons for making a different decision. This is because they are working to their own agenda, e.g. seeing the additional needs of a service user but being unable to release the additional care required because of the increased cost involved, as they have been told by management to reduce expenses.

congenital disorders: disorders which are present at birth, e.g. congenital dislocation of the hip.

connective tissues connect other tissues and *organs*, protect and support organs and allow movement between the different organs. Connective tissue consists of *cells* supported in a fluid or semi-fluid substance called matrix which is produced by the tissue cells. There are different types of connective tissue:

- Areolar tissue – found all over the body: beneath the skin, connecting organs together and filling the spaces between organs. This tissue consists of a transparent semi-fluid matrix containing fibres and cells. There are two types of fibre: unbranched flexible, strong, non-stretchable white collagen fibres which occur in bundles and a loose network of yellow elastic stretchable fibres. The cells include the fibroblasts which produce fibres, mast cells which secrete an anti-coagulant, fat-filled cells and phagocytic histocytes which are important in defending the body against disease.

- Fibrous tissue – there are two types. White fibrous tissue consists almost entirely of closely packed, white collagen fibres. The bundles of white fibres are bound together by areolar tissue. Such tissue is found where strength with limited flexibility is required (e.g. tendons which attach muscles to bone). Yellow elastic tissue consists mainly of yellow elastic fibres. It is found where strength with great elasticity is required (e.g. *ligaments*, which join bones). This tissue is also found in the walls of *arteries* and in the bronchioles.
- *Adipose tissue* – areolar tissue with a matrix of closely packed fat-filled cells. It is important for storage. It is found in the dermis of the skin where it prevents heat loss, above the kidneys and in older people around the heart.
- Skeletal *cartilage* tissue – tissue which contains cartilage cells called chondroblasts. Cartilage is found at the end of bones, in the spine and in the walls of the windpipe. Skeletal tissue has more solid matrix.
- Bone – tissue which consists of cells supported in a solid matrix containing calcium, phosphate, carbonate and fluoride minerals.

consciousness: a state of being fully awake, alert and aware of the surrounding environment. Consciousness is controlled by the nervous system which co-ordinates the functions of all the body systems. When a person is involved in an accident or is injured in some way, he or she may lose consciousness and become *unconscious*. (See *coma*.)

consent: the agreement of a client to treatment or therapy. There are different ways of obtaining consent:
- oral consent – the client gives their spoken agreement
- written consent – the client gives consent in writing
- informed consent – information given to the client enables them to come to a decision
- capacity to give consent – when a person has the ability to give consent and no-one else is allowed to withdraw that consent
- consent for minors – consent for children under the age of 16 years is given by a parent or guardian. (See *age of consent*.)

consent form: a method of recording the agreement to, or the giving of, *consent*.

Contact a Family: a national charity which offers support to any parent or professional who is caring for a child with *special needs*. This support is offered through a *network* of local, national and *self-help* groups which offer advice. (See *children with disabilities*.)

contact tracing: methods used to find out the number of people with whom a person has had contact. This occurs when a person has contracted an infectious disease. To avoid the disease spreading to others, the doctor or health worker may ask the person concerned who their contacts were. Contact tracing is used in cases of *HIV, sexually transmitted diseases* and other potentially fatal infections.

contagious diseases: those diseases which are transmitted from one person to another. Examples include influenza and impetigo, a skin infection which is contracted by others when the infectious part of the body is touched.

content analysis is a research method. Researchers define a set of categories and then classify various materials in terms of the frequency with which they appear in the different categories. Content analysis involves a systematic study of different sources of material such as government reports, photographs and biographies relating to the issues which form the common themes or categories relevant to the **research**. For example, research into **child abuse** using content analysis may consider categories such as **race, class** and **gender**. In this way the researcher would be able to determine the different type of perpetrator or child abuser and details of the child and their background.

continuum of care: a **care** service which is continuous, each part blending smoothly with others (a **seamless service**). Clients experiencing a continuum of care should feel that each service works together to meet their different health and social care needs. This can involve:

- care at home such as **care provided by domiciliary services**
- care in a **residential home**
- care from home, such as visiting a **day centre** or hospital clinic
- transport which may also be provided.

(See **multi-disciplinary teams**.)

contraceptives are methods used to prevent **conception**. They are an important aspect of a sexual relationship where an unwanted **pregnancy** may cause **stress** and other problems. The use of a condom is also an effective means of preventing sexually transmitted diseases such as gonorrhoea and HIV.

contrast media techniques are methods used to give more detailed information on **X-ray examination**. They involve injecting a radio-opaque dye into the appropriate part of the body. This outlines any space or soft tissue. There are different techniques used on different parts of the body. Examples of contrast media techniques are **angiograms**, which investigate blood vessels and barium meals which help visualise the digestive tract.

Control of Substances Hazardous to Health (COSHH) Regulations 1993: regulations set up by the Health and Safety Commission which require all employers to carry out a **risk assessment** with regard to hazard and **risk**. A **hazard** can be any item, piece of equipment, chemical or biological agent which has the potential to cause harm. Risk is any harm which is likely to be caused by a hazard. For example, an unlocked cupboard containing cleaning materials in a day nursery could be assessed as a risk, because children could open the cupboard and interfere with the **chemicals**. The risk assessment procedures need to meet certain requirements:

- identifying any hazardous substance or equipment which is to be used or is being used in the workplace
- identifying those who use the substance or equipment
- evaluating any risk to the person or persons who use the substance/equipment and assessing any likely damage to health
- deciding on a procedure which will introduce systems of control when using the substance/equipment
- recording the risk assessment
- reviewing the risk assessment.

The **Health and Safety Commission** is responsible to the Health and Safety Inspectorate. Health and safety inspectors visit a workplace to check that the COSHH requirements are adhered to. (See **environmental health**.)

Control of Substances Hazardous to Health (COSHH) Regulations 2002:
regulations which have been set up to protect workers from the health *risks* which arise from
exposure to hazardous substances at work. These regulations relate to controlling substances
such as soldering fumes, sawdust, flour and grain dust and biological agents, all of which can
give rise to disease. To comply with COSHH, employers need to ensure that they:
- carry out risk assessments
- set up and maintain a framework of precautions
- monitor exposure and carry out regular disease surveillance
- have plans of action in place in the event of an accident or emergency
- ensure that staff are supervised and trained in the use of hazardous substances.

control systems of the body: the way in which different parts of the body are
co-ordinated to perform different functions. *Communication* between the different parts is
via the nervous system and/or chemical reactions brought about by the *hormones* of the
endocrine system.

convenience sampling or non-representative sampling: a *sampling* method
where the researcher uses the subjects or number of people who are available and the most
convenient. For example, a student studying health and social care issues may choose a
subject such as *drug misuse* and their sample group may be a number of students in their
college or school.

conventional therapies are treatment and therapies available in mainstream health and
social care, e.g. treatment given by a *general practitioner (GP)*.

conversational skills are ways in which individuals can use *language* to communicate
with each other. They are a means by which a carer can:
- introduce themselves to a client or patient and get to know the client. Talking is a way of
gaining relevant information such as address and health history
- build rapport with clients by finding out their hobbies, interests and their favourite subjects,
such as television 'soaps'
- sustain a relationship, asking a client how they feel, or remembering previous
conversations. All this can be a way of introducing security and trust as the client feels that
the carer has listened to them; reminding a client of positive and familiar topics can provide
positive reinforcement and can build self-esteem.

It is important to remember that the art of conversation has to be learned and developed.
Questioning should be structured in such a way that the client/patient does not feel
intimidated or threatened.

The development of language and conversation is the way in which babies and young
children learn to relate to the world in which they live. When language is delayed, or
there is a speech impairment, other methods of making conversation are used such
as *sign language, body language* and *gestures*. (See *communication, effective
communication, communication skills, building confidence, building a positive
relationship, interpersonal skills, strategies for effective communication, interaction*.)

co-ordination: the way in which different parts of an organisation or the body work
together in an efficient and organised manner. For example, changes in the *NHS (National
Health Service)* have led to co-ordination of care through *strategic health authorities*.

coping is the way in which individuals learn to live with *changes* occurring in their everyday lives. These changes can be predictable or unpredictable. Change can bring happiness or heartache to an individual's life. In order to cope with change people develop different strategies. These help them to understand themselves as they experience difficult and painful situations. Coping strategies can include:

- identifying the reactions, thoughts and feelings that the change is bringing to the surface
- being aware that change has happened and that there is something that can be done to support that change
- coming to terms with life after the change.

It is important to remember that different people cope with change in different ways. Some people may react with anger, frustration, depression and helplessness. Whatever the reaction, people going through change may need *support* and help. There are different methods of coping, which include using:

- the individual's own initial and immediate response through denial and the use of defence mechanisms
- problem-focused strategies such as discussing the situation with a counsellor or care professional who will help the individual deal with the situation they face one step at a time
- emotion-focused strategies such as diverting the negative and painful thinking into different activities such as keeping busy, thinking of things which are far worse, or through strategies such as prayer and meditation.

There are various support mechanisms available to help individuals cope. These include:

- family and friends and a *network* of support
- *counselling* using a professional agency
- support or *self-help* groups provide empathy and advice
- information services such as *Citizens Advice Bureaux*.

cornea: the transparent area at the front of the *eye*. The function of the cornea is to focus light onto the retina. When light rays pass from one medium to another with a different density they are bent. This process is called refraction. Refraction occurs in the eye when light rays pass from the air into the cornea and through the lens. The angle through which rays of light are bent by the cornea is always the same. This creates a potential problem because light rays from objects which are close to the eye need to be bent more if they are to be focused. Therefore the lens is able to change shape. It is the lens, therefore, which alters the amount of refraction, allowing both close and distant objects to be brought into focus on the retina. This process is called *accommodation*. The cornea consists of living cells which are supplied with nutrients (such as glucose) from the aqueous humour – a liquid which lies directly behind it. There are medical conditions which can affect the cornea and so affect an individual's sight. Sight can be clouded or sometimes lost completely. Such problems can be treated by a corneal transplant where a small piece of cornea is transplanted from a donor.

coronary arteries are *blood* vessels which carry oxygen to the muscles of the *heart*.

coronary heart disease: disease affecting the *coronary arteries* which supply the muscle of the *heart*. When one of these arteries becomes blocked, the area of heart *muscle* that it supplies is deprived of oxygen. The muscle therefore dies and gives rise to what is known as a heart attack or a myocardial infarction. There are three main reasons why blockages occur in the coronary arteries:

- atherosclerosis – this is due to the build-up of fatty material or *atheroma* in the lining of the artery wall. Eventually this material, along with fibrous tissue and calcium salts, forms hard plaques which lead to the narrowing of the lumen of the artery
- thrombosis – the presence of a *blood* clot in one of the coronary arteries. This is often associated with atheroma. It is thought that the blood clot forms when the surface of one of the plaques breaks away. The clot blocks the lumen of the artery
- spasm – the muscle in the wall of the coronary artery contracts and goes into a spasm. The reasons for this are not really understood but it again produces a narrowing of the lumen.

cot death: see *sudden infant death syndrome (cot death)*.

Council of Europe: an organisation which produces legislative frameworks which affect the lives of individuals in the *European Union (EU)*.

counselling: the process or interaction by which one person helps another person to help themselves. It is a way of relating and responding to another person so that they are helped to explore their thoughts, feelings and behaviour, in order to reach a clearer self-understanding. This enables the person to find and use their strengths and draw on their resources so that they can cope more effectively with their lives. Counselling has basic principles which are applied when a counsellor works with a client. These principles include providing:

- an opportunity for a client to work towards behaving in a more satisfying and resourceful way in dealing with a problem or difficult situation
- a voluntary service for the client
- an opportunity for the counsellor to clarify with the client the basis on which counselling is to be given
- the client with reassurance that their rights and decisions are respected
- the means whereby a counsellor may continue to monitor and develop their own skills, experience, resources and practice
- a service which ensures that counsellors are properly trained for their roles and are committed to maintaining their *competence*
- relevant support to counsellors so that they have regular and appropriate supervision/ consultative support
- a confidential service so that all information which passes between counsellor and client is treated with discretion.

The British Association for Counselling is a national voice for counselling. (See *active listening*, *communication*, *communication skills*, *conversational skills*, *listening skills*.)

'crack' is a stimulant which is a form of *cocaine* usually smoked or mixed with *heroin* and injected.

creating a PowerPoint presentation is a method of using supporting resources to develop an oral presentation, i.e. *giving a talk*. When creating a presentation it is important not to use more slides than are necessary. A few basic rules apply when using PowerPoint:

- the 6/6 rule – no more than 6–8 lines per slide and no more than 6–8 words per line. Only enter key words onto the slides, not full sentences. This is important if the audience is going to listen to what is being said

- use voice pitch and tone to vary what is being said – it may be necessary to pause and emphasise some words. This will make the presentation more interesting for the audience
- keep animations simple – lots of words whizzing round the screen, and eye-catching transitions between slides, may seem like fun but they are very distracting to the audience
- keep colours simple – using the templates and colours provided will make for an attractive and professional-looking presentation
- remember – the PowerPoint presentation should be used to support the oral presentation, not the other way around. It is important to know the subject well and to practise at least three times before the actual presentation. This will enable the presenter to speak much more naturally and only use the PowerPoint slides to prompt what they need to say
- nerves – nerves before giving a presentation are part of the experience. Just before the start of the presentation, imagine it is over and everyone is clapping and smiling, saying what a good presentation it was and that there appeared to be no nerves. (See *target group/audience*.)

creative play: a way in which children learn about the world around them. This involves exploring, experimenting and imagining. Creative *play* makes a major contribution to the way in which children develop. It reinforces the enjoyment and satisfaction that children achieve through making objects and through discovery. It is creative play that enables children to explore the function of materials and to find out how things work. This develops their senses and also encourages their fine motor skills and *hand/eye co-ordination*. Examples of creative play are painting, collage, sand play, water play and imaginative play or make believe. Creative play is identified in the *early years curriculum* and integrated into the early learning goals as creative development.

crèche: a form of childcare provision which offers informal, short-term, group care for children while their parents attend courses or classes, or go shopping. If crèches are provided for more than two hours a day or for more than six days a year, they must be registered with *OFSTED.*

crime involves breaking the legal codes set up in society and supported by the judicial system. This can include burglary, theft, violence and other acts against a person or their property. The criminal is the person who has carried out the crime. The victim is the person on the receiving end of the crime. People are often asked to declare any past criminal offences when they apply for employment within the health and social care sector (see *victim support*). Criminology is the study of crime and reviews its extent, and the nature of offenders within society.

Crime and Disorder Act 1998: an Act of Parliament which makes provision for preventing crime and disorder. It deals with issues such as:
- racially aggravated offences
- the rebuttable presumption that a child is '*doli incapax*', that is, incapable of committing an offence.

crime prevention: procedures or methods used to educate the general public about ways of avoiding becoming victims of crime. For example, local *police education officers* work with **schools** and colleges and talk to pupils about crime. Local neighbourhoods may join together with the police to set up neighbourhood watch schemes. In this way local groups can take part in crime prevention by watching for any suspicious behaviour in the area.

criminal justice system: a range of professional groups whose roles and responsibilities are to enforce law and order in society. Professionals involved in law and order include police forces, the Probation Service, youth justice workers, Crown Prosecution Service and victim support.

Criminal Record Bureau: (CRB) an agency which carries out police checks on all prospective workers involved in education, health and social care, e.g. teachers, child care workers, **volunteers** and **social workers**. (See **Vetting and Barring Scheme – Every Child Matters.)**

crisis: an episode in an individual's life which may be difficult to cope with. Examples include an accident, sudden death, redundancy, unemployment, diagnosis of illness or abuse. When the episode is found to be difficult or impossible to handle, then voluntary or statutory workers can support or organise a routine to help the individual involved.

culture relates to a way of life. All societies have a culture or common way of life. A society's culture includes the following:
- **language** – the spoken word and verbal communication
- customs – **rights**, rituals, **religion** and **lifestyle**
- shared system of values – **beliefs** and morals
- social **norms** – patterns of behaviour which are accepted as normal and right (can include dress and diet).

The different cultures evident in society reflect the richness of cultural diversity, where they live and work together but retain their individual identity.

curriculum vitae (CV): a summary of the main aspects of a person's previous experiences. A curriculum vitae may be used by individuals when they are applying for employment or voluntary work. There are usually four main areas covered in a CV:
- personal data – name, address, telephone number, email address and driving licence
- education and training – the level of education, including the names of schools and colleges attended with dates and a list of qualifications gained. Any further training courses attended should be included, with details of certificates or diplomas achieved, written in chronological order putting the most recent qualifications first
- work experience – name and details of previous employers with dates of employment. There should be a list of each job held with details of the skills and abilities required to carry them out, and wherever appropriate, the level of responsibility attained and a description of any specialist achievements and skills
- leisure activities – general interests and positions held (e.g. club secretary, youth club leader, membership of any groups). Any particular skills that have been acquired through leisure activities can also be mentioned here.

cycle of disadvantage or oppression is a theory which is based on the idea that **poverty**, low-paid employment or unemployment runs in families and that children brought up in poverty under-achieve in education and have limited opportunities as they grow older. In addition to this, it is more likely that their children will also grow up in the same situation and so the cycle reinvents itself.

cystic fibrosis: a *genetic disorder* affecting children. It leads to the *exocrine glands* becoming defective. The production of thick mucus obstructs the intestinal glands including the pancreas and the bronchi. *Signs and symptoms* of the disease include *failure to thrive*, weight loss, coughing and a gradual deterioration of the *respiratory system*. Some children display the symptoms at birth, while others may not develop symptoms for weeks or even years. Cystic fibrosis is progressive and incurable. It can be detected through the 'sweat test' when a sample of the child's sweat is analysed.

cytotoxic drugs are used to combat and treat malignant disease such as *cancer*. Such drugs inhibit cancer cells by slowing down cancer cell division. However, they can also have harmful side effects such as damaging and destroying white blood cell growth. Some patients may also suffer from hair loss, baldness, vomiting and sickness as a result of the treatment. Use of such drugs should be carefully monitored. (See *chemotherapy.*)

Do you need revision help and advice?

Go to pages 292–304 for a range of revision appendices that include plenty of exam advice and tips.

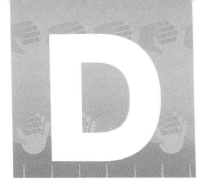

daily living tasks: see *activities of daily living*.

data: facts and information collected by a researcher during a course of study. Data can be *qualitative* or *quantitative*. Qualitative data is descriptive and is often about attitudes, beliefs or feelings. Quantitative data is measurable and is expressed in numerical form.

data analysis: the methods used to examine *data* which has been collected by a researcher. The results are sometimes compared with other *research*.

data collection is the way in which researchers gather the information necessary to support their *research*. The researcher decides whether the data will be *quantitative* or *qualitative* or a combination of both. To collect the data a representative sample of the population is usually selected. Careful *sampling* is crucial to the research findings, particularly if they are to be applied to the population as a whole. Evidence can be collected from primary sources such as interviews and questionnaires or from secondary sources such as books, journals and the internet. After collection, the data is analysed and evaluated to reach a conclusion. (See *research*.)

Data Protection Acts 1984 and 1998: Acts of Parliament giving people the right to access information about themselves contained in personal records stored on a computer or on paper. (See *access to information*.) Under the Data Protection Act individuals have rights which include:

- the right to know what information is collected, stored and processed. They can see the information and correct it if necessary
- the right to refuse to provide any information
- the right to ensure that data is accurate and up to date
- the right to confidentiality and that information should not be made accessible to any unauthorised person
- the right that information should not be retained for longer than necessary.

day care is the provision which is available to young children, older people and the disabled during the day. In day care, the physical, emotional, social, intellectual and cultural needs of the client are supported. Carers are available to supervise and support the clients as their individual needs arise. Examples of day care are *day nurseries, pre-school groups* and *day centres*.

day centre: a care setting which people can attend between one and five days a week. The centre provides:

- meals and snacks
- *leisure* and recreation

- supervised care activities
- *respite care* for carers
- opportunities to meet and socialise with others.

Day centres are a valuable means of support for clients with physical, mental and *learning disabilities*, for older people and for families in need of support and care. Day centres can be statutory, voluntary or private sector provision.

day nurseries provide full- or part-time day-care for children up to five years of age. Only a few nurseries take children under six months. Day nurseries are staffed by trained *nursery nurses*, and untrained childcare workers. Private and council day nurseries must conform to national standards, and be registered and inspected by *OFSTED*.

day surgery is the provision offered by a hospital or health centre which involves treating a patient within a single day. Patients are admitted for an operation and return home the same day. Day surgery is a cheaper form of treatment than longer-term admission to hospital.

deafness or hearing impairment is the temporary or permanent loss of hearing which can occur in one or both ears. The updated term for deafness is hearing impairment. Temporary deafness can be caused by an ear infection or a build-up of wax in the external canal. Permanent deafness is usually caused by damage to the ear, the *auditory nerve* or the hearing centre in the *brain*. Deafness can be:

- total – which means that no sounds can be heard
- partial – which means some sounds can be heard but not others; it is often difficult for sufferers to understand what others are saying.

The nature of deafness may vary as follows:

- outer ear deafness – usually caused by a build-up of wax which blocks the ear canal or when a bead or small object has been pushed into the ear blocking out sound waves
- middle ear deafness – repeated infection damages the middle ear. The minute ear bones or ossicles become stuck together. This is termed 'glue ear'. The sound waves no longer cause the ear ossicles to vibrate and sound impulses are not transmitted to the brain
- inner ear deafness – is due to damage to the cells in the cochlea. This inhibits the conversion of vibration into sound impulses.

deamination: the process of breaking down surplus amino acids to produce urea.

death is the result of the total shutdown in the systems of the body. The number of deaths per year is measured and compared locally, nationally and globally. These are called *mortality rates*. Mortality rates are usually recorded in an HMSO publication 'The Social Trend', or are provided by the *World Health Organisation (WHO)*. *Local authorities* keep their own local mortality rate records. *Infant mortality* rates are the number of deaths of babies under one year old in a given year as a proportion of the number of babies born that year. A death certificate is issued after death, following a medical examination of the body.

death rate is the number of deaths per year per 1000 people in the population. Age-specific death rate is the number of deaths of people within a specified age range per year per 1000 people in that age range. This is termed the crude death rate. (See *demographic trends*.)

decision making: a process which involves the client or patient discussing their treatment and *care* with their professional carers. This relates closely to *consent*. It should be acknowledged that the client, patient or service user has the individual right to make a decision with regard to their care. (See *care value base, autonomy, rights and choices, empowerment*.)

defence mechanisms: unconscious strategies that protect the conscious mind from *anxiety*. According to Freudian theory, defence mechanisms invoke a distortion of reality in some way so that we are better able to cope with a situation. There are different mechanisms including displacement, projection, identification and repression. (See also *Freud*.)

Defence mechanism	Behaviour
Identification	Person subconsciously copies the behaviour or lifestyle of a person she/he secretly envies.
Repression	A person may repress a negative feeling from their consciousness. If this causes anxiety then they will choose to ignore the situation. They may forget to go for cervical smear checkup, because they do not want to think about the implications of the smear results if they are not negative.
Projection	A person blames everybody else, the place where they work or the management system. This is a way of covering over their own inadequacies.
Displacement	When a person is annoyed or frustrated by a situation they will often take this out on someone else. The feelings are displaced onto an inappropriate situation.

deficiency diseases are the result of a person not eating a healthy and varied *diet*. Deficiency diseases cannot be transmitted to other individuals and can usually be cured by adding the missing substance to the diet. A *vitamin* deficiency disease is one which develops as a result of a shortage of vitamins. A person who lacks vitamin C may develop scurvy; scurvy can be cured by eating oranges which contain vitamin C.

degenerative disease: a disease or illness which affects the body in such a way that it causes physical or psychological deterioration which cannot be rectified. An example of a degenerative disease is *Parkinson's disease*.

dehydration: the loss of fluid or water from the body. This can have serious side effects. Dehydration occurs when an individual has lost more water than he/she has taken in through food and drink. This may happen if they have:

- a severe *infection* which causes sweating and vomiting
- drunk a large amount of *alcohol*
- taken vigorous exercise
- spent time in a hot and dry environment without drinking.

When dehydration occurs the fluid must be replaced as soon as possible. This can be done by giving the person a mixture of 1 teaspoon of salt and 8 teaspoons of sugar to 1 litre of water. This replaces the water and minerals lost through sweating, vomiting or diarrhoea. Medicines such as Dioralyte can be bought over the chemist's counter to produce the same effect. In severe cases, a person may be admitted to hospital and given extra fluids by intravenous infusion or drip.

dementia: a range of illnesses involving the *degeneration* of the *brain*. This can lead to a serious decline in mental faculties including loss of *memory*. There are a number of different types of dementia, but the most common are:

- cortical dementia – memory impairment, personality changes, loss of speech (e.g. *Alzheimer's disease*)
- sub-cortical dementia – memory impairment, personality deterioration which can result in degeneration of cognition, emotion and movement (e.g. *Huntington's disease*).

There are different methods of treatment for dementia, and the process of diagnosis forms an important part of how the patient/client will be treated. If the dementia is due to some underlying disease such as HIV/AIDS, or a brain tumour, then these conditions will be treated. However, if there is no apparent cause for the dementia then the level of the dementia itself will be assessed. *Drugs* such as neurotransmitters are the main type of treatment for dementias. It is important to remember that dementia is not part of normal ageing. Most older people show no signs of dementia. (See *Admiral Nurse Service*.)

demographic changes: changes that are brought about by variations in the factors affecting population, for example *birth rate, death rate*, emigration, immigration and *life expectancy.*

demographic trends: a collection of data that locates, identifies and describes the characteristics of a population in terms of age, disability, geographical data, etc. It is influenced by health needs, disability, average age of the population, employment and unemployment, different family structures, numbers of older people, and provides information about the way in which society is changing. Government bodies review statistics so that they can construct social policies relevant to the needs of the population. For instance, the rising number of older people in the UK population is an indicator of the increasing need for health and social care provision for the elderly. Examples of different types of demographic trends are:

- age profiles – birth and death rates, numbers of children, older people, etc.
- the geographical distribution of the population, for example the numbers of people who live in towns, cities or in rural areas
- patterns of health and disease, for example the numbers of people who suffer from different diseases, children who suffer from different types of infectious disease, the number of cases of meningitis which are reported in geographical areas
- ethnicity – the different ethnic groups which make up society such as Chinese, Welsh, Afro-Caribbean
- social and economic groups, for example, the unemployed, persons on benefit, lone parents.

Demographic trends are based on local, regional, national and global statistics.

demography: the study of population, especially with reference to distribution and size. The information or *data* on which the study of demography is based is obtained by *census*. The registration of births, marriages and deaths also provides a continuous flow of information. Demography is a useful tool for those delivering and administering services, both at national and local level as it enables them to predict and plan for future needs in society. (See *demographic trends*.)

denial is a common type of *coping* mechanism. It is a way in which people manage different events, circumstances and situations in their lives. Denial is a mechanism often used in the following circumstances:

- *death* of a family member or friend
- news of *terminal illness*
- redundancy
- sudden incident or *accident*.

In order to cope with a situation the person tries to ignore or refuse to believe what is happening. To deny the occurrence of an event can make the situation unreal. It is part of the process of *grief* and the person needs support to accept what is happening and to work through the different dimensions of the incident and its impact on their relationship with others.

dentists: professionals who treat the *teeth* and gums. They also promote dental health and oral hygiene. Dentists work in their own practices or in hospitals:

- as orthodontists giving specialist advice on straightening teeth
- on oral and maxillofacial surgery, correcting facial defects as well as damaged features, resulting from accidents and disease to jaw and face
- for the community dental service – providing a service to young children, expectant mothers and people with *special needs*.

Dentists either work in the National Health Service or in private practice. Dentists qualify as Bachelors of Dental Surgery after training which takes five years.

There are other careers within dental health, including technicians who make dental appliances, therapists and hygienists who advise people on how to look after their teeth and gums, and dental nurses who work with dentists in hospitals and private practice. Such nurses prepare fillings and dressings, pass instruments to the dentist and generally attend to patients.

deoxyribonucleic acid (DNA): a nucleic acid mainly found in the *chromosome* of cells. It is the hereditary material of all organisms except some viruses. DNA can be extracted from small samples of tissue and examined (DNA 'fingerprinting'). Such testing is used in situations such as:

- solving crime, through forensic science investigations – fingerprints or body fluids are often left at the scene of a crime, and are unique to a given individual
- detecting inherited diseases, where signs and symptoms have not appeared – DNA profiles can sometimes identify those members of the family who have inherited a given disease (this method may be used in forecasting the occurrence of the disease in a family)
- monitoring bone marrow transplants – DNA fingerprinting can predict whether new bone marrow is likely to be accepted or rejected
- revealing family links – DNA can indicate whether claimants are part of a given family.

Department for Children, Schools and Families is the government department responsible for education and support for children, the schools they attend and the families that they live in. It is responsible for children's services and schools, 14–19 education and the *Respect Task Force*.

Department for Work and Pensions: (formerly the Department of Social Security, DSS) the central government department responsible for policies with regard to welfare *benefits* and how they are distributed to the client. It also offers support and guidance with regard to benefits.

Department of Health: the central government body responsible for the administration of health and social care. It is presided over by the Secretary of State for Health.

Department of Health and Social Services Northern Ireland: the department responsible for health, social services and social security in Northern Ireland. The department co-ordinates the different services in association with four boards. A junior minister is responsible for this department and he or she reports to the Secretary of State for Northern Ireland.

dependant: a person who relies on another person for physical, social, emotional, intellectual or economic support. For example, a child or young person under the age of 16 years is dependent upon his or her parents or primary care giver.

dependence describes the reliance that a service user has on a carer to carry out particular tasks. It can also refer to reliance on drugs or illegal substances which can cause withdrawal symptoms if the individual stops taking the drugs or substance.

dependency ratio: the proportion within a population of those under 15 years and over 65 years to those between 16 and 65 years (i.e. of working age). Those under 15 make up the 'young dependants', and those over 65 the 'elderly dependants'. Together they are referred to as the 'dependent population'. (See *demography*.)

depression is a mental health disorder. Depression may be indicated by the loss of social and emotional functioning which can either be biologically based (endogenous depression) or related to life events (reactive depression). Those with depression experience a feeling of sadness, worthlessness and guilt. They find the challenge of living overwhelming. Depression is probably the most widespread of mental disorders affecting 1 in 20 people.

determining patterns of health relate to social and statistical trends with regard to health and ill health. It is supported by academic, medical and governmental research. This includes *World Health Organisation (WHO)* statistics, *public health* observations, *demographic trends* as well as national and local reports.

devaluing: having a fixed attitude which *stereotypes* views and beliefs held by others as being of no importance, for example, disregarding a person because of their *culture*, their religious belief or their personal *lifestyle*.

development: the evolution of different skills and abilities through the ages and stages of life, e.g. movement in a baby evolves into rolling, crawling and walking. There are factors which can affect and influence development. These include:

- behaviour problems – aggression, attention deficit disorder, attention seeking
- biological – through the mother to foetus link, e.g. foetal alcohol syndrome
- environment – the location of housing or community – are conditions overcrowded, is the neighbourhood safe to live in, are the surroundings polluted by traffic, etc.
- family life – family relationships, child rearing practices of parents or parent, siblings, whether the child's basic needs are met, e.g. child abuse
- inherited factors – genetic and inherited diseases and disorders, e.g. cystic fibrosis

- lifestyles – nutrition and choices of diet, e.g. malnutrition
- psychological – bonding and separation issues, sibling rivalry, fears and insecurity, e.g. separation anxiety
- social and economic factors – social class, gender, culture, education, discipline, socialisation (see *disability*, *developmental delay*, *social factors, economic factors*).

development theories: theories which seek to explain and describe human development. They relate to how an individual develops. They include psychodynamic, humanistic, cognitive and behavioural theories. (See *behaviour theories*.) Theorists vary in the emphasis which they place on a particular stage of development. Some theories studied on health and social care courses are as follows:

- genetic and biological approaches – which explore genetic influences as well as effects of the endocrine and nervous systems (e.g. *Gesell*, *Eysenck*)
- the importance of early experience and stages of development (e.g. *Freud*, *Erikson*, *Bowlby*)
- the impact of the environment and the development of modified behaviour (e.g. *Skinner*, *Pavlov*)
- the interaction between social influences – social constructivism (e.g. *Vygotsky*, *Bruner*)
- developmental stages as they relate to the environment (e.g. *Piaget*)
- social learning – which explores the effect of other individuals, groups, cultures and society (e.g. *Bandura*).

The study of these different theories with regard to development, behaviour and learning is a means whereby health and social care workers can understand how individuals develop and grow. It is possible to explore reasons for an individual child's or adult's behaviour and to learn strategies for the management of development, behaviour and learning. For example, an understanding of biological theory will determine an understanding of how genes affect the individual in terms of their vulnerability to certain diseases and disorders. (See *learning theories*.)

developmental delay is a term used to describe a child who has not reached his or her *developmental norms or milestones*.

developmental norms or milestones: the average or typical skills and behaviours that might be present in a child of a particular age. These are established by studying large numbers of children of the same age. (See *human growth and development*.)

developmental tests: see *child health surveillance programmes*.

deviance: a person's *behaviour* which breaks the rules of normal conduct and norms of behaviour within a particular social group. Deviance very much relies on the concept of majority rule, i.e. the way that most people behave in a group. For example, most nurses wear a uniform when working on a hospital ward. If one nurse chooses to work on the ward in shorts and T-shirt this would be viewed as deviant behaviour. However, deviance is a relative term which can change from time to time and from place to place.

diabetes mellitus is a condition in which the amount of glucose in the body cannot be properly controlled. Glucose comes from the digestion of starchy foods such as bread or potatoes and sugary foods, and from the liver. Glucose levels are controlled by insulin, a hormone produced in the *pancreas* which lowers such levels by converting glucose into glycogen which is then stored in the liver. The main symptoms of untreated diabetes are thirst, the passage of large amounts of *urine*, extreme tiredness, weight loss, genital itching and blurred vision. The main aim of treatment is to restore near normal blood glucose levels. Together with a healthy lifestyle this will help improve well-being and protect against long-term damage to the eyes, kidneys, nerves, heart and major arteries. There are two different types of diabetes mellitus.

- Type 1 is insulin-dependent diabetes. This develops when there has been a severe lack of insulin in the body because most of the pancreatic cells which manufacture insulin have been destroyed. This type of diabetes usually appears before the age of 40 years. The cause is not known but viruses may play a part. It is treated with insulin replacement and diet.
- Type 2 develops when the body can still make some insulin, though not enough for its needs, or when the insulin that the body does make is not used properly. This type of diabetes usually appears in people over the age of 40 years. It is most common among the elderly and overweight. The tendency to develop this form of diabetes may be passed from one generation to the next. It is usually treated by diet alone. It is estimated that between 75% and 90% of people with diabetes are Type 2 dependent. Between 1,035,000 and 1,242,000 (around 2%) of the UK's population have diabetes.

diagnosing disease: methods used by a doctor or professional person to detect the cause of signs and symptoms with which a patient or service user is presenting.
A doctor will:
- take a medical or case history
- carry out a physical examination
- conduct special tests such as blood tests, X-ray examinations, urine tests.

diagnostic imaging techniques: methods used to detect and assess the condition of a disease or disorder using images. Examples are *X-ray examination* and *computed axial tomography* or CAT scanning.

diagnostic techniques or tests: methods used to detect and provide evidence of *disease* or disorders which are affecting an individual. Examples are *blood tests*, *X-ray examinations* and *diagnostic imaging techniques*.

diaphragm: a thin, tough sheet of *muscle* and fibrous *tissue* which separates the trunk of the body into two parts. The upper part is called the thorax (chest) and contains the heart and lungs, while the lower part is called the abdomen and contains the main organs of digestion, excretion and reproduction.

diarrhoea: loose and watery stools forming part of the *faeces*. When a person suffers from diarrhoea they pass frequent watery stools. *Babies* with diarrhoea may quickly suffer *dehydration* because the fluid lost is greater than the amount of fluid which they are taking in.

diet: the amount and type of food and drink which is regularly consumed. A person's diet will often depend on:
- the different types of food available
- cultural and religious influences
- personal preference
- how physically active a person is
- the amount of money available to spend on food.

A balanced diet is one which contains the appropriate amount of all the essential nutrients, i.e. carbohydrate, fat, protein, vitamins, minerals, fibre and water. Diets should be designed to meet the specific needs of individuals, i.e. babies and young children, adolescents, adults and older people. Other requirements need to be taken into account such as whether the individual is sedentary or active, their lifestyle, culture, religion, beliefs, pregnancy, as well as diet-related disorders such as diabetes. (See *balanced diet*, *nutrition*, *nutrients*.)

dietary reference value (DRV): dietary standards which refer to different foods and *nutrients*. This also includes the estimated average requirements (EAR) in the diet. These are related to age, gender, activity levels and state of health (See *Committee on Medical Aspects of Food Policy*.)

dietetics: the study of the scientific principles of nutrition, i.e. the study of food and how it is applied through diet, feeding and disease.

dieticians are trained professionals who advise others with regard to food and *nutrition*. Their special skill is to translate scientific and medical knowledge relating to food and health into terms which everyone can understand. Dieticians, as part of a team, care for people in hospital or in the community. They also work to promote good health by teaching the public and other health professionals about *diet* and nutrition. Qualified dieticians join the British Dietetic Association following a recognised degree or two-year postgraduate diploma. Degree courses in dietetics, which include state registration, last four years.

differential growth rate: this measures how different parts of the body grow and develop at different times and rates. For example, the *nervous system* grows rapidly in the first few years of life, the reproductive organs hardly grow until *puberty*, while general bodily growth occurs steadily throughout childhood. (See *centile charts*.)

diffusion: the movement of substances, molecules or ions from where they are high in concentration to where they are in lower concentration. It is an important means of transport of substances through *cell* surface membranes. The rate at which substances move in and out of cells can be affected by a number of factors such as:
- temperature
- surface area of the membrane
- difference in concentration on either side of the membrane
- thickness of the membrane.

An example of diffusion can be seen in the way that oxygen is passed from the alveoli to the blood in the capillaries of the *lungs*.

Food and oxygen move by diffusion from the *blood* or *tissue* fluid into the cells. *Carbon dioxide* and other waste materials diffuse in the opposite direction, from the cells into the blood. Therefore an exchange of materials takes place.

digestion: a process which breaks down food from a solid form. Large molecules of food are broken down into soluble matter so that they can be absorbed into the bloodstream for transport to different parts of the body. The *digestive system* is responsible for the process which begins as soon as food enters the mouth. Food then proceeds through the oesophagus to the stomach, into the duodenum, the rest of the small intestine, the large intestine, the rectum and out through the anus. During digestion, food is broken down by both physical (including mechanical) and chemical means.

digestive system: the organs associated with the ingestion, digestion and absorption of food. Also called the alimentary system. The main parts of the digestive system include:

- mouth – food is introduced into the mouth and chewed by the teeth which break it down and mix it with saliva. **Enzymes** in the saliva start breaking down starch. The taste buds on the **tongue** ensure that food is enjoyed but they can also give the person warning of anything which is unpleasant or harmful to the body. The tongue rolls the food into a bolus and pushes it to the back of the throat where it is swallowed and enters the oesophagus
- oesophagus – this is a long muscular tube which links the back of the throat to the **stomach**. The movement of food through the oesophagus is by **peristalsis** which enables the food to be pushed down into the stomach
- stomach – the stomach is a muscular pouch which acts as a reservoir for food collection. Food is stored in the stomach and after a period of time the muscular activity of the stomach churns up the food and mixes it with gastric secretions. These consist of mucus, hydrochloric acid and the enzyme precursor pepsinogen. The pepsinogen is converted into pepsin which then begins to break down the proteins. Hydrochloric acid is responsible for activating pepsinogen and also kills any harmful bacteria which may have been swallowed with the food. The mucus which is mixed with the food lubricates it. The food passes from the stomach to the duodenum, through the pyloric sphincter, in a liquid form called chyme
- duodenum – this is the first part of the small intestine which is C shaped and is approximately 20 cm long. The chyme goes into the duodenum where digestive juices from the **pancreas** are secreted on to the partly digested food. **Bile** is sent from the **liver** to break down (emulsify) fat into smaller droplets
- ileum – the food passes on into the ileum where further enzymes are secreted from the intestine wall to complete the conversion of all **carbohydrates** to sugar, all **proteins** to **amino acids** and all fats to **fatty acids** and glycerol. Absorption of food takes place in the small intestine, although a small amount of water, glucose, alcohol and other substances which do not need to be broken down further may be absorbed in the stomach. The wall of the small intestine provides a large surface area through which absorption takes place. From the small intestine the food is passed into the colon
- colon – the colon (large intestine) is the final part of the muscular tube which carries semi-liquid digested food or chyme. Here 90% of the remaining water is absorbed from the chyme and the semi-solid faeces remain. When the lower part of the colon (the rectum) is full of faeces pressure is put on the walls of the rectum which contain nerve endings. These send messages to the brain which inform the person that they need to open their bowels. The food is passed out through the anus, an opening at the end of the rectum which is controlled by a ring of muscle called the anal sphincter.

It is necessary for health and social care workers to have a basic understanding of how the digestive system works. For example, when helping older clients or children with toileting it is important to observe the faeces for colour, formation and amount. Such **observation** can lead to early recognition of disease or disorder. For example, stools which are pale, putty-coloured and fatty can indicate a malabsorption disorder of the intestines, for example gallstones. The appearance of fresh **blood** in stools, or of **diarrhoea**, can also indicate some disease or disorder of the alimentary system (see also **vomiting**). Dysfunctions of the digestive system include ulcers, irritable bowel, Crohn's disease and bowel cancer.

dignity: a carer should ensure that their clients are given the type of care which enables them to feel that they are worthy of respect and should have pride in themselves and positive *self-esteem*. (See *care value base*, *building confidence, respect*.)

direct care: see *caring*.

direct payment: payments designed to allow people to manage and pay for their own care. This enables them to organise their own care rather than having it organised by their local social services department. This method of payment is supported by relevant legislation. The process was updated in 2003 to give guidance to local councils on how to make direct payments. Then in 2008 the government published 'A guide to receiving direct payments from your local council – a route to independent living', which offers advice to those already receiving payments and to those who are thinking about applying for payment.

Disabilities Trust: a charity set up in 1979. Its aim is to provide an imaginative concept of personal care and specialist housing for people with severe physical disabilities.

disability: a substantial and long-term learning, mental or physical impairment of a person's ability to carry out normal everyday activities for living. There are different causes of disability which include genetic and chromosomal factors such as ***Down's syndrome***, birth injury such as cerebral palsy, infectious diseases such as meningitis, lifestyle-related disease such as breathing problems due to heavy smoking, accidents causing severe injuries, nutritional effects on the foetus such as ***foetal alcohol syndrome*** as well as age-related disorders such as arthritis, and sensory impairments such as sight and hearing loss. There are three types of disability:

- learning disability which relates to cognitive development and intelligence. This can be a result of brain injury or some other form of disease or inherited or genetic disorder, e.g. Down's syndrome
- physical disability which relates to loss of motor skills and co-ordination which affects mobility, e.g. multiple sclerosis
- sensory disability which relates to impairments in hearing, sight and loss of sensation or numbness in the skin, e.g. partially sighted and vision disorders.

There are barriers for those with disabilities such as limited access to education, employment and transport although legislation is trying to make access easier. Disability affects the lives of a large proportion of our society. There are over 6.5 million people with disabilities living in the UK – together with millions more involved as family carers. According to the latest national estimates, two-thirds of those with disabilities are living in or on the edge of poverty. Unemployment is much higher amongst the disabled, with three out of four relying on state benefits as their main source of income. (See ***benefits***, ***informal carers***, ***Disability Alliance Educational and Research Association***, ***Royal Association for Disability and Rehabilitation***, ***National Disability Advisory Council***.)

Disability Action is a development agency working to ensure that people with disabilities attain their full rights as citizens. Disability Action has over 180 member groups covering every aspect of disability from learning to physical, sensory and hidden, i.e. those disabilities which are not obvious to others.

Disability Alliance Educational and Research Association is a national, registered charity which has the principal aim of relieving ***poverty*** and improving the living standards of disabled people. Founded in 1974, DAERA brings together over 300 member groups, from national organisations covering all aspects of disability, to local **self-help** groups. Such a wide membership base plays an active role in shaping policies, in developing services and in influencing a highly effective campaign strategy. Only voluntary organisations can act as full voting members of DAERA but **local authorities, strategic health authorities** and departments of local authorities can become affiliated members. The aims of the alliance include informing the disabled and their carers about their rights to state benefits and services. The alliance also undertakes research into their needs – with particular emphasis on income and, through its campaigning, promotes a wider understanding of the views and circumstances of all those with disabilities, looking to end the link between disability and poverty. (See **pressure groups**.)

Disability Discrimination Act 1995 and 2005 is an Act of Parliament which makes it unlawful to discriminate against disabled persons with respect to employment or the provision of goods, facilities and services. The Act established the **National Disability Council**. The Act incorporated the Disabled Persons Employment Acts 1944 and 1958 and the Disabled Persons Act 1981 and 1986. The 1944 Act implemented recommendations following the Tomlinson Report 1943 which aimed at ensuring that those with a disability were given a fair chance of employment. Three key features were:

- the Register of Disabled Persons
- a duty placed on employers to recruit a percentage of people with a disability (quota scheme) into their workforce
- the provision that certain jobs were to be reserved for those with disabilities.

The Disabled Persons Act 1981 placed a duty on the providers of buildings and premises to comply with standards of access for those with a disability. This Act was updated in 2005 with regard to additional requirements for public authorities and the promotion of equal opportunities for disabled people. The updated version:

- includes multiple sclerosis, HIV and cancer within the disability remit
- makes it unlawful if transport operators discriminate against disabled people such as by limiting their access
- makes it easier for disabled people to rent property and make the necessary adjustments to the property to meet the daily living needs of their disability
- makes it unlawful for local authorities to treat disabled people less favourably.

Disability Living Allowance: a tax-free benefit for those under the age of 65 years with care and **mobility** needs, or for those who are terminally ill and need help with personal care. It is:

- not dependent on **national insurance** contributions
- not affected by any savings or (usually) by any income that the person or their partner may have
- usually ignored as income for those on income support or on jobseekers' allowance.

There are two qualifying components:

- care component – where an individual needs help with personal care because they are ill and disabled, for example with activities such as bathing, dressing, or using the toilet
- mobility component – where a person between the ages of 5 and 65 years needs help in getting around, for example if they cannot work or have difficulty in walking because they are ill or disabled. If they can work but need help with walking then they can also apply for financial support. (See **benefits**.)

Disability Wales is an independent charity working to promote the rights, recognition and support of all disabled people in Wales. Disability Wales operates a central unit which can provide general information on a wide range of subjects such as:

- access
- aids and equipment benefits
- education
- employment
- holidays
- housing
- leisure activities
- transport and mobility.

The organisation actively campaigns for greater awareness and understanding of disabled people in Wales and, in particular, Disability Wales works to establish a disabled person's right to be treated as an individual.

Disabled Living Foundation: a national charity providing practical, up-to-date advice and information on many aspects of living with disability. It offers support for disabled and older people and their carers in the following ways:

- the Hamilton Index – a comprehensive directory of daily living equipment with different aids and adaptations
- courses and training – which focus on practical issues surrounding disability
- an equipment centre – this houses a display of over 1000 items of disability equipment with experienced therapists available to provide supporting information and advice for anyone who would like to learn, update or expand their knowledge of equipment
- a database which is the most comprehensive in Europe on disability equipment containing details of over 14,000 items, including currently available and discontinued products, with suppliers' names and addresses and self-help groups
- a consultancy service which can be tailored to meet the needs of a wide range of organisations involved in the design, building, management and operation of facilities for the disabled.

disadvantage refers to the limited opportunities that individuals may have in the community that they live in. For example, children who live in a poor economic community have fewer opportunities than those who live in a more affluent area. This affects health, housing, education, income, lifestyle and life choices. (See *cycle of disadvantage or oppression*.)

discipline: the setting of boundaries for positive behaviour. This addresses codes of behaviour in a variety of health, social care and educational settings. *Codes of practice* are written procedures which outline how professionals should address discipline issues. They are an integral part of professional care and education practice. A code of practice in a care provision should include procedures for:

- clients and their behaviour in different settings
- carers and how they relate to the clients
- teams with appropriate reporting and communication mechanisms.

disclosure is the revelation of information to another person. It takes place when a client informs another person that abuse has taken place. For instance, in an interview with a childcare professional, a child may say that they have been abused. Disclosure can be particularly distressing when the abuse has involved a father or a familiar family friend or relative.

discrimination is unfair treatment based on prejudice. In health and social care settings, it may relate to a conscious decision to treat a person or group differently and to deny them access to relevant treatment and care. There is anti-discriminatory legislation in place to cover areas such as *race, disability, gender* and some aspects of employment legislation relates to health status.

Discrimination can take three forms:

- internal – a person develops negative stereotypical and fixed ideas and attitudes about individuals or groups in society
- individual – a person develops negative and discriminatory attitudes towards a person because that person is, for instance, black or gay, religious or old
- institutional – a group, organisation or company can reinforce discriminatory practice by the way in which they treat their staff; an example of this would be the attitude towards women and their prospects of promotion to management.

Discrimination can be:

- direct (overt) – as in the behaviour of an individual who openly discriminates against another by making racist jokes or name calling
- indirect (covert) – as in the behaviour of an individual which is less obvious but whose actions can show a subtle form of discrimination; this may happen in employment where there are clear *equal opportunities* policies but a disabled person may still be continually bypassed for promotion.

discriminatory practice relates to negative and inappropriate discriminatory *behaviour* within a care setting. This can take the form of *abuse* of power, *bullying* and *harassment*, *infringement of rights*, *labelling* and *stereotyping*.

disease is a condition of the body that has been diagnosed because of the presenting *signs and symptoms*. Diseases can be divided into three types:

- physical disease which affects parts of the body, e.g. coronary heart disease
- psychological disease which affects the mind. These are called mental health disorders, e.g. depression
- social disease which is associated with lifestyle or the environment, e.g. alcoholism, eating disorders.

There are other factors which can contribute to disease. These are:

- allergies, i.e. when an individual has a severe reaction to something, e.g. asthma can be a reaction to animal hair
- infections, e.g. coughs which can have long-term effects on the lung.

There are different methods of treatment for diseases, such as medication (see *drugs*) and surgery which can be major or minor, *complementary therapies*, *radiotherapy*, *chemotherapy* and *counselling*.

Disease can also be:

- Communicable – passed from one person to another. This includes infections caused by viruses (influenza), bacteria (meningitis), fungus (athlete's foot) and parasites (head lice). They can be transmitted in a number of ways, e.g. droplet infection, touch and physical contact. They can occur at any age.
- Non-communicable – caused by some breakdown in bodily function resulting in disease and dysfunction such as degenerative (arthritis), deficiency (lack of vitamin C causes scurvy), inherited disease (cystic fibrosis), lifestyle or environmental disease (lung cancer due to smoking).

Many diseases can be prevented by:
- adequate health and safety precautions at home and in the surrounding environment
- a healthy and balanced diet
- a healthy lifestyle, moderate alcohol intake, no smoking and the taking of exercise
- immunisation and screening programmes
- a pollution-free environment, clean water and food supplies and safe sewage disposal. (See *acquired disorder*.)

disease surveillance: consistent monitoring of key *infections* or incidence of disease in order to:
- detect and determine trends which could be developing, e.g. the growing incidence of tuberculosis
- review and evaluate how to reduce future incidence
- implement methods of infection control, e.g. the surveillance of measles. For example, recent controversy over a purported link between the MMR injection and autism meant that some parents stopped having their babies immunised against measles. Consequently there has been an increase in the incidence of measles.

disempowerment: the denial of the *rights and choices* to which clients are entitled. This includes withholding relevant information from the client and not involving them in any form of *decision making* with regard to emotional, physical, intellectual, social and cultural aspects of their lives. (See *empowerment*.)

disinfection: the process of eliminating *infections* or *bacteria* and *viruses*. Infection can be picked up from equipment, instruments, clothes and the surrounding environment. Liquids, sprays and solutions, which are made from chemicals (disinfectants), are used to treat contaminated areas.

disorder: see *acquired disorder*.

district nurse/community nurse/practice nurse: qualified nurses who work specifically with patients or clients in their homes in the community in which they live. They form part of the *primary health care* team. They work closely with GPs and are usually based in a health *clinic* or *health centre*.

diversity reflects practice which benefits a multicultural care environment because it positively supports different cultures, lifestyles, beliefs, religions and traditions. Diversity promotes *respect*, tolerance and social cohesion and builds positive self-esteem because individuals feel valued.

divorce: the legal dissolution of a marriage. Over the last 50 years there has been a major change in social attitudes towards marriage and family life. In recent years there has been a fall in the number of couples getting married and a rise in divorce rates. Divorce is a stressful time for families, especially young children who find the breakdown in relationship between parents distressing. (See *family support worker* and *conciliation*.)

divorce rate: a statistical measure of the number of divorces, usually expressed as the number of divorces in any one year per thousand married couples in the population.

doctor: a health professional who gains a qualification through medical school which is recognised by the General Medical Council.

Doctors:

- detect and diagnose *disease*, disorders and *dysfunctions* with regard to the human body
- treat disease, disorder and dysfunction and monitor recovery
- prevent disease, disorder and dysfunction through *health promotion, child development* and *immunisation programmes*.

Once qualified a doctor has many choices. He/she may decide to:

- work in an NHS hospital in specialist areas such as medicine, surgery, pathology or psychiatry
- work in the independent sector, i.e. private hospital, voluntary organisations
- complete further training to become a GP.

To qualify as a doctor, an individual completes clinical training which enables them to register with the General Medical Council; training takes five or six years.

domestic roles: the roles which are played by the man and the woman within a home environment. A stereotypical role of a woman is that she cooks, cleans and brings up the children, while a man goes out to work and does not wash up or clean. However, the domestic division of labour has changed in recent years with the emergence of 'new man', that is the man who helps with housework, childcare and other domestic tasks.

domestic violence is physical *abuse* within a relationship. One partner in the relationship might use physical, emotional, economic, sexual or psychological means to exercise control over the other. Domestic violence is a criminal offence. It takes place in partnerships irrespective of age, race, class, culture or religion. In a majority of cases the violence is committed by a man against a woman. The Domestic Violence and Matrimonial Proceedings Act 1976 has been reinforced by new initiatives which were introduced by the Government in 1997. This should mean:

- much stronger protection for child victims of domestic violence
- that there will be a recognition of the different relationships in which domestic violence can arise (this is viewed by many as a major improvement in the law). (See *Women's Aid Federation*.)

Domestic Violence, Crime and Victims Act 2004: an Act of Parliament relating to criminal justice, which was introduced to increase the protection, support and rights of those who are victims of or witnesses to *domestic violence*. It also brings in new rules for trials of those charged with causing the death of a child or vulnerable adult.

domiciliary services are health and social care services which are available in the home. One example of these is the *home care service*. These services may be *means tested* so some clients may be required to pay a contribution towards the service provided. Such services may be provided by *local authorities*, private or *voluntary sector* organisations. (See *community care*.)

Down's syndrome: a genetic condition caused by the presence of an extra chromosome; those with Down's syndrome have 47 chromosomes instead of the usual 46. About one baby in every 1000 has Down's syndrome. They are usually born below average weight and length and have distinguishing features such as a face which appears flattened. They often have large, sometimes protruding tongues in small mouths, their eyes slant and they have broad hands with short fingers. An increasing number of children with Down's syndrome are now attending mainstream schools and are going on to gain employment and lead semi-independent lives as full members of the community. The Down's Syndrome Association is the only national *charity* working exclusively for children with Down's syndrome and their families.

drop-in centres are usually part of a larger scheme or service. They offer an informal facility for clients to 'drop in' for a chat and a cup of tea; older clients, for example, may drop in to a church hall for coffee. Parents with young children may drop in to a *health centre* or *family centre*. Another term used for drop-in centres is 'pop in' centres. They provide short-term sessions which offer support and the opportunity to meet others.

droplet infection: a way in which infection is spread. It involves tiny droplets containing pathogens (disease-causing organisms) being sneezed, coughed, talked or breathed out and sprayed on to people nearby. Droplets can stay in the air and be breathed in later. The 'common cold' is spread in this way.

drug dependence is addiction which can cause:
- uncontrolled craving for a particular drug
- harmful side effects causing deterioration of physical, emotional, social and intellectual well-being
- withdrawal or severe physical reactions when the person stops taking a drug.

There are different types of dependence which include:
- physical dependence – the continual use of drugs leads to physical reactions as the body craves a particular drug
- psychological dependence – the continual use of a drug in order to 'feel good' and to support a sense of well-being, a feeling that is short-term, which disappears as the effect of the drug wears off. Therefore more of the drug must be taken to promote the effect for more of the time.

(See *drug misuse*.)

drug misuse and drug abuse are terms to describe the use of *drugs* which are taken for non-medical reasons. Taking drugs in this way is harmful to the body and is generally considered to be socially unacceptable. An example of the misuse or abuse of drugs is taking *amphetamines* or 'speed' to produce feelings of pleasure and excitement.

drugs are chemicals taken to alter the way in which the mind or body works. They can be used in the treatment of *infections* and *diseases*. Drugs can be divided into three types. These are:
- medicines – used to treat and prevent diseases. They can be either bought over the counter at a chemist shop or obtained by prescription from the GP or dentist
- social or recreational drugs – those drugs which are considered to be socially acceptable because they are being taken by a large part of the population. These drugs include caffeine which is found in tea and coffee, alcohol, and nicotine which is found in cigarettes and tobacco
- illegal drugs – these are controlled by *legislation* and are taken to produce feelings of pleasure and excitement but possessing and using them is against the law. (See *drugs and legislation*.)

drugs and legislation: certain drugs are controlled by *legislation*. Controlled drugs are classified into three categories which are differentiated according to the penalties that can be imposed.

- Class A. These drugs are the 'hard' drugs of addiction such as *heroin, cocaine, morphine*, pethidine, *methadone*, opium and *LSD (lysergic acid diethylamide)*.
- Class B. Those most likely to be encountered are *cannabis*, cannabis resin, amphetamine, dexamphetamine and methedrine.
- Class C. These drugs are also considered to be addictive but not as dangerous as Class A or B. The drugs referred to are, as far as the police are concerned, relatively uncommon.

dying: the process that a person goes through when all the systems in the body begin to slow down in the approach to *death*.

dysarthria is a speech disorder. It occurs when the mechanisms which are involved in speech are limited due to sensory malfunction or tumours, damage or injury to the *muscles* and *nerves* surrounding the *throat* (e.g. in Parkinson's disease).

dysentery: an infection of the intestines. The organism causing it may either be a particular type of protozoan or a bacterium. The infection usually occurs as a result of living in overcrowded and poor living conditions. The disease can spread and can reach *epidemic* proportions. It also causes severe *diarrhoea* and can lead to *dehydration* and weight loss.

dysfunction: impairment, abnormality or disorder affecting a person's physical, emotional, intellectual, cognitive or mental functioning. Such breakdown can affect any body system and/or organ.

dyslexia: a specific learning difficulty caused by a defect in the part of the *brain* which processes *language* and affects the skills that are needed for learning in either or both of the following areas:

- literacy – reading, writing and spelling
- numeracy – arithmetic, problem solving and calculation.

This does not mean that individuals with dyslexia cannot become fully literate or numerate. With suitable help they can succeed and often have different and valuable problem-solving abilities.

dyspraxia: a neurological disorder which affects children. Messages are not transmitted to the *brain* in the normal way. The cause is not known. However, there are signs and symptoms which can include the child being:

- slow to reach milestones, for example, speaking
- inhibited by movements which are uncoordinated, e.g. they cannot run, hop or jump; throwing and catching a ball is difficult; they can be clumsy and accident prone
- unable to hold a pencil properly and drawing is difficult; later on they find maths, reading and writing difficult
- excitable, with temper tantrums and a poor concentration span
- affected by poor memory and difficulty grasping concepts.

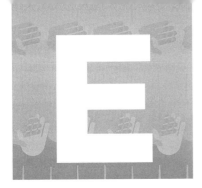

E. coli (Escherichia coli) are bacteria which live in the large intestine, colon or bowel of humans. They are found in large numbers in human **faeces**. *E. coli* is a harmless bacterium when it lives in the large intestine but when it contaminates water (or food) through sewage or poor hygiene it can cause diseases such as dysentery and **gastroenteritis**.

E numbers are *food additives* which have been identified and given a serial number. Foods which contain only additives with E numbers can be supplied in countries within the European Community. Such additives were originally tested and recognised by the EC as being safe for human consumption.

early years: a term used to describe the care and support for learning of pre-school children, for example, *day nurseries, playgroups* and *childminders*.

early years curriculum: the curriculum that all children follow, providing a foundation for learning from birth to five years. This is called the Early Years Foundation Stage and was updated in 2008 as part of the 10-year childcare strategy set out in the **Childcare Act 2006**. The principles are grouped into four themes. These are:

- a unique child – this includes child development, **inclusive practice**, keeping safe, and health and well-being
- positive relationships – this includes children learning to respect each other, working with parents as partners, and the need for a **key worker** or named person to support learning for each individual child (see **partnership with parents**)
- enabling environments – this includes **observation**, **assessment** and planning, supporting every child, the learning environment, the wider context such as working towards the implementation of **Every Child Matters**
- learning and development – this includes **play** and exploration, active **learning**, creativity and critical thinking. This is covered in six areas of learning, i.e. the early learning goals.

The early learning goals last until the end of the reception year in primary school. The curriculum ensures continuity for children as they progress from their **early years provision** to primary school. The early learning goals are:

- **communication, language and literacy**
- mathematical development (see **numeracy**)
- creative development (see **creative play**)
- personal, social and **emotional development**
- knowledge and understanding of the world
- physical development (see **motor skills, physical growth and development**).

early years provisions are those which support the care and learning of pre-school children. They are registered and inspected by **OFSTED**. They can also cater for children with *special education needs*.

There are different types of early years provision with varying specified numbers of staff to the number of children. The provisions include:

- local education authority nursery schools – open ten half-day sessions a week, for 40 weeks each year. The schools may take up to 50 children per session, and staff must have teacher or **nursery nurse** training
- independent nursery schools – with opening times similar to **local authority** establishments, with up to 30 children per session
- nursery classes – childcare provision situated within primary schools with up to 30 children per session
- *day nurseries* – provision for children which offer full-time day care for children from three months to five years
- independent day nurseries – similar to those operated by the local authority except they are privately owned
- *pre-school groups* – childcare provisions which are supported by the Early Years Alliance, formerly the Pre School Playgroup Association. Children usually attend for morning or afternoon sessions (see *early years curriculum*)
- childminders
- parent toddler groups which are usually run by voluntary organisations.

early years workers are those who work with young children and their families. They may be **childminders**, pre-school workers, **playworkers**, **nursery nurses** and nursery assistants, teachers, **social workers**, **family support workers**, play leaders and babysitters.

ears are the organs of hearing and balance. The position of the ears at the side of the head is important as this enables a person to know the direction from which sounds come. Sound waves reach the ears and produce **nerve impulses** which are transmitted to the **brain** via the **auditory nerve**. The structure of the ear is made up as follows:

- the outer ear is a visible flap of **cartilage** called the pinna. This collects sound waves and passes them through the ear canal to the eardrum (tympanic membrane). The eardrum is a thin sheet of tissue which covers the entrance to the middle ear
- the middle ear contains the three small **bones** (ossicles) called the malleus (hammer), incus (anvil) and stapes (stirrup). When sound waves reach the eardrum or tympanic membrane they cause it to vibrate and the vibrations are transmitted through the ossicles to the inner ear
- the inner ear contains fluid-filled tubes called the cochlea and semi-circular canals. The cochlea contains sensory cells which convert vibrations of sound into nerve impulses. The semi-circular canals are concerned with balance. The cells in the semi-circular canals are very sensitive to movement of fluid. When a person moves their head, impulses are sent to the brain so that the brain is aware of the person's position. If they make a sudden movement and lose their balance then impulses are again sent to the brain which in turn sends an impulse to the appropriate muscles to bring about a correcting movement.

Dysfunctions of the ears include tinnitus and glue ear. (See *deafness or hearing impairment*.)

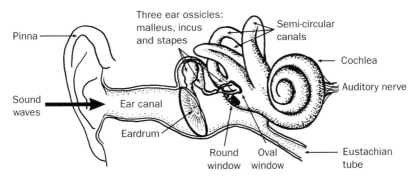

The ear

eating disorder: a disruption in the eating habits or appetite of an individual. This may relate to the amount and the type of *food* that an individual eats or chooses not to eat. These disorders are closely associated with the emotional, psychological or physical *well-being* of a person. Examples include a teenage girl who may overeat, binge and make herself sick. Weight loss can also be caused by physical illness, however; for instance, a young child may lose weight due to poor absorption of nutrients in the small intestine. This is called malabsorption syndrome. (See *anorexia nervosa, bulimia nervosa*.)

echocardiography: a procedure using *ultrasound* as a means of studying the structure and movement of the *heart* in order to diagnose any disease, disorder or dysfunction.

economic factors are factors which affect family finances. They include income, employment and the cost of living. These factors have an influence on the health and well-being of the individual.

economy, efficiency and effectiveness are the three major aspects alongside social, demographic, technological and political reform which have determined change in the *NHS (National Health Service)* in the last 20 years. These aspects of change are defined as follows:
- economy: relates to the different methods and strategies used in funding and in the management of resources within the health service, i.e. the cost of NHS staff, buying necessary equipment and maintaining NHS buildings
- efficiency: explores how the health service is working in terms of results and competence, i.e. are there positive results in terms of the number of patients being treated?
- effectiveness: looks at the ways in which the needs of service users are being met, e.g. are hospital *waiting lists* being reduced?

Enshrined in these major aspects are *equity* and accessibility, which review the quality of fair and equal treatment of service users. (See *trends in health care, quality assurance*.)

ecstasy: a Class A *drug* in the same category as *heroin* and *cocaine*. It is an illegal drug and other names include 'Disco burgers', 'Dennis the Menace', 'Fantasy' and 'E'. It is taken as white, brown, yellow or pink tablets and acts as a stimulant, producing its effect after 20 minutes. It gives a sense of prolonged *well-being* with a heightened perception of colours and sounds. It has potentially harmful side effects including *anxiety*, panic attacks and insomnia (inability to sleep). It is usually taken at clubs and 'raves' and in this atmosphere may cause severe **dehydration** which can lead to heat stroke.

ectopic pregnancy is the implantation of the fertilised egg outside the uterus. Instead of being implanted in the uterus the egg is implanted in the Fallopian tube. As the embryo grows it puts pressure on the walls of the Fallopian tube. At approximately six weeks into the **pregnancy** the growing embryo can rupture the wall of the Fallopian tube. This is a surgical emergency and the woman needs immediate hospital treatment. (See **fertilisation**.)

eczema is one of the commonest reasons for dry and sensitive **skin**. There are different types of eczema:

- atopic eczema – is found in babies and young children. It is thought to be hereditary as it runs in families. There are links with conditions such as **asthma** and hay fever. Common symptoms include an overall dryness of the skin usually accompanied by extreme itchiness. The skin may become inflamed, cracked and split and may be prone to infection
- seborrhoeic eczema – there are two types of this condition, one which is most commonly seen in babies and the second type seen in young adults. Areas affected tend to be the oily parts of the body such as the scalp, face, groin and chest. Seborrhoeic eczema is not normally itchy
- discoid eczema – this condition is usually confined to the arms and legs and consists of scaly, itchy, coin-shaped patches that can blister and weep
- varicose eczema – this condition is confined to the legs, commonly found in older people and in those with varicose veins
- contact eczema – there are two types, irritant and allergic. Irritant eczema is caused by exposure to substances such as soaps, detergents, engine oils, hair dyes and bleaches. Allergic eczema is caused by specific sensitivity to a material such as nickel, chrome or rubber.

education: the process of learning, it involves acquiring and developing knowledge and skills in formal settings such as **schools** and informal settings such as sports and leisure clubs. The government has set up a comprehensive programme to improve schools in England. In the White Paper 'Excellence in schools', a programme of school reforms is based on a series of strategies to improve standards. These include:

- expanding **early years** or **pre-school group** education
- campaigning to improve **literacy** and **numeracy** in primary education to ensure that children have the tools for learning
- reducing class sizes in infant schools.

Education Act 2005: an Act of Parliament which ensures that all children's services and schools are inspected by **OFSTED**. This includes **childminders**, **day nurseries**, **pre-school groups** and careers services.

educational psychologist: a trained professional who is responsible for assessing and supporting children with **special education needs**. Educational psychologists are members of a team or panel of professionals who review and monitor a child's education needs and play a responsible role in the statement process. They monitor ongoing special needs children who are integrated into mainstream schools. They may also explore issues such as **intelligence**, management of children in a classroom setting, dealing with children's **behaviour**, psychometric testing, teacher training and any other agency working in direct contact with the education process. (See **special needs** and **statementing**.)

effective care practice: implementation of the *care value base* in support of clients, patients and service users. (See *empowerment*.)

effective communication is dependent on various factors. Some factors enhance communication and others inhibit it.

Type of factor	Enhancing factors	Inhibiting factors
Physical	Non-verbal communication, the environment, privacy, good personal grooming and dress, appropriate touch and proximity	Invading *personal space*, noise, distractions, inappropriate environment, ignoring changes in the body language of others, having a closed position
Emotional	A relaxed manner, understanding, warmth, sincerity, respect, responsiveness, *empathy*	A high degree of distress in the situation, imposing own agenda, minimising importance of feelings, blocking, giving inappropriate advice, being patronising, off-loading own experience
Social	Attentiveness, common interests, respecting identity, appropriate language, *self-awareness*, receptivity, encouraging others	*Stereotyping, labelling,* lack of respect for individuality, ignoring or excluding, having a defensive or aloof attitude
Spoken	Clarity, pace, tone of speech, prompts, reflection of content, asking open-ended questions, respecting silence, *assertive skills*	Inappropriate language for the setting (such as jargon, dialect or slang), inappropriate closed questions, interrogating, being overly aggressive or submissive
Working with those with special needs	Attending specifically to individual difficulties and disabilities by using preferred form of *interaction*, including sign language, *Bliss system* and different technologies, the role of *advocacy*	Lack of awareness or disregard of individual difficulties and disabilities

egocentrism occurs when the individual is unaware that others may have a different view or opinion from their own. (See *Freud*.)

elderly people: see *older people*.

electrocardiogram (ECG): a test which traces the electrical activity of the *heart*. The tracings form a pattern which is shown on an electrocardiograph (see next page). When the heart beats, electrical activity forms a wave which moves from the top to the bottom of the heart. Electrodes are placed on the skin and these register the electrical activity as a tracing onto a screen or sheet of paper. This method of testing is a way of detecting whether the heart is working properly and efficiently. For example, after a heart attack the tracing of the waves will indicate damage to the heart muscle.

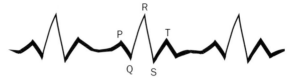

P wave is due to atrial contraction
Q, R, S and T waves are due to ventricular activity

A healthy ECG trace – a small section is shown

electroencephalogram (EEG): the tracing of the electrical activity of the brain forms a pattern, measured on an electroencephalograph. When messages are taken to and from the brain they are transmitted by electrical charges called impulses. Electrodes are placed on the head and these register the electrical activities in the brain as a tracing onto a screen or sheet of paper. This method of testing the brain is a way of detecting electrical activity defects such as *epilepsy*.

embolism: a *blood* clot which breaks away from the place where it has formed and is transported in the bloodstream until it becomes trapped in an *artery* and is unable to move any further. An embolism is often responsible for:
- *cerebrovascular accident (CVA) or stroke* – a clot in the cerebral artery in the *brain*
- pulmonary embolism – a clot in the pulmonary artery in the *lung*
- myocardial infarction or *heart attack* – a clot in the *coronary artery*.

embryo: the product of *fertilisation*; a sperm has penetrated an egg and the embryo is formed, usually in the Fallopian tube. It then moves into the *uterus* where it becomes implanted. The embryo develops all its main organs in the first eight weeks. After this, the embryo becomes known as the *foetus*.

emergency services (999): services such as police, fire brigade and ambulance services, mine, mountain, cave and fell rescue, and HM Coastguard.

emotional development: see *human growth and development*, *bonding*, *attachment* and *separation*.

emotional maturity: the development of a stable *self-concept* or *identity*, which enables an individual to become *independent* and take responsibility for his or her own actions.

emotions are feelings that individuals experience in the relationships that they have with themselves, with others and with the world they live in. Emotional growth is an important aspect of a child's personal development. Emotional needs include love, affection, consistent care, security, praise and encouragement. Meeting these needs in a supportive way enables a child or client to develop positive *self-esteem*. Providing emotional support is a key responsibility for a carer working in health and social care.

empathy: a person's awareness of the emotional state of another person and their ability to share an experience with them. It might take the form of a common feeling of sadness and pain in an unhappy situation. It is a reason why *support groups* are successful: they are set up by people who have been through similar situations in their lives. An example is CRUSE, where those who have been through the **bereavement** process can share feelings and relate with others who have themselves been recently bereaved.

employment: working in an occupation in exchange for wages or a salary. (See **work**.)

Employment Equality (Age) Regulations 2006: legislation that makes it unlawful to discriminate against a person because of his/her age. (See *Age Concern – the National Council on Ageing*.)

empowerment: the way in which a carer encourages an individual client to make decisions and take control of her/his own life. A carer should involve a client in conversations which relate to their care and lifestyles, giving them the opportunity to reply and respond. Empowerment is a process which builds a client's *self-esteem* and confidence in their ability to make decisions. Sharing information enables a client to make informed choices. (See *building confidence, strategies for effective communication, active listening*.)

enablement: methods used by health and social care workers to support their clients and encourage them to be as *independent* as possible in their daily lives. Methods include:

- teaching life skills or social skills to help them to care for themselves; an example is *activities of daily living*
- helping clients to live as independently as possible, e.g. moving clients into their own accommodation
- helping clients to make decisions about their care and different aspects of their daily lives
- helping clients to take up suitable employment
- encouraging clients to attend support or user groups
- providing relevant *information* and *advice*. (See *normalisation*.)

endemic disease: a *disease* which is present only in a certain part of the world (such as malaria in the tropics).

endocrine system: a system made up of a number of ductless *glands* found in different parts of the body. The glands secrete hormones which travel in the blood to target organs where they have a chemical effect on the body. Examples of the main endocrine glands are the *pituitary*, *thyroid*, *parathyroid, pancreas, gonads* (ovaries and testes), *adrenal glands* and *hypothalamus*.

endocrinology is the study of the *endocrine system*. The endocrine system produces *hormones*.

energy is the capacity to carry out different activities to live, *work* and *play*. There are thousands of chemical reactions which take place in the body cells in order to release or acquire energy. Energy cannot be destroyed.

English as a second language: when a child or person's first language is not English. (See *bilingualism*.)

enquiry methods: methods used as part of the *research* process. They involve using primary sources of *data* which are collected through experimentation and *observation*.

enteritis is the inflammation of the intestine due to a disease or food poisoning. (See *gastroenteritis*.)

entitlement: a person's right to receive the relevant health and social care, e.g. free health care which is available to everyone through the **NHS (National Health Service).**

environment is the totality of surrounding conditions which affect and support an individual. The living environment should be safe, secure and promote health. Factors which promote the health and well-being of individuals are enshrined in the Green Paper *Our Healthier Nation – a Contract for Health*. These factors include:

- air quality – monitoring and controlling *pollution* (i.e. poisonous gases emitted into the air) through legislation such as the Clean Air Act 1993. Measures such as no *smoking* policies in organisations including department stores, offices, public transport and hospitals were subsequently extended in the *Health Act 2006* to all public places.
- *housing* – monitoring *legislation* and policies to improve quality of housing and housing management
- *water* quality – monitoring pollution of rivers and streams according to relevant legislation; ensuring that *public health strategies* are in place to protect drinking water
- social environment – the people who may influence an individual's *quality of life*, for example family, friends, colleagues, medical and educational services, neighbours, etc.

In addition to this, there are procedures which should be in place to support the *health and safety* of staff and service users, such as routines for:

- *food hygiene* and the application of relevant legislation
- protection from fire with fire safety and fire precaution regulations such as *fire drills*
- controlling working environments including legislation relating to *health and safety at work*
- *health and safety* regulations including control of hazardous and poisonous substances (such as *Control of Substances Hazardous to Health (COSHH) Regulations 2002*)
- regulations concerning disease
- health, such as immunisation and *health screening*.

Issues concerned with the environment are also covered in the Environmental Protection Act 1990. (See also *care environment and care context*.) Environmental factors, such as pollution, can affect the health, well-being, growth and development of an individual.

environmental health relates to the healthy status of the environment in which we live. It covers issues such as risks and potential problems to the health and safety of an individual including risks from the activity of nature such as the weather, and risks from human activity such as the use of electricity and gas which generates high levels of energy. There is legislation in place to support environmental health. (See *environment*, *pollution*.)

environmental health officers are employed by the local authority and have received specialised training. Their role is to protect public health by monitoring the environment with regard to food, fire, working environment and pollution.

environmental health services are services which are based within local authorities. Their role is to:

- assess, control and correct any risk which might be present in the local community
- monitor risk so that it does not increase
- prevent the various factors which have the potential to cause harm or affect the health of different individuals and groups in society.

These services include safety services, public health services, as well as the licensing of lotteries, fair grounds, public houses, pet shops, pest control, noise pollution and housing. (See *Health and Safety at Work Act 1974*, *health and safety*, *risk assessment*.)

Environmental Protection (Duty to Care) Regulations 1991: legislation that requires manufacturers of waste to dispose of that waste themselves in a safe way.

enzymes are chemicals which speed up chemical changes within the body without any change occurring to the enzymes themselves. They are a type of catalyst.

epidemic: episodes of *disease* which spread rapidly and affect large numbers of people. Epidemics occur when:

- there is a lack of *immunity* in a population and people are in a poor state of health
- there are conditions in which germs can spread easily
- a particularly virulent strain of disease arises, e.g. the flu virus.

epidemiology: the study of the nature, prevalence and spread of *disease*. It explores the causes of particular diseases in order to develop an appropriate approach to prevention and cure. For example, the discovery of the link between cholera and infected drinking water was an important advance in controlling the incidence of cholera.

epilepsy: a disorder or dysfunction affecting the electrical activities in the *brain* which results in recurrent epileptic seizures or fits. Epilepsy is an abnormal electrical discharge in the brain. Epilepsy may be caused by brain tumours, drugs, cerebral disease such as dementia, systemic illness which affects brain function (e.g. kidney failure), head injuries. It may also be hereditary. There are different types of epilepsy. The most common forms are:

- grand mal epilepsy, where fits cause the individual to lose consciousness, and to fall to the ground with twitching and jerking of the limbs. There may be frothing at the mouth and, in some cases, the individual will pass urine
- petit mal epilepsy, which causes the individual to lose consciousness for a few seconds. They may suddenly lose concentration, stop talking and appear blank. As soon as this phase passes the sufferer returns to what they were doing. The individual does not fall to the floor or seem any different except for a blank expression and an inability to respond during the attack.

Epilepsy is diagnosed by a number of tests such as an *electroencephalogram (EEG)* and brain scans which examine the electrical activity of the brain. Treatment of epilepsy is by anti-epileptic drugs. Those who suffer from epilepsy have to make appropriate career choices as some occupations would be deemed unsuitable, for example, working in the fire or police service. Some people with epilepsy are not allowed to drive a car. *Cognitive development* and *intellectual development* are not impaired, neither is the ability to learn. However, some sufferers feel self-conscious about their medical condition because of the fits, particularly as they do not always know when these will happen. There are some epileptics who have an 'aura', a feeling or sense that they are going to have a 'fit'. Babies and young children sometimes suffer from 'fits' when they have a high temperature; these are called convulsions and are not an indication that the individual will suffer from epilepsy in later life.

epithelial tissues: groups of specialised *cells* forming layers which cover or line the surfaces of organs. There are different types of epithelial tissue as shown in the diagram.

1 Ciliated epithelium – found in nasal passages

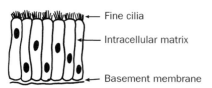

- Fine cilia
- Intracellular matrix
- Basement membrane

2 Stratified epithelium – found in skin

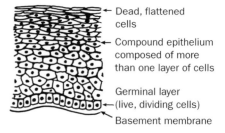

- Dead, flattened cells
- Compound epithelium composed of more than one layer of cells
- Germinal layer (live, dividing cells)
- Basement membrane

3 Columnar epithelium – found in lining of stomach

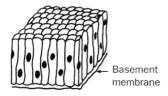

- Basement membrane

4 Cubiodal epithelium – forms the duct of a gland

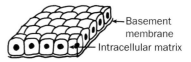

- Basement membrane
- Intracellular matrix

5 Glandular epithelium

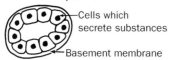

- Cells which secrete substances
- Basement membrane

6 Squamous epithelium

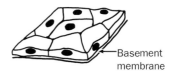

- Basement membrane

Epithelial tissues

equal opportunities are principles which reinforce policies contained in legislation. They are the result of anti-discriminatory practices and ensure that every individual has:
- a right to employment and *access to services*
- rights to non-discriminatory medical treatment, independent of race, gender, class, religion, culture, age and sexual orientation.

equal opportunities policies are statements which are written to ensure *anti-discriminatory practice*. They are implemented at every level in health and social care. They are applied in:
- staff recruitment, selection, training and professional updating
- staff knowledge and understanding of how the policies work in their care of service users
- fostering positive anti-discriminatory attitudes amongst staff and service users and their families by ensuring that adequate support systems are in place, e.g. communicating care plans, and any changes in care, and explaining procedures in a way that the service user understands. (See *care value base*.)

Equal Pay Act 1970 and Equal Pay (Amendment) Regulations 1983: Acts of Parliament which are aimed at eliminating *discrimination* between men and women in terms of payment for work of equal value and contractual conditions. The 1983 legislation brought Britain into line with the European Directive on equal pay for equal work.

equality is giving individuals the right to equal value and care. This creates opportunities and values *diversity* in the wide range of differences amongst individuals.

Equality Act 2004: an Act of Parliament which was introduced to address *equal opportunities* and *discrimination*. It has three main functions, which are:

- to replace the Equal Opportunities Commission, the Commission for Racial Equality and the Disability Rights Commission with a single Commission called the *Equality and Human Rights Commission*
- to make it unlawful to discriminate on the grounds of *religion*, *belief* or *sexual orientation* in the provision of facilities, goods and services
- to ensure public and *local authorities* promote equality of opportunity between men and women and prohibit sex discrimination in the workplace. (See *equal opportunity policies*, *anti-discriminatory practice*.)

Equality and Human Rights Commission was set up in October 2007. Its main objectives are to:

- build positive relationships
- eliminate discrimination
- protect human rights
- reduce inequality.

It replaces, reinforces and builds on the work developed by the three previous equality commissions, that is:

- Commission for Racial Equality
- Disability Rights Commission
- Equal Opportunities Commission.

The role of the Commission is to create a voice for the disadvantaged and to add other aspects of equality to this such as *age*, *human rights*, *sexual orientation*, *belief* and *religion*.

Equality Commission for Northern Ireland is an independent national body with responsibility for promoting awareness of and enforcing anti-discriminatory law in Northern Ireland.

equality in care practice: see *care value base*.

equity: the quality of being fair and reasonable in a way that gives equal treatment to everyone.

Erikson, EH (1902–1994): an American psychoanalyst. He believed that a stronger emphasis should be placed on the lifelong relationship between the individual and the social system in which they develop. Erikson suggested that there are eight stages in a person's life, with each stage presenting challenges that are characteristic of that particular period. For example, in mid-life, 'generativity versus stagnation', those without children or without jobs or *lifestyles* that have significant meaning to them may experience a feeling of stagnation. Psychologically healthy individuals meet the challenges of each stage while psychologically unhealthy individuals may fail to meet such challenges and must therefore deal with the conflicts that emerge in the stages that follow.

Erikson's stages of development

Stage		Relationships	Age
1	Basic trust versus basic mistrust	The baby with the mother or primary care giver	0–1 years
2	Autonomy versus shame and doubt	The young child and its parents or primary care giver	1–3 years
3	Initiative versus guilt	Family units including extended family	3–6 years
4	Industry versus inferiority	School and out of school	7–12 years
5	Identity versus role confusion	Different groups such as peer groups	12–18 years
6	Intimacy versus isolation	Partnerships in different relationships, friendships, family	20s
7	Generativity versus stagnation	Building interest in society or 'Just the home front'	Late 20s–50s
8	Ego integrity versus despair	'Human kind' or my kind	50s and over

erythrocytes or red blood cells are cells in the *blood* whose main function is to carry *oxygen* from the *lungs* to the *tissues*. They do not have a nucleus and only exist for approximately 100–120 days. They are manufactured in the *bone marrow*. They are disc-shaped and are able to fold and bend as they pass through blood vessels. Red cells contain *haemoglobin* which carries oxygen. The haemoglobin readings in blood relate closely to an individual's iron count.

ethical issues are those issues which relate to moral and responsible ways of working to promote *independence*, *autonomy*, *equal opportunities*, justice, *confidentiality* and *anti-discriminatory practice*.

ethics: moral codes of practice which are concerned with:
- behaviour (moral conduct), e.g. unprofessional behaviour such as direct *discrimination*
- issues such as legal, religious, social and personal concerns (moral issues), e.g. *abortion*
- debates within society about different codes of practice, e.g. the issue of prolonging life in a terminally ill person versus euthanasia.

(See *care value base, code of ethics*.)

ethnic groups: groups of people who share and belong to the same cultural tradition, racial origin, sometimes with distinguishing physical features, common language or religion.

ethnic minorities are groups of people from different cultural or religious or racial backgrounds who make up only a small proportion of a country's population. Examples of ethnic minorities in the UK are the Vietnamese, Irish, Turkish, Pakistani and Bengali communities.

ethnicity is a term which expands on the term race to include *culture*, *lifestyle*, *religion*, traditions, dress code and language (see *race*).

ethnocentrism: an individual's assumption that their society's *lifestyle* and *culture* is the norm and the right way of living with any other culture or lifestyle being regarded as inferior or misguided.

eurocentrism: a belief held by those individuals who view the world from the attitudes of white European *culture* and *society*. This way of thinking or value base does not acknowledge issues of diversity of culture or *race*, believing that the holder's views are superior.

European Convention on Human Rights: an international treaty signed by 12 member countries of the Council of Europe on 4 November 1950. It ensures that fundamental human rights are supported. The Court of Human Rights can change laws. For example, its intervention led to the abolition of corporal punishment in state schools.

European Court of Human Rights: set up under the Convention of Human Rights in November 1998. It is composed of a number of judges equal to that of the contracting states (currently 41). Judges are elected by the Parliamentary Assembly of the Council of Europe for a term of six years. (See *Human Rights Act 1998*.)

European Union (EU): a group of 25 countries in Western Europe and Scandinavia representing more than 400 million citizens. The European Union has developed a number of key institutions responsible for determining policy and legislation such as a Council of Ministers, European Parliament, European Commission, Economic and Social Committee, European Council and the European Court of Justice.

euthanasia: the killing of someone who is enduring extreme suffering, for example from an incurable disease. The individual involved may give clear directions as to what should happen in the event of their own faculties deteriorating, resulting in limited and restricted *quality of life*.

- Passive euthanasia involves a decision which is made on behalf of an individual who has severe limitations and restrictions on their quality of life, such as a patient or client in a permanent vegetative state or state of permanent unconsciousness. It is the act of letting a person die.
- Active euthanasia involves a deliberate act to end a life.

All aspects of euthanasia provide health and social care workers with ethical and moral dilemmas. A person may be suffering from a particularly painful form of cancer and their loved ones have had to watch them endure considerable discomfort. This may lead to discussion and heartache. Euthanasia is a difficult and contentious subject but, in each area of health and social care, professionals have codes of ethics which act as guidelines forming a framework for practice. (See *codes of practice*.)

Every Child Matters: a set of measures to reform and improve the care of children and young people from birth to the age of 19. It is part of the framework of change laid out in the *Children Act 2004*. The aim of these measures is to increase and develop the opportunities open to young people to improve their lives and reach their full potential. Every Child Matters is about opportunities for each child to:

- be healthy
- stay safe

- enjoy and achieve
- make a positive contribution
- achieve economic well-being.

All organisations working with children and young people are required to work together to enable children to achieve more through these measures.

excretion: the removal of waste products resulting from metabolic processes in the body. Excretion includes loss of urea through the *kidneys* and *carbon dioxide* from the *lungs*. (See *waste disposal* and *urinary system*.)

exercise: an activity which is necessary for the body to keep healthy and in good working order. Regular exercise is beneficial to the body in the following ways:

- it controls *stress* and reduces *blood pressure*
- it keeps the *joints* supple and mobile, preventing stiffness
- it enables the *muscles* to maintain their strength, tone and healthy condition
- it maintains body stamina, which results from greater efficiency in the different organs, such as the heart
- it helps to develop the *bones* and muscle co-ordination
- it raises self-esteem by releasing a feel-good factor
- it improves health, rehabilitating muscles following illness or surgery
- it maintains good health, improves appetite, induces sound sleep and prevents excessive body weight
- it has social benefits, as exercise is a means of meeting others, e.g. at the gym.

Exercises which allow a person to breathe in sufficient *oxygen* to oxidise glucose to provide the necessary energy are called *aerobic exercises*.

Exercise should be safe, so before an exercise programme is started a person should have a medical check. It is important to wear appropriate clothing. Ensure that correct monitoring equipment is available to check pulse, blood pressure and lung function. There should be opportunities for warming-up and cooling-down exercises. Barriers to participation in regular exercise include cost, fitness levels, location of gym or leisure centre, work and travel commitments, and lethargy, i.e. can't be bothered. (See *monitoring health and fitness*.)

exercise programmes are designed to meet the exercise needs of the service user. They should be carefully planned, monitored and evaluated. This should include:

- *assessment* of fitness level
- safe environment
- correct equipment
- suitable clothing
- correct preparation in terms of warming up and cooling down
- suitable exercises to match the person's needs.

exocrine glands: glands which have ducts or channels which secrete fluids 'externally'. For example *sweat glands* secrete sweat and *salivary glands* secrete saliva.

expiration: breathing out air. It involves the following process:

- intercostal muscles relax and the rib cage moves downwards and inwards
- the *diaphragm* muscle relaxes, moving upwards to become more dome-shaped
- the volume of the thorax becomes smaller so increasing the pressure in the thoracic cavity

- the natural elasticity of the *lungs* and increased pressure on them causes the lungs to decrease in volume and air is forced out.

extroversion: an aspect of the *personality* which is characterised by a number of different traits such as impulsiveness and sociability. *Eysenck* developed the Eysenck Personality Inventory, a method of testing people along the continuum of *introversion* to extroversion. The more sociable, impulsive and willing a person is to take risks, the higher they score on extroversion. Extroverts have a lower level of cortical activity, and therefore must seek stimulation to maintain their psychological state.

eye contact: maintaining eye contact is a way of reading messages in the eyes. It can be a means of giving positive support and is an important part of individual and group communication. Many emotions are mirrored in the eyes. Feelings of happiness, joy, sadness, anger and mistrust can be seen. However, it is important to note that in some *cultures* eye contact is viewed as a negative way of behaving. (See *communication, building confidence*.)

eyes are the organs of sight, sending nervous impulses to the *brain* when stimulated by light rays from external objects. The brain interprets the impulses to produce images. Each eye consists of an eyeball made up of several layers and structures. It is set into a socket in the *skull* and is protected by eyelids and eyelashes.

The eye consists of the:
- sclera or sclerotic coat – the 'white' of the eye. This is tough, fibrous and opaque, with blood vessels
- choroid or choroid coat – a layer of tissue with blood vessels and dark pigment. Pigment absorbs light to stop reflection within the eye
- iris – an opaque disc of tissue, with blood vessels and central hole (pupil). It contains muscle fibres, some of which are in concentric circles, while others radiate out from centre to edge. The former contract to decrease pupil size (in bright light) while the latter contract to increase it (in dim light). The iris has various amounts of pigment producing eye colours
- cornea – a transparent continuation of the sclera. It protects the front of the eye and 'bends' (refracts) light rays onto the lens
- conjunctiva – a thin mucous membrane. This lines the eyelids and covers the cornea
- ciliary body – a ring of smooth muscle around the lens. This contracts to make the lens smaller and fatter. It relaxes to make the lens larger and thinner. The ciliary body and the muscles of the iris are known as intrinsic eye muscles
- lens – the transparent body whose role is to focus the light rays passing through it (i.e. 'bend' or refract them) so that they come to a point, in this case on the retina. A lens consists of many thin tissue layers and is held in place by the fibres of the suspensory ligament. These join it to the ciliary body, which can alter the lens shape so that light rays are always focused on the retina, whatever the distance to the object being looked at. This is known as *accommodation*. The rays form an upside-down image, but this is compensated for and corrected by the *brain*
- retina – the innermost layer of tissue at the back of the eyeball made up of a layer of pigment and a nervous layer consisting of millions of sensory nerve cells or sensory neurones and their fibres. These lie in chains and carry nervous impulses to the brain. The first cells in the chains are receptors, i.e. their end fibres or dendrons fire off

impulses when they are stimulated by light rays. These cells are called rods and cones because of their shape. The receptors are photoreceptors, that is they are stimulated by light

- macula lutea or yellow spot – an area of yellowish tissue in the centre of the retina. It has a small central dip, called the fovea or fovea centralis. This has the highest concentration of cones and is the area of acute vision
- blind spot or optic disc – the point in the retina where the optic nerve leaves the eye. It has no receptors and so cannot send any impulses
- **aqueous humour** – a watery liquid containing sugars, salts and **proteins**. It fills the space called the anterior cavity, protecting the lens and nourishing the front of the eye. It constantly drains away and is replaced
- vitreous humour – a fluid similar to aqueous humour, but stiff and jelly-like. It fills the space called the posterior cavity and keeps the shape of eyeball, protects the retina and helps 'bend' or refract the light.

Dysfunctions of the eyes include myopia (shortsightedness), hypermetropia (longsightedness), astigmatism and **squint (strabismus)**.

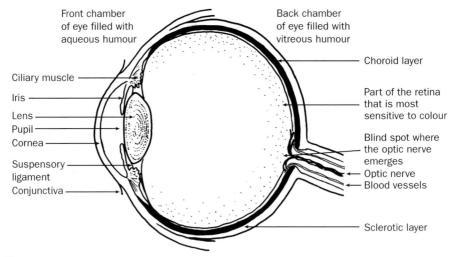

Front chamber of eye filled with aqueous humour

Back chamber of eye filled with vitreous humour

Ciliary muscle

Iris

Lens

Pupil

Cornea

Suspensory ligament

Conjunctiva

Choroid layer

Part of the retina that is most sensitive to colour

Blind spot where the optic nerve emerges

Optic nerve

Blood vessels

Sclerotic layer

The eye

Eysenck, HJ (1916–1997): a psychologist who studied the personality. He believed that much of the personality was determined by biology in terms of its development. He produced the Eysenck Personality Inventory (EPI) as a way of measuring personality. It measures the degree of introversion–extroversion, and of neuroticism–stability. Participants are asked a series of questions. The responses to these questions provide the relevant information sufficient to construct a score for extroversion and neuroticism. As some may falsify their answers in a way they consider socially desirable, the inventory includes a lie scale of questions that can only be answered in one way.

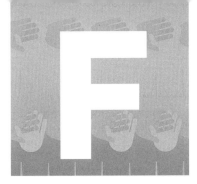

failure to thrive: the description used for a baby who does not grow at the expected rate and develops slowly. (See *centile charts*.) Reasons for failure to thrive include:

- genetic make-up – comparisons with the size of parents and grandparents
- food and feeding – the baby may be 'a slow feeder' and finds feeding difficult; they may tire easily when sucking
- food absorption – difficulty in digesting milk feeds
- food allergies – they may be allergic to milk
- loss or lack of appetite – the baby turns away from the food provided
- *infection* – the baby may be vulnerable to infections, especially of the ears, nose and throat, and these can affect feeding
- home *environment* – this may affect how the baby grows. For instance the baby may lack attention, may be left alone for long periods or may receive no stimulation from its surroundings.

When babies are not thriving, their growth should be carefully monitored and recorded at regular intervals. Different strategies can be introduced to promote the baby's growth. An example of this is changing milk feeds to soya milk in small amounts for short regular periods. (See *human growth and development, developmental delay*.)

family: a group of individuals who are related by blood, *adoption* or marriage. (See *family structures*.) The role of the family is influenced by moral issues, because it is a social as well as a biological formation. Some support for selected family groups can be found at:

- Families Anonymous – a self-help fellowship for families and friends of drug abusers
- Families Need Fathers – this is primarily concerned with the problems of maintaining a child's relationship with both its parents during, and following, a *divorce*.

A government Green Paper 'Supporting Families' was introduced in November 1998 as a result of the rise of lone-parent families in modern-day Britain. Following this:

- the National Family and Parenting Institute has been set up to provide advice and information which meet the needs of the multicultural diversity which is present in society
- the roles of *health visitors* and school nurses are being explored and extended to provide programmes of training involving parent and toddler groups, and groups working with teenagers
- the role of grandparents – older people are able to volunteer to be surrogate grannies and support young parents
- paternity leave has been made available for fathers as well as mothers. (See *family structure*.

family centres: centres which offer a range of services to children, their parents or any other person looking after children. Family centres may provide recreational activities, counselling, advice and self-help support. These facilities may be purpose-built or attached to a school or day nursery.

family credit: extra state income benefit to support working families on low incomes. It is *means tested* and benefits those families with children where wage-earners are in low-paid work. It replaced family income supplement following the Social Security Act 1988.

family life describes the relationships which exist within the family. In the last fifty years there have been significant changes which include:

- a change in *family structure* with an increase in *lone-parent families*, dual-worker families (both parents having jobs outside the home)
- an increase of births outside the formal arrangement of marriage
- more couples choosing not to marry but to live together as a couple without the formal and legal formalities of marriage
- changes in conjugal roles within the family.

Family Policy Studies Centre: an organisation which researches issues of family trends and public policy. It is particularly concerned with the understanding of contemporary family structures and patterns. This includes changes that are taking place within family structures, and the implications of these changes in terms of policy and practice. The Family Policy Studies Centre acts as a forum which:

- analyses issues with regard to the study of family and related policy using its own research staff
- provides information for dissemination and debate, aiming to serve as a bridge between policy makers, academics and practitioners and to produce a range of material which is available to the public.

family size: the number of children born to a couple. Factors which affect family size may include:

- the availability and reliability of affordable contraception
- social norms governing the 'ideal' family size
- economic decisions by the family regarding the cost of rearing children and its impact on the family's standard of living.

family structure: a group of individuals who live together to form a *family*. There are different family structures:

- a nuclear family is regarded as a man and woman and their dependent children living at the same residence (they co-operate together socially and economically)
- an extended family is one in which the basic nuclear structure has been added to, or extended, either vertically (e.g. grandparents, parents, children) or horizontally (e.g. two or more brothers living together with their respective spouses and children)
- reconstituted or step families – a couple who have divorced and remarried to include the different children from previous relationships
- *lone-parent families* – one adult living with children; this family structure can be due to divorce, partnership break-up or death
- dual-worker families – both adult parents have jobs outside the family home
- *gender* families – couples from the same gender group who have chosen to rear children together.

Changes in family structures have led to differences in service provision, such as increased demand for child care, *child protection*, out-of-hours services from GPs in the case of dual-worker and lone-parent families, and demand for *after-school clubs*.

family support worker is a professional who works with families. They provide practical help and support as well as providing the necessary emotional support for families experiencing short- or long-term problems and difficulties. For example, they may give support to a family with young children, when there are marriage or relationship stresses between the parents, or there is a child with a *disability*.

fat-soluble vitamins are *vitamins* such as vitamins A, D, E and K which will dissolve in lipids, and only slightly, if at all, in water.

fats (lipids) are made up of *carbon, oxygen* and hydrogen. The proportion of oxygen to hydrogen is less in lipids than in carbohydrates. Lipids/fats are insoluble in water but can dissolve in other organic solvents such as ether and ethanol. Lipids are made up of glycerol and *fatty acids*. Fatty acids can be saturated or unsaturated depending on the presence of double bonds between carbon atoms. The functions of fats are to:
- provide a source of *energy*
- enable the fat-soluble *vitamins* A, D, E, and K to be absorbed
- provide layers of protection around the vital organs of the human body
- provide layers of heat insulation around the body.

(See also *adipose tissue*.)

fatty acids are the major components of *fats*. They are made up of a hydrocarbon chain and a terminal carboxyl (acid) group (COOH). If there are no double bonds in the hydrocarbon chain they are saturated. If there is one double bond they are called monounsaturated. If there is more than one double bond present they are called polyunsaturated.

fear: an emotional state which is brought on by a feeling of impending danger. It has a number of characteristics such as increased heart rate, sweating, behaviour changes, dry mouth and occasionally a feeling of numbness or immobility. There are natural fear mechanisms in the body which are activated by the 'fear, fright and flight' functions of the hormone *adrenaline*. However, there are other situations which can cause irrational fears and which may relate to emotional, psychological, mental and physical disorders, diseases and dysfunction. (See also *anxiety*.)

feedback: a method of reflecting on information and giving a view or opinion. Feedback can be written or spoken and is related to any discussion, task, activity or role in which a carer has taken part. (See *reflective practice*.)

feedback system: a 'circular' system where the output is used to control the input. A negative feedback system is one in which the rise in the output is used to reduce the input. Control of the level of thyroid hormone in the blood is an example of negative feedback – when the level of thyroid hormone is too high, it suppresses thyroid-stimulating hormone production by the anterior *pituitary gland*. (See *homeostasis* and *biofeedback*.)

feelings: see *emotions*.

female reproductive system: the part of the female body responsible for reproduction. The female reproductive system consists of the following:
- *ovaries* – two female *gonads* which are held in place by *ligaments* in the lower abdomen, below the *kidneys*. The ligaments attach the ovaries to the walls of the pelvis. The female gametes or sex cells (ova, or one ovum) are produced regularly in the ovarian follicles of the ovaries after puberty

- ovarian follicles – a fluid-filled ovum and its coating of follicle cells each contains a maturing ovum. The follicles gradually get larger and begin to secrete hormones. Each cycle of follicle production results in only one fully mature follicle which is called a Graafian follicle
- fallopian tubes – narrow, muscular tubes linking the ovaries to the uterus. These allow the ovum's passage from the ovary to the uterus through muscular movement known as *peristalsis*
- uterus or womb –a hollow organ inside which a developing baby or foetus is held, or from which the ova are discharged. Once discharged, the ova pass out of the reproductive system. The womb has a lining of mucous membrane (the endometrium) covering a muscular wall with many blood vessels (see *menstruation*)
- *vagina* – a muscular canal which leads from the uterus out of the body. During *sexual intercourse* the penis ejaculates semen, containing sperm, into the vagina
- vulva – the outer part of the female reproductive system containing the labia which are folds of skin surrounding the opening of the vagina and the urethra.

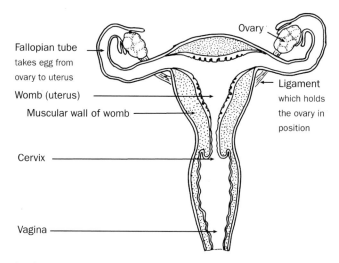

Female reproductive system

feminists: those who believe that in society women:
- should have equal rights to men
- are entitled to the same financial rewards in employment as men
- should be viewed by society as equal to men in terms of status, employment and access to opportunities.

Women's groups have campaigned for women's rights in society. (See *Equality and Human Rights Commission, Sex Discrimination Acts 1975 and 1986*.)

fertilisation is the biological process which involves the fusion of a sperm with an egg. This usually takes place in the fallopian tube. Many sperm may reach the egg but only one will penetrate the membrane which surrounds it. Following penetration the membrane changes in structure to form a barrier against any other sperm. The head of the sperm moves through the cytoplasm towards the nucleus of the egg and the nucleus of the sperm and egg fuse together. This produces a fertilised egg (zygote) which now starts to divide, first into two cells, then into four, then into eight and continues to divide as it journeys along the fallopian tube. By the time it reaches the uterus it is a ball of cells called an **embryo**. (See **conception**.)

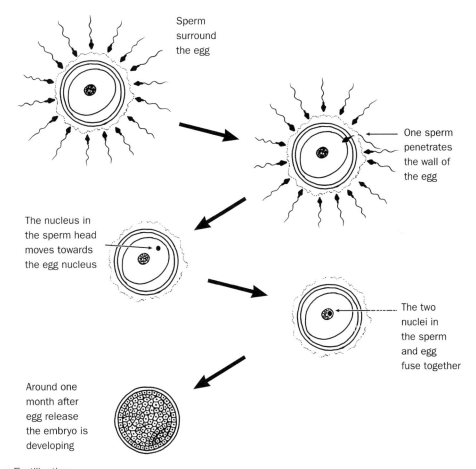

Sperm surround the egg

One sperm penetrates the wall of the egg

The nucleus in the sperm head moves towards the egg nucleus

The two nuclei in the sperm and egg fuse together

Around one month after egg release the embryo is developing

Fertilisation

fertility rate: the number of live *births* in a population per 1000 women of childbearing age, which is usually between 15 and 50 years of age. The figure is often broken down still further into age-specific fertility rates.

fire drill: all institutions are required to implement a procedure which enables people to have practice at finding the best available exits from a building in the event of fire. Under the Fire Precaution Act 1971 all types of institutions, organisations and settings should review and implement precautions such as:

- providing a means of escape in the event of fire
- providing appropriate equipment to fight a fire
- a method of giving fire warnings to staff, service users, clients and patients
- training new employees with regard to fire drill.

Every organisation should practise fire drills to simulate the events of a 'real fire'. The local fire brigade will advise any organisation with regard to risk from fire. A fire safety officer will visit organisations and give any advice considered necessary. (See *Health and Safety at Work Act 1974*, *Fire Precautions Workplace (Amended) Regulations 1997*.)

Fire Precautions Workplace (Amended) Regulations 1997 are regulations which relate to fire safety in the workplace. They were put in place to protect employees, visitors and property from the risk of fire. Employers are required to:

- carry out, monitor and review a fire *risk assessment*
- provide firefighting equipment and ensure it is maintained and tested
- ensure there is emergency planning and staff training
- ensure there are means of escape
- nominate and train fire marshals. (See *Regulatory Reform (Fire Safety) Order 2005*.)

first aid is immediate assistance given to a person who has been injured or taken ill. According to St John Ambulance the aims of first aid are:

- to preserve life
- to limit worsening of the condition
- to promote recovery. (Source: *First Aid Manual*.)

Individuals can be trained to be qualified first aiders. Organisations such as the British Red Cross and St John Ambulance run programmes of first aid training. The term 'first aider' is used for those who have been trained and have received a first aid certificate. (See *health and safety and first aid*.)

Five-A-Day campaign is a campaign to encourage people to eat five portions a day of fruit and vegetables, and so reduce their risk of heart disease, some cancers and other chronic conditions.

foetal alcohol syndrome: this is a combination of *signs and symptoms* which occur in a newborn baby as a result of the mother's high intake of *alcohol* during pregnancy. These defects can take the form of growth retardation, and heart and limb abnormalities. Stimulants other than alcohol can also affect the *foetus* or unborn baby in a similar way. These include:

- nicotine – *smoking* may affect the growth of the foetus in the womb
- *drugs* – e.g. when the mother takes heroin, the baby can be born with an addiction to heroin
- some therapeutic drugs (see *thalidomide*).

foetal growth and development: stages of growth of the developing *foetus* in the uterus from conception to 40 weeks. The *placenta* provides oxygen and the essential nutrients which are passed into the bloodstream of the foetus from the mother's bloodstream via the umbilical cord. The foetus grows in a sac of fluid (the amniotic sac) which gives it protection from injury and infection. Just before the birth the membranes in the amniotic sac rupture. This is known as 'the waters breaking'. The development of the foetus is as follows:

- age 8–9 weeks: the foetus is approximately 20 mm long. The eyes and mouth are formed. The hands and feet are forming. The heart, brain, lungs and other organs are developing. The heart beats from about 5 to 6 weeks
- age 10–14 weeks: the foetus is approximately 60 mm long; it is fully formed. The heartbeat is strong. Pregnancy may begin to show
- age 23–30 weeks: the foetus is approximately 30–35 cm long. Fat begins to form under the skin. Its skin is covered with lanugo (a fine covering of hair) and vernix caseosa (a layer of greasy substance). The foetus is 'viable' from 24 weeks. This is the legal term which

means that the baby is capable of surviving outside the womb. Some babies now survive birth at an even earlier age

- age 31–40 weeks: by about 32 weeks the baby is usually lying head downwards ready for birth. Some time before birth, the head may move down into the pelvis and is said to be 'engaged', but sometimes the baby's head does not engage until labour has started.

foetus: the developing embryo becomes a foetus after the first eight weeks of development in the womb. The foetus develops and grows in the womb until **birth**.

food: substances which are eaten by all humans and other living organisms in order to provide nourishment. Foods contain a number of nutrients such as **carbohydrates, proteins** and **fats, water, minerals** and **vitamins**. Roughage or fibre is also necessary to help to move food through the gut. (See **balanced diet, malnutrition**.)

food additives are chemicals which are added to food to:
- improve its appearance and make it more appealing to the consumer
- prevent **food poisoning**
- reduce the growth of bacteria and mould
- improve the nutritional value of food
- prevent food deteriorating.

Additives in food are regulated to ensure that they are used safely (see **E numbers**).

food allergies: a reaction to food that has been eaten or touched. This can be mild or severe. Food allergies include those to nuts, shellfish, gluten, lactose and fruits. Possible reactions include **asthma**, skin rashes and breathing difficulties.

food hygiene: the study of the food handling methods which are used in the production, preparation and presentation of food. The aim of food hygiene is the production of food which is both clean and safe to eat. There are four main aspects which support food hygiene practice. These are the:
- introduction of hygiene regulations with regard to raw meat, cooked meat and certain other foods before it is delivered to shops, homes, canteens and restaurants
- care and hygiene practice of those handling the food during production and service
- storage arrangements for food
- design and cleanliness of cooking equipment, kitchens and food preparation areas.

(See **food safety regulations**.)

food poisoning: an illness caused by eating food which has been contaminated with **bacteria** or their toxins. Symptoms include **vomiting, diarrhoea**, nausea or feelings of sickness, or abdominal pain. Some of the organisms responsible for food poisoning are *Salmonella*, *Listeria*, *Staphylococcus* and **Clostridium**.

food preservation: methods of processing which prevent the growth of harmful **bacteria** and fungi and slow down the rate of food deterioration (e.g. pickling and freezing).

food safety is the safe handling and cooking of food to prevent **food poisoning** and unhygienic food production. It is underpinned by **food safety regulations** and the **Food Safety Act 1990**.

Food Safety Act 1990: an Act of Parliament which aims to control safety at all stages of food production. This is to ensure that food is safe to eat, reaches quality expectations and that its description does not mislead customers. The Act also sets out powers of enforcement and penalties for those who do not comply.

Food Safety and General Food Hygiene Regulations 1995: regulations aiming to ensure common food hygiene rules across the *European Union (EU)*. The main purpose of the Act is to ensure that food poisoning is prevented. (See *food hygiene*, *food safety regulations*.)

food safety regulations: regulations which support legislation on food preparation and handling. Food handlers must:

- keep clean, cover cuts with blue waterproof dressings (so they are easily seen if they fall into food), wear suitable protective over-clothing, and must not smoke or spit
- report to the person managing the food business if they are suffering from food poisoning or a food-borne disease
- ensure that food preparation areas have a separate basin for washing hands, a good supply of disposable paper towels or an electric hand drier, a clean nail-brush and plenty of soap. Hands should be washed before handling food or when changing from handling uncooked to cooked food
- implement building regulations with regard to toilet facilities; these should be provided well away from the main food production or food preparation area, with notices reminding staff to wash their hands. This is to ensure that food is not contaminated with the harmful bacteria which are present in human faeces
- be encouraged not to wear heavy make-up which can contaminate food
- ensure that long hair is covered with a hat or tucked into a hairnet so that flakes of skin or hairs do not fall into the food
- not wear strong-smelling perfume or aftershave which can taint delicately flavoured food
- not smoke or eat while on duty; they can be permitted to do this when having regular rest breaks but must, of course, wash their hands again before resuming work.

The food hygiene regulations, introduced in 1970, were amended in 1991. Under the *Food Safety Act 1990* the training of all those involved in food handling was recommended.

Food Standards Agency: set up by the government in 1998 to monitor standards of food manufacture and to promote healthy eating. It has taken over some of the responsibilities of the Ministry of Agriculture, Fisheries and Food.

foodborne disease: a disease that can be transmitted via food (e.g. *Salmonella*).

foster care is the care of a child or children by a *local authority*. The child is looked after by a qualified foster carer who has been screened by the local authority. The needs of children and the role and responsibilities of the local authority, or recognised voluntary organisation, are set out in the *Children Act 1989* and Foster Placement (Children) Regulations 1990 and 2002. Children in foster care remain the responsibility of the local authority. Where there is more than one child in a family every effort is made to keep the children together. Children are fostered for a variety of reasons. These include situations where the:

- parents have been deemed unfit to care for their children; this occurs in some cases of *child abuse*
- parents are unable to cope because of illness
- parents are in prison and not in a position to care for their children.

Foster carers have statutory roles and responsibilities which include:
- providing day-to-day care
- helping and supporting a child as they return home to their parents
- allowing access for parents to visit their child or children
- allowing a parent to remove the child if the child has been in care for less than six months, otherwise the parent has to give 28 days notice of removal
- working closely with the child's social worker.

foundation trusts are a type of NHS hospital trust which is administered by local managers, members of staff and the general public. It is designed to meet the needs of local communities.

formal care: see *caring*.

fracture: the cracking or breaking of a *bone*. The fracture may be caused by a hard blow or fall. Treatment involves supporting the break in its normal position, either with a plaster-of-Paris splint, fibreglass splint or bandage. There are different types of fracture such as:

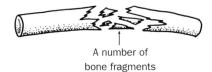

Site of fracture

Simple fracture – this is a clean break or crack in the bone

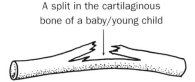

A number of
bone fragments

Comminuted fracture – this produces multiple bone fragments

A split in the cartilaginous
bone of a baby/young child

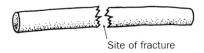

Greenstick fracture – produces a bend in the bone because it is cartilaginous (usually occurs in children)

Fracture has perforated the
surface of the skin

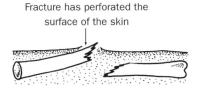

Open fracture – part of the broken bone penetrates the outer surface of the skin and so can cause bleeding

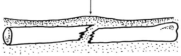

Fracture is contained and the
surface of the skin remains intact

Closed fracture – the bone is broken but it does not penetrate the surrounding skin

fragile X syndrome: a disorder which is caused by an abnormality of the *X chromosome* in human cells. It predominately affects males and may lead to learning disability and retardation.

frail and elderly: *older people* who have been affected by an injury or trauma, disease, dysfunction, psychological or psychiatric disorder which makes them more vulnerable. For example, *Alzheimer's disease* affects a person's personality and memory. *Arthritis* affects a person's physical well-being. An *accident* can have psychological as well as physical effects.

Framework for the Assessment of Children in Need and their Families 2000: (often referred to as the Assessment Framework) a systematic way of collecting, analysing and recording information, which relates to what is happening to children and young people within their families and the community they live in. The information is then used to support professional decisions on how to help these children and their families.

Fraser competence: (previously known as Gillick competence) relates to the rights of children under the age of 16 years old. It gives children the right to make decisions about medical treatment without parental consent as long as the child is thought to be legally responsible by a doctor. One example is being able to use contraception without parental consent.

free play: the way that children *play* using their initiative and imagination without any guidance from adults. This form of play encourages a child's independence and develops positive *self-esteem*.

free-basing: this is the illegal manufacture of the drug *crack*. It involves the heating of *cocaine* with a chemical which produces hard rocks of various sizes. (See *drugs*.)

Freedom of Information Act 2000: an Act of Parliament which deals with how public authorities provide access to information. The Act gives rights of access to a range of information, regardless of how it is stored, to all organisations and individuals.

Freud, Sigmund (1856–1939) invented psychoanalysis which relates both to the body of theory about the unconscious and his therapy based upon it. Freud's theories include:
- *personality* theory which covers the three aspects of the personality, the id, the ego and the superego, which interact and relate with each other
- *defence mechanisms* which are methods used by the ego to cope with conflict
- the different psychosexual stages of the personality based on the theory that the driving force behind personality is the sex drive or the need to express sexual energy.

Friedreich's ataxia: an *inherited disorder* which causes *degeneration* of the nerve cells in the *spinal cord*. This leads to muscular weakness and *ataxia* which makes walking and movement difficult. It starts in early childhood and, as the disease progresses, the child's *mobility* is greatly reduced until by adulthood he/she is confined to a wheelchair.

funding: sources of money which are required to provide health and social care services. Resourcing of health and social care provision is an important influence on the type of provision which is supplied. Funding can come from:

- central government
- local government (local authorities)
- charities
- business and commercial sources
- public donations
- covenants/bequests.

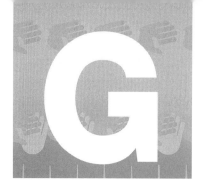

gall bladder: an organ of the body which stores *bile*. Gallstones develop in the gall bladder as a result of the build-up of *cholesterol* which is excreted in the bile.

games are periods of *play* which have instructions or rules enhancing the enjoyment of those taking part. There are different types of play including:

- ball games (e.g. football)
- court games (e.g. tennis)
- board games (e.g. Monopoly)
- games involving song and rhyme (e.g. 'ring-a-ring-o'-roses').

Some games such as football are competitive. They may be a satisfying experience for both children and adults alike. Childhood games encourage team spirit and working with others in a positive way. They can develop cognitive skills such as problem solving. For example, playing Monopoly can involve counting and the concept of buying and selling property.

gaseous exchange: the process in which *oxygen* is taken into the body and *carbon dioxide* released from the body during respiration. Air containing oxygen enters the lungs. The oxygen passes through the walls of the lungs into the blood. Carbon dioxide passes out of the blood, through the walls of the lungs and into the air contained within the lungs. It is then breathed out. The lungs form a large surface area for air and oxygen to be breathed in and carbon dioxide to be breathed out. The actual gaseous exchange takes place in the air sacs or *alveoli* of the lungs. (See *mechanism of breathing*.)

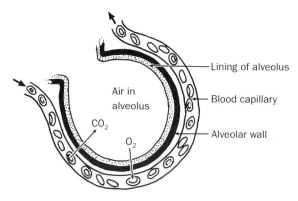

Gaseous exchange

gastric glands are situated in the *stomach*. They are responsible for secreting gastric juices. When food enters the mouth, gastric juice is produced in the stomach and additionally as the food enters the stomach. Gastric juice contains:

- hydrochloric acid – which acts as an antiseptic, kills off *bacteria* and promotes the action of the *enzymes*, pepsin and rennin
- pepsin – the enzyme responsible for digesting proteins by breaking them down into peptides
- rennin – the enzyme responsible for clotting milk.

(See *digestion*.)

gastroenteritis: inflammation of the lining of the *stomach* and intestine which can be caused by:

- *disease*, such as dysentery, when there has been contamination of the water supply with sewage
- *food poisoning* when food preparation and hygiene practices have been inefficient; causes include *infections* such as *salmonella*, bacterial toxins such as that of Clostridium, allergy to certain foods such as shellfish or poisoning due to eating toxic chemicals.

gastro-enterology is the study of the *digestive system*.

gays: see *lesbians/gays*.

gender: the social identity of male and female not restricted to biological differences.

Gender Recognition Act 2004: an Act of Parliament that allows transsexual people to change their legal *gender*, i.e. a man can become a woman and a woman can become a man.

gender role: attitudes, behaviours, personal development and interests that are considered appropriate for one *gender* and inappropriate for the other.

gender stereotypes: fixed beliefs about what it means to be male or female. Examples of gender *stereotyping* are the varying beliefs about which occupations are suitable for men and women.

general practitioner (GP): a *doctor* who is qualified and registered to work within a surgery practice or health centre. General practitioners are involved in ongoing changes in the NHS. They play an active part in *primary care trusts*.

General Social Care Council: a government organisation set up in 1998. The function of the General Social Care Council is to enforce standards of conduct and practice within the social care workforce. The council ensures that service users, carers, practitioners, employers and the general public have confidence in the standards which are set for social care. These include service standards and occupational standards of *competence*. The Council is accountable to the Secretary of State for Health. The *Care Standards Act 2000* requires that codes of practice are consistently updated and reviewed.

genes: unit of the *chromosome* containing a code or characteristic pattern which is inherited (passed on) through generations. Genes influence hair and eye colour, blood group, etc. Chromosomes contain thousands of genes. Different chromosomes contain coded instructions which dictate the way in which an individual will grow and develop. (See *deoxyribonucleic acid (DNA)*, *genetics*.)

genetic counselling: special *counselling* given to people where there is any likelihood that the baby they have conceived or are about to conceive may inherit a *genetic disorder* or disease. This is likely if the disease or disorder is one which has:

* affected any other children in the family
* affected other members of the family (i.e. grandparents or close family).

For example, there can be a heart-breaking debate if a mother has conceived and is carrying a child with *Down's syndrome* as to whether she should go ahead with the pregnancy or have an *abortion*. A professional genetic counsellor is available to provide a means of support, and the opportunity to discuss options. Furthermore, genetic counselling sometimes takes place after the birth of a baby with a genetic disease or disorder. The questions then are, will future babies be affected and should the parents try for more children?

genetic disorders and diseases: disorders, disease or dysfunction which occur when there is a deficiency in a whole *chromosome* or in part of a chromosome. If there is a deficiency in a whole chromosome or more/fewer chromosomes than normal are produced in each cell then the individual being formed will be affected. For example, a child with *Down's syndrome* has 47 chromosomes instead of 46. Genetic disorders are those which are inherited or passed on from one generation to another. Examples include disorders caused by a:

* defective and dominant gene, e.g. *Huntington's disease*
* defective and recessive gene that a child receives from each parent, e.g. *sickle cell disorders*
* defective gene which affects a sex chromosome, e.g. *haemophilia*. This is where the gene is carried on the X chromosome.

genetics: the study of the factors which relate to inheritance. It involves the study of the effects of *genes* on a child's development and growth. Children inherit genes from their parents. Inherited characteristics influence the development of the different and distinguishing features of each individual (e.g. height, hair colour, shape of the body, appearance) and even types of behaviour. The genetic make-up of a child is called the genotype. The genes influence the appearance (or physical characteristics) of a person and this is called the phenotype. It is important to recognise that genes occur in pairs and that two sets of genes which are inherited occupy the same position within their respective *chromosomes* as they do in the parents.

Gesell, Arnold (1880–1961): a psychologist who believed in the notion that human growth and development can be measured in terms of biological growth. During the 1920s and 1930s Arnold Gesell observed hundreds of children in order to identify and establish age and stage '*norms*' for what children were achieving at given ages. He devised two sets of scales, one for infants and one for pre-school children.

gestures are non-verbal messages which are communicated using arms, hands and fingers. It is important to remember that the meanings of gestures differ from one culture to another. (See *communication*.)

giving a talk is the process involved in carrying out an oral presentation to a group or interview panel. This involves:

- deciding on a topic – consider the audience, taking into account their age and knowledge of the presentation topic
- choosing the content – it is important to allow time to research the topic and be selective as to what is included
- planning the structure – the talk should have an introduction that informs the audience about the content of the talk. Next comes the body of the talk, making sure that the audience know the points that are being made, and if possible use images to reinforce each or some of these points. At the finish, include a conclusion which summarises what has been talked about and brings the talk to an end. There should be time for questions from the audience. Finally, thank the audience for their participation
- rehearsing the talk – take time to rehearse, using cue cards to remember the main points. A rehearsal will give the opportunity to identify strong points and possible weak points and will indicate how long the talk will take
- considering the timing – this includes thinking about whether to use PowerPoint or an overhead projector. Check that the appropriate equipment is available and ready to use. (See *creating a PowerPoint presentation*, *target group/audience*.)

glands are special organs (or sometimes groups of *cells* or single cells) which produce and secrete a variety of substances vital to life. There are two types of human gland – exocrine and endocrine:

- exocrine glands are those which secrete substances through tubes, or ducts, onto a surface or into a cavity. Most body glands are exocrine, e.g. the digestive glands. Exocrine glands can secrete fluids, for example digestive juices into the digestive system. Such juices contain enzymes which cause the breakdown of food. Other examples of exocrine glands are the *salivary glands*, the *pancreas* and *liver*
- endocrine or ductless glands are those which secrete substances called hormones directly into the blood (there are blood vessels in the glands). These glands may be separate bodies or cells inside organs such as the *pituitary gland* which is situated at the base of the brain and is directly influenced by the hypothalamus. The pituitary gland is made up of an anterior (front) lobe and a posterior (back) lobe. Many of the *hormones* in the pituitary stimulate other glands to secrete hormones.

glycolysis: a series of reactions in the body which is part of cell respiration. It takes place in the cytoplasm of cells. Glycolysis involves a number of stages and links with the *Krebs cycle* (see diagram overleaf).

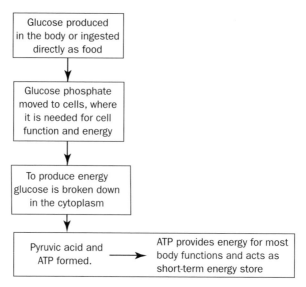

A diagram to show glycolysis

gonads are the male and female reproductive organs in which sex cells (gametes) and hormones are produced. Sex hormones are required for the body to develop normally. In the *male reproductive system*, the reproductive organs are the testes. The main *female reproductive* organs are the ovaries. An important female hormone is oestrogen as this promotes the development of the characteristic female physical shape. The hormones oestrogen and progesterone regulate the menstrual cycle. The male hormones are called androgens and include testosterone. Androgens are responsible for the physical and muscular development of the male as well as the distribution of body hair and the deepening of the voice. (See *endocrine system*.)

government: the state *organisation* which has overall responsibility for managing the nation. It makes policy decisions which affect the lives of individuals and communities. There are different types of government such as:

- central government – nationally elected and formed by the political party which wins the majority of Parliamentary seats in a general election. It is led in the UK by a Prime Minister and cabinet ministers. It is the over-riding organisation which develops *policies* and *legislation*
- government departments – these are departments which are developed from central government and controlled by the appropriate cabinet minister, e.g. by the Secretary of State for Health who is responsible for the *Department of Health*
- local government – are the locally elected councillors in *local authorities* who administer policies at local level
- *European Union (EU).*

GP: see *general practitioner (GP).*

Gram staining is a method of using a blue dye to help identify *bacteria* microscopically. If the bacteria have certain surface features the blue stain is retained and the micro-organism will be gram positive (+). If they are unaffected by the stain they will be gram negative (–).

graphs: a diagrammatic method of presenting *data*. These may take the form of line graphs in which two variables are plotted on a *chart*. The relationship between them can be compared.

grief is a response to *loss*. This includes loss of a person, relationship, job, pet or any aspect of a person's life which is important to their daily living. Grief is a painful process with the loss of a child, husband, wife or partner particularly difficult to cope with. The process of grief often goes through different stages. These are:

- shock and disbelief ('it must be someone else, it isn't true'). A person might feel numb, shocked and locked into a state of isolated disbelief
- *denial*, at this stage the bereaved person behaves in an unreal way. They live as though the person has not died; or as if they did not really lose their job. This stage can last for hours or days
- despair, as there is a growing awareness of what has happened. In addition to this, the person is filled with longing to know the reasons why. There may be feelings of depression, guilt and anxiety which mingle with despair. A sense of unfulfilled dreams adds to the feelings of despair. During this stage individuals need care and support. This will involve listening and allowing the person to express their anger and their feelings of deep pain
- acceptance, the person begins to pick up the aspects of their life and learns to live with the loss they have suffered.

It is important to remember that the timescale between each stage will depend on the loss and the circumstances of that loss. (See *bereavement, coping*).

grievance: a formal term for a complaint which one individual or group will make against another individual or group. There are procedures in place within organisations so that if a person has a grievance they can go to their supervisor and make a complaint, e.g. a group of workers may report a grievance against a manager for *bullying* staff. This would often involve *trade unions* which have representatives who give support on these occasions.

groups: a number of individuals who are linked by common characteristics such as hobbies, culture, lifestyle or appearance. A group has shared *beliefs* and interests within which it functions. These are called group values. The way in which individuals relate and interact within this structure is called group dynamics (see *team* and *sociogram*).

group communication: the way in which members of a group communicate and interact with each other. Effective *interaction* within a group is about:

- developing positive relationships within a group
- ensuring each member of the group has an opportunity to contribute, with each member showing respect and enhancing group cohesion
- negotiating with others and seeking advice from group members
- valuing the contribution that each group member makes, with each member being encouraging and inclusive.

Communicating in groups is important in setting up programmes of care, planning support, managing others and carrying out tasks and working together. Positive group or team working is an essential tool in providing effective care and support to service users. (See *effective communication*, *strategies for positive communication*, *interpersonal skills*, *active listening*.)

group stages: stages which suggest how a group is formed from beginning to the end of the process. The stages are:

- stage 1 – the introduction or forming of a group. The group has come together but no common goal or purpose has been established
- stage 2 – the storming stage, which is where people establish themselves in the group. There may be some power struggles here as the more dominant personalities try to exert their influence
- stage 3 – the norming stage, which is when people form common objectives as to how the group should function in order to complete tasks effectively
- stage 4 – the performing stage, which is about how people work together to meet objectives by carrying out their tasks effectively
- stage 5 – the adjourning stage, which is about how the group members, having completed their tasks and having met their objectives, are able to discontinue the group.

It is important to add that these stages will vary in time frames and that in some cases a group may hover between the forming, storming and norming stages until they have established roles and responsibilities and are able to function effectively.

group types are different collections of people who come together for formal or informal purposes. They are defined as:

- formal groups who meet to discuss and carry out tasks related to work, and professional support, e.g. *multi-disciplinary teams*, *support groups* and committees. These groups work within an agreed format with meeting agendas and minutes
- informal groups who meet for leisure or hobbies, e.g. a group of friends, or family members, going on a trip.

growth: the increase in physical size and changes in shape of an individual as they progress through the life stages.

growth and development: see *human growth and development*.

growth hormone is produced in the anterior lobe of the *pituitary gland*. It controls the physical growth of the body and is produced mainly during childhood when physical growth is rapid. A child's growth rate needs to be monitored regularly (see *centile charts*). Deficiency of this hormone can lead to stunted growth. Excess secretion of this hormone can lead to gigantism. Growth hormone can be given to a child who has a growth deficiency due to a malfunctioning pituitary gland. (See *human growth and development*.)

Guthrie test: a test used to detect diseases and disorders such as phenylketonuria (PKU) and hypothyroidism. PKU is an inherited condition which affects a baby's ability to metabolise part of the protein contained within foods. Hypothyroidism is a condition which occurs when the thyroid gland is underactive. The Guthrie test is carried out when the baby is about six days old and has been taking milk feeds for several days. Blood is collected from a heel prick to cover four circles on a specially prepared card which is then sent to the laboratory. Early detection and dietary treatment of PKU enables the child to develop in a normal way.

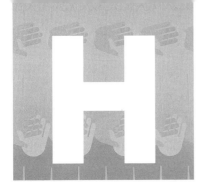

haematology is the study of the *blood*. Haematologists study the formation, composition and the functions of the blood. This helps them to detect and diagnose any disorder, dysfunction and disease which may be present. Blood diseases such as leukaemia and blood deficiency disorders such as anaemia can be detected through the study of a blood sample.

haemoglobin: iron-containing pigment in *blood*. It is found in the *red blood cells*. It carries *oxygen* in the form of oxyhaemoglobin. Carboxyhaemoglobin is formed when haemoglobin combines with *carbon monoxide*. It does this readily, which makes carbon monoxide a powerful respiratory poison, as the carbon monoxide combines with haemoglobin at the sites normally occupied by the oxygen molecules.

haemophilia: an inherited sex-linked recessive condition. Generally only males suffer from haemophilia, but it is passed on through female members of the family. The defect causing haemophilia is on the *X chromosome*. The daughter of a man with haemophilia may inherit his X chromosome and so be a carrier. Haemophiliacs suffer from a bleeding disorder because they lack a clotting factor in the plasma. Any cut, knock or injury can therefore be life-threatening. The Haemophilia Society provides support for haemophiliacs, their families and friends.

hallucinogen: any type of substance which is capable of causing hallucinations. Examples include *LSD* and 'magic mushrooms'. These *drugs* give a person short-term experiences which can be either pleasant or confusing and very frightening. In some cases these drugs can trigger a psychosis or some form of *mental health disorder*.

hand–eye co-ordination is what a young child develops while learning to control his/her hands and fingers. The hand–eye movements enable a child to bring an object into their line of vision. When a child holds a spoon and lifts it to the mouth this movement is dependent on hand–eye co-ordination. This fine muscle control develops gradually throughout childhood. (See *motor skills*.)

harassment is behaviour which is similar to *bullying*. It can be defined as the unwanted conduct of a person affecting the dignity of another person. Such conduct can be physical or verbal, e.g. making offensive sexual or racial remarks.

hazards are anything in the workplace, community or family that can cause harm to an individual or individuals. A health hazard is one that affects an individual's health and leads to illness, e.g. unhygienic food preparation. A safety hazard is one that leads to injury or accident, e.g. no safety gate on the stairs would be a risk to young children. A security hazard could be one that leads to intruders entering buildings, resulting in the theft of information and property. Lack of entry restriction devices in care homes could put vulnerable service users at risk from unwelcome intruders.

Hazards within health and social care relate to
- the work **environment**, which reviews working conditions such as exposure to harmful substances
- work practices and working methods
- the general environment which reviews practice with service users in their homes. (See **risk**.)

Hazardous Waste Regulations 2005 are rules which government has set out with regard to the production, disposal, carrying or receiving of hazardous waste.

headaches are associated with pain in the membranes around the brain. This pain can be caused by:
- tension in the muscles of the head and neck
- interrupted blood flow to the head
- stress
- dehydration and hangover
- food allergies and hunger
- airless, crowded and hot environment.

There is a form of headache called a migraine which has accompanying signs and symptoms such as visual disturbances, nausea and vomiting, and tremors.

health is defined in different terms such as the:
- positive approach – when health and physical **well-being** is achieved and maintained. This includes the psychological well-being of an individual
- holistic approach – when the physical, psychological, cognitive, emotional, social and spiritual aspects of the body are functioning in a positive way
- negative approach – when good health is maintained because of the absence of **disease**.

There are different models of health which include the:
- medical or biomedical model – explores the role of medicine and medical care in the maintenance of health. It explores the effective treatment of disease through medication, surgery and the use of research and technology
- social model – explores the role in the reduction of illness by using preventive measures, e.g. health education.

There are various factors which affect health such as:
- environmental – which relates to an individual's surroundings
- social economic – which relates to social class and poverty.

Health is measured by morbidity/mortality rates, incidence of disease, disease prevalence, disease surveillance, and patterns and trends of health determined by age, social class, gender, ethnicity and locality.

Health Act 1999: an Act introduced with the aims of:
- breaking down the barriers between health and social services
- funding older people's care services
- tackling health inequalities.

Some sections of the Act were updated by the National Health Service Act 2006, which has consolidated earlier NHS **legislation**. This includes:
- pooled funds – where **resources** from different agencies are pooled together to provide care
- integrated provision – where agencies link up staff, resources and management structures.

Health Act 2006: an Act of Parliament that makes provision for the banning of *smoking* in enclosed public places. This includes:

- places of work
- places that the public access to obtain goods and services. This also includes public vehicles.

health and safety is about safe practices within the workplace and the environment (which includes use of public buildings such as schools, churches, public houses, etc). These are underpinned with regulations, *legislation* and guidelines (a health and safety statement that an individual is expected to comply with in their work).

There are a number of requirements which organisations are expected to follow. These are policies and practices which are integrated into health and safety legislation. Examples are:

- carrying out regular *risk assessments*, which are recorded, reviewed and evaluated and reported to a designated health and safety officer
- displaying health and safety information such as a health and safety law poster listing the names of the employee representative, the manager responsible, details of the enforcing authority, first aider's availability, location of *accident book*, location of health and safety policy document
- dealing with waste and spillage which is either hazardous or non-hazardous in a safe way such as mopping up blood and vomit
- ensuring that equipment and resources are correctly labelled and stored
- following security requirements by checking rights of entry so that service users are safe
- dealing with clients with *challenging behaviour* who can cause harm to themselves or to others
- reporting any health and safety issues such as accidents to the designated person
- training staff in health and safety and *first aid* in their individual organisations (see *ABC of resuscitation*). This includes lifting and hygiene practices such as hand washing to combat *MRSA* and *Clostridium difficile*.

health and safety and first aid describes the requirements for *first aid* within an organisation. There should be a poster with the following details on it placed in appropriate locations. Such posters should contain details of:

- named and trained first aider to take charge in an emergency. If there are a number of first aiders, then a rota of responsibilities
- availability of first aid box and where it is located
- location of first aid room
- availability of *accident book* to record accidents.

Health and Safety at Work Act 1974: an Act of Parliament which regulates health and safety of employees in the workplace. The Act makes recommendations which include:

- all employers and their employees being made aware of *health and safety* issues: personal responsibility is an important requirement
- a comprehensive framework involving *legislation* and regulations with regard to *hazards* and potential hazards, *fire regulations* and *codes of practice*
- the setting up of the Health and Safety Commission to ensure the implementation of the Act
- regular health and safety reviews to be carried out by external inspectors.

The commission may instigate legal proceedings, give help and advice and set up advisory committees to support employers and employees. This Act has been regularly updated. (See also *Control of Substances Hazardous to Health (COSHH) Regulations 2002*.)

Health and Safety (Display Screen Equipment) Regulations 1992: regulations which govern the use of computers at work. These should be applied to any person who uses computer screens for a significant part of their work day.

Health and Safety Executive: a major department which was set up within the Health and Safety Commission. The Health and Safety Inspectorate is responsible to the executive as it carries out inspections of premises, etc. It ensures that the Reporting of Injuries, Diseases and Dangerous Occurrences Regulations, policies and codes of practice within Health and Safety Acts are implemented and that *accidents* are investigated.

Health and Safety (Signs and Signals) Regulations 1996: regulations that implement the standardising of safety signs at work.

Health and Social Care Act 2001: an Act set up to introduce free *nursing care* to older people being looked after in residential care homes.

Health and Social Care Act 2008: an Act of Parliament which sets out measures to integrate and modernise health and social care services. This includes regulation of the professions involved in health and social care.

health and social care organisations: see *care organisations*, *care settings* and *community care*.

health and social care structures: a framework of health and social care provision which is arranged to complement the needs of the different client groups. Examples of health and social care services supporting older people would include *residential care, home care, respite care, occupational therapy, day centres, domiciliary services*, *social workers*, parking concessions and voluntary support.

health and social care workers are professionals who work within the health and social care sectors. Their responsibilities are to:
- provide active support to enable service users and patients to communicate their needs and preferences
- use positive and effective *communication skills* to support dignity, self-esteem, diversity, equal opportunities and respect
- work within *confidentiality* and disclosure requirements as well as to maintain accurate records and take responsibility for the secure storage of data
- deal with any tensions between staff and service users in a sensitive manner and to refer when and if necessary. This also applies to tensions which can arise in staff teams or groups.

health and well-being relates to the physical, emotional, intellectual, psychological, social and spiritual well-being of an individual. Factors which promote health and well-being include:
- a balanced diet
- regular exercise
- weight monitoring
- limited alcohol intake and not smoking cigarettes
- regular medical check-ups.

(See *health*.)

health authority: see *strategic health authority*.

health care is care which is provided through the *NHS (National Health Service)*. Health care is available through a combination of statutory, voluntary, private and informal health provisions. Health care provision operates at three levels:

- primary care – health care offered to individuals through GPs and their teams in general practice. Primary care also includes dentists
- secondary care – health care offered through hospitals, *national health trusts* and private hospitals in the *independent sector*
- tertiary care – specialist health care offered through special hospitals including cancer hospitals such as the Royal Marsden Hospital. The Royal Marsden treats people with cancer from all over the world.

health care assistants or clinical support workers provide nursing support in hospitals or other health care settings such as nursing and care homes. They carry out general duties for patients which include:

- recording temperature, pulse, respiration and blood pressure
- assisting with toileting and bathing
- encouraging mobility, helping with exercises
- supporting a patient's self-esteem, talking, reading, listening and sharing information
- carrying out 'domestic' duties, such as tidying up, sorting laundry, etc.

Health Care Commission (The Commission for Health Care Audit and Inspection) was set up under the Health and Social Care (Community Health and Standards Act) 2003 with the aim to encourage the improvement of health care provision throughout England and Wales. It was replaced in 2009 by the *Care Quality Commission*.

health centre: a community-based organisation which accommodates the *general practitioner (GP)* and the *primary health care team*. It may offer other services such as support group sessions for the elderly, back pain clinics and *screening programmes*.

Health Development Agency: a *special health authority*. It was set up to improve the health of people in England, exploring in particular how to reduce inequalities in health. It works closely with the government, the public sector, private and professional organisations. This authority commissions research and advises on the setting of standards and provides developmental support to those working in public health at regional and local levels.

health education: a programme which informs the general public about issues relating to healthy lifestyles. This allows individuals the benefit of making informed choices. These programmes are designed:

- to improve the health of the population as a whole by increasing the length of people's lives and the number of years people spend free from illness
- to improve the health of the worse off in society and to narrow the health gap.

Health education programmes have three different levels:

- primary health education aimed at healthy people. For example, giving presentations and targeting people with information on healthy diets
- secondary health education aimed at those people who already have a health condition. For example, exploring strategies to encourage a heavy smoker with lung problems to give up smoking, or an overweight person with a heart condition to reduce their weight

- tertiary health education aimed at those individuals who have a disorder, dysfunction or disease which could not have been prevented and for which there is no cure. The information issued relates to rehabilitation and specialist support programmes.

Health education relates closely to **national health targets**. Health education may explore issues such as:

- reducing the likelihood of disease by promoting **immunisation** programmes, or healthy eating to prevent heart disease
- minimising the risk of potentially harmful lifestyles, e.g. smoking, drinking, taking **drugs**, certain sexual practices, all of which may be associated with medical conditions (e.g. heart disease, cancer, HIV)
- promoting healthy living practices through diet and exercise
- promoting personal safety and security in relation to the safe use of equipment, safety in the home and at work.

health education campaigns: methods used to communicate health information to the general public. They allow individuals to become aware of the health issues which can affect them. Such campaigns cover a number of issues which link closely to **national health targets**. The aim of such campaigns is to provide knowledge by supplying appropriate information which enables individuals to make choices about their health. An example might be encouraging people to give up **smoking**, or to look at fat content when buying **food** in order to maintain a low fat diet. Health education campaigns can encourage individuals to take more control of health issues in their lives. In some cases this can lead to changing **lifestyle** habits, such as taking more **exercise** and learning to manage **stress**.

health improvement programmes: programmes set up in localities to support the **national contracts for health**. The functions of such programmes are to:

- give a clear description of how national aims, priorities, targets and contracts are tackled locally
- set out a range of locally determined priorities and targets to address issues and problems which are judged important with particular emphasis on areas of major **inequalities in health** in local communities
- support specific agreed programmes of action to address national and local health improvement priorities
- show that the action proposed is based on evidence which is known to work from research and best practice reports
- indicate which local organisations have been involved in drawing up a plan, what their contributions will be and how they will be held to account for delivering it
- ensure that the plan is easy to understand and accessible to the public
- be a vehicle for setting strategies in the shaping of local health services.

(See also *Our Healthier Nation – a Contract for Health, national health targets*.)

health inequalities: see *inequalities in health*.

Health of the Nation 1992: a government report presented in the House of Commons in July 1992. It was designed to set out a national strategy for health in England. The key areas selected in the report are coronary heart disease and strokes, cancers, mental illness, HIV/AIDS, sexual health and accidents. These are all areas identified as major causes of premature death or avoidable ill health. The report was updated in **Our Healthier Nation – A Contract for Health** (1998). However, Our Healthier Nation 1998 does not highlight HIV/AIDS and sexual health. (See **national health targets, Acheson Report 1998.**)

health promotion is about raising awareness of a wide range of health issues such as healthy eating and sensible drinking. Certain factors influence health promotions such as:

- **demographic** data which provide information on patterns of disease, and risk-associated lifestyles such as binge drinking and obesity
- updated scientific evidence which relates different aspects of **health and well-being** to individuals
- reviewing concerns with regard to health issues which have been raised by the government, pressure groups, mass media and the general public.

There are different approaches to health promotion. All are used to activate a health promotion campaign which aims to develop knowledge about health issues, getting individuals to improve their health and prevent them from becoming ill. These approaches have a focus on disease prevention and include:

- biomedical – intervention by medical professions. Examples are **immunisation** programmes
- behavioural – intervention which works with the educational approach in order to change the **behaviour** of the individual, e.g. available information on how to give up **smoking**
- educational – intervention by promoting knowledge and understanding of health and **lifestyle** issues, e.g. healthy drinking limits
- service user centred or empowerment – intervention by increasing self-awareness of different health issues so that an individual is able to identify choices and take action, e.g. a service user explores eating and **exercise** patterns and feels empowered to join a gym
- social change – intervention by seeking to change society's attitude to a health issue, e.g. **healthy eating plate, Five-A-Day campaign**.

Methods used to communicate the message can come from numerous sources such as the **mass media** (television, local and national radio, internet, newspapers, etc), leaflets, community presentations, advertisements, **pressure group** campaigns and posters.

health protection: strategies used to safeguard populations against ill health through different means such as legislation, finance, or social. For example using health and safety legislation to reduce the number of accidents, using taxation policies to reduce smoking and drinking by putting additional tax on cigarettes and alcohol, targeting groups in society who are at risk, e.g. cervical screening and breast screening. (See **health screening.**)

Health Protection Agency: an independent agency whose role is to protect the **health and well-being** of the population.

Health Protection Agency Act 2004: an Act of Parliament that established the *Health Protection Agency*.

health screening: a way of checking an individual's health to ensure that various parts of the body are functioning as normal. Methods of screening include:

- breast screening – early detection of breast cancer
- cervical screening – early detection of cervical cancer
- prostate screening – early detection of prostate cancer
- testicular screening – early detection of testicular cancer.

In some cases, screening the blood (i.e. *blood tests*) can identify the likelihood of certain cancers such as leukaemia and ovarian cancer.

health targets: see *national targets for health*.

health visitor: a registered *nurse* who qualifies through further training as a health visitor. A health visitor is employed by a health authority and is based in a health centre or GP surgery. The health visitor offers support and guidance, monitors the growth and development of babies and young children, and takes part in *child abuse* procedures as well as working with older people. Their main concern is *health education* as well as the direct care and welfare of their clients.

healthy eating plate: a visual tool to help people eat more healthily by showing the types and proportions of foods they need in order to have a well-balanced and healthy *diet* (also called the eat well plate).

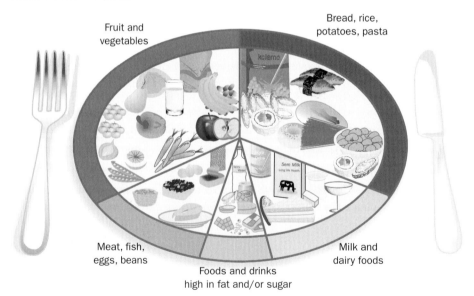

A healthy eating plate

hearing impairment: see *deafness or hearing impairment*.

heart: a muscular organ which pumps *blood* round the body. The heart consists of:

- *atria* (auricles) – the two upper chambers. The left atrium receives oxygenated blood, i.e. blood with fresh oxygen from the *lungs* via the pulmonary veins. The right atrium receives deoxygenated blood from the rest of the body via the superior and inferior vena cavae

- **ventricles** – the two lower chambers. The left ventricle receives blood from the left atrium and pumps it into the aorta. The right ventricle receives blood from the right atrium and pumps it via the pulmonary arteries to the lungs.

(See **cardiac cycle**.)

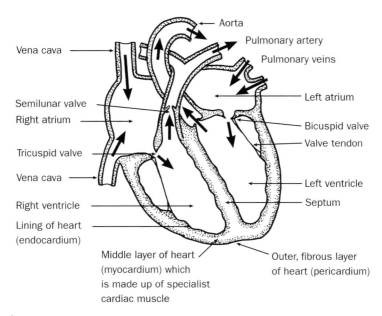

The heart

heart attack: also known as myocardial infarction, is the result of a blockage in the **coronary artery**. This can lead to the death of a segment of heart **muscle**. The person suddenly experiences severe pain in the centre of the chest. The pain extends to the throat and down the left arm. The person needs calm reassurance and emergency treatment. A person complaining of chest pain should never be left on their own and an ambulance should be called as soon as possible.

heart disease and strokes: a priority health target area identified by the government in 1998. Heart disease and strokes were selected as a priority area because:

- they are a major cause of early death, accounting for about 18,000 deaths (one-third of all deaths) in men and 7000 deaths (one-fifth of all deaths) in women under 65 years of age
- deaths from **coronary heart disease** alone account for more than a million years of life lost amongst those under 75 years
- heart disease and stroke can often be prevented
- there are marked inequalities of incidence; for example, women born in West Africa and the Caribbean have a higher risk of a stroke than other women. Men of working age in the bottom social class are at least 50% more likely to die from coronary heart disease than men in the overall population.

Although death rates from heart disease and strokes have been decreasing, the health target is to reduce the death rate from heart disease, stroke and related illnesses amongst people under 65 years, by at least a further third by 2010 from a baseline. This is the basic mortality target established in 1996.

heart rate is the rate at which the *heart* beats, usually expressed as beats per minute. At rest an adult heart beats approximately 70 times a minute. It beats faster in a child. Heart rate increases when exercise is being taken as the heart supplies the muscles of the body with extra oxygen and food to maintain the exercise. Heart rate increases during times of excitement, fear and *anxiety*. (See *pulse*.)

hepatitis: inflammation of the *liver*, which is caused by *infection*, or damage due to chemicals or *drug* treatment/misuse. The inflammation affects the liver, interfering with *bile* production. Yellow pigments of bile circulate in the bloodstream causing yellowing of the skin and the whites of the eyes and dark yellow *urine*. The most common forms of hepatitis are:

- hepatitis A – transmitted by food and water which is contaminated with faeces due to lack of hygiene precautions in food preparation. It is also transmitted from person to person or by injecting with unclean hypodermic needles. It can often occur in institutions or amongst large groups of people where food is not adequately prepared. There is *vaccination* available against this disease
- hepatitis B – this is transmitted by sexual contact or from a mother to her unborn baby or foetus. It can be transmitted through injections, *blood transfusions* using contaminated or unclean needles for either injecting drugs or following *acupuncture* and tattooing. It is caused by a virus which can be present in other body fluids such as saliva, vaginal fluid and semen. There is vaccination available in the form of gamma globulin containing antibodies to the virus
- hepatitis C – this is a non-A and a non-B hepatitis mainly transmitted through infected blood and syringes which have been contaminated with the virus. It is said to be the most common form of hepatitis transmitted through blood transfusion. There is a vaccination available for this
- hepatitis E – as with hepatitis A this is transmitted through drinking water contaminated with faeces. It can reach *epidemic* proportions in tropical areas. There is no vaccination available.

heredity: the transmission of *genetic* characteristics from one generation to another, i.e. parent to child.

heroin: a *drug*, a derivative of morphine, which is derived from the opium poppy. The plant is harvested in order to be processed into a painkilling or analgesic drug. The drug is most effective when given by injection to patients suffering from severe pain, e.g. those patients suffering from advanced cancer. One of its side effects is that individuals can develop tolerance, or physical and psychological *dependence.* When the medication of heroin is reduced or a patient is taken off the drug, *withdrawal symptoms* can be unpleasant and can last for up to two weeks.

Heroin has addictive properties and individuals can become addicted to the euphoric effects of heroin and become 'mainliners'; mainliners use the injection method to 'rush' or intensify the euphoric experience. Some addicts now choose to smoke heroin and heat it on a strip of tinfoil until it gives off smoke ('chasing the dragon'). Heroin addicts have a mortality rate which is 18 times higher than normal. *Death* is not normally due to the direct effects of heroin use. Death may be due to:

- an overdose
- illness resulting from the use of 'dirty' or unclean needles and injection techniques, including venous thrombosis, *HIV/AIDS*, septicaemia or *hepatitis*
- mixing heroin with other substances
- associated health-related illness due to physical *neglect*.

heterosexuality: an attraction to persons of the opposite sex which may lead to sexual contact.

histograms: a method of representing data which has been collected as a result of a research project. The method represents the frequency distribution of the data diagramatically in the form of a *chart*. A histogram consists of a series of blocks or bars with a height proportional to the frequency of an item or event. (See *bar chart*.)

histology is the microscopic study of *tissues*. When, for example, a *tumour* develops in a part of the body a sample of the tissue is sent to the histology department within a pathology laboratory for examination. The method is used to detect many different disorders, dysfunctions and disease. (See *pathology*.)

HIV (human immunodeficiency virus): a virus which can cause *AIDS*. The *virus* gradually breaks down the *immune system* of an infected person.

holistic care involves caring for the whole person. This means that the physical, intellectual, emotional, social, religious and cultural needs of the client are taken into account and care for that person is implemented accordingly. It is based on the belief that all these aspects are interlinked and should not be considered separately. (See *care value base, complementary and alternative medicine, homoeopathy*.)

holistic health: the development of the person as a whole. It takes into account the spiritual, physical, intellectual, emotional, social and environmental aspects of *health and well-being*.

home care service: *community care* teams which provide care for older and disabled clients in their own homes. The care includes shopping, cooking meals, helping clients with washing, dressing and cleaning. The carers are usually employed by the social services department, voluntary or private organisations. In some cases, this is a *means-tested* service.

Home Life 1984: a code of practice introduced to improve the standards of care for clients in residential care. It was conceived by the *Centre for Policy on Ageing* and recommended that:
- special provision be made available for individual client groups
- all *residential homes* for the elderly should be registered with the *local authority*
- all local authorities should be involved in carrying out inspections on private and statutory homes for the elderly under the Registered Homes Act 1984
- all clients have rights and choices which should be respected including those of *confidentiality* and *privacy*
- client admission procedures should be standardised
- building, room and staffing requirements should be identified.

In 1990 a policy called Community Life developed this further by adding that all care packages, i.e. all aspects of care required by a client, should reflect his or her informed choice. Each client should know their individual *rights and responsibilities* with regard to their care and treatment. (See *Better Home Life 1996*.)

Home Office: the central government department responsible for the administration of the justice system including the police, the probation and prison services.

Home Start UK: a voluntary organisation set up across the country to help young families under stress. It deals with single mothers and broken marriages. Help is given through a network of experienced parents who support young families under stress.

homelessness: the condition suffered by a person who has no home. Under the Housing (Homeless Persons) Act 1997, *local authorities* are required to help homeless people who have priority *housing* needs, i.e. persons who have become homeless when they are pregnant, or have young and dependent children.

homeostasis: processes within the body which maintain its steady state. Conditions outside the body (the external environment) are continuously varying, but the body has mechanisms (homeostatic controls) for adjusting factors within the body so that the internal environment surrounding the *cells* is kept steady. Cells are surrounded by *tissue* fluid. This maintains an environment around the cells which allows them to function well and the body to remain healthy. For the homeostatic mechanism to work there must be:

- receptors capable of detecting changes
- a control mechanism to co-ordinate appropriate corrective mechanisms
- effectors which actually bring about the corrective mechanisms.

Their effectiveness depends on negative *feedback*.

Examples of conditions kept constant within the internal environment of the body by homeostatic mechanisms include:

- pH – the body's internal pH has a natural range of 7.33–7.42
- body temperature
- respiratory gases
- blood sugar levels.

homoeopathy is a complementary system of medicine that regards physical, emotional and mental symptoms as being intimately connected. Minute doses of natural substances are prescribed according to a complex pattern of symptoms in every area of the body. Individual likes and dislikes and the family history of each individual are also taken into account. People suffering from all kinds of illnesses, from depression to arthritis, migraines to ulcers, and now the 'modern' illnesses, such as AIDS and myalgic encephalomyelitis (ME or chronic fatigue syndrome), can be helped to regain a better level of health. Homoeopathy treats the individual person rather than the disease. This means that the homoeopath will want to build up a complete picture of a patient and their medical history, as well as all their symptoms, in order to find the remedy that provides the closest match. (See *complementary and alternative medicine, holistic care*.) Treatment is carried out by homoeopathic doctors who are qualified doctors with specialist training in homoeopathy, or by homoeopathic consultants who have attended a course in homoeopathy at a college associated with the Society of Homoeopathy.

homosexuality: sexual contact with members of the same sex, or a sexual preference for one's own sex. (See *lesbians/gays*.)

hormone replacement therapy (HRT): oestrogen administered to women when the natural production of sex hormones has been reduced or stopped for some reason, such as at *menopause*, or after a total hysterectomy (surgical removal of the *uterus* and ovaries). In some cases the hormone progesterone is given as part of hormone replacement therapy to women who are experiencing the symptoms of menopause and who still have a uterus.

hormones: chemicals secreted directly into the bloodstream by the *glands* which form the *endocrine system*. They travel in the *blood* to target *organs*. The effects of hormones are slower and more general than *nerve* action. They control long-term changes such as:

- the balance of *water* and salt levels within the body thus maintaining *homeostasis*
- the different stages involved in reproduction
- the rate of *growth and development*
- *sexual maturity*
- the rate of activity.

hospice: an institution set up with the main purpose of caring for the dying. The most famous hospice is St Christopher's in London. A hospice may provide the following:

- *holistic care*: explores the social, intellectual, emotional, spiritual and physical needs of the patient
- *palliative care*: supportive and total care to those who are dying
- short- or long-term care: as the need arises
- home care: teams from the hospice support the patient in their own home
- *counselling*: enables the patient and their families to discuss their feelings about the illness.

hospitals are large institutions which treat people who have health disorders, dysfunctions and disease. In 1998, new measures for hospitals were introduced based on *clinical governance*. They included:

- success and failure rates after certain types of treatment to be monitored, including *deaths*, complication rates following operations, deaths after *heart* attacks, deaths after a fractured neck of femur or with *MRSA* or *Clostridium difficile*
- a national performance framework to be set up focusing on the quality and not just the expense of NHS services
- sophisticated measures of clinical quality to be developed on a specialty by specialty and hospital by hospital basis
- details of each hospital's performance in operations to be monitored
- doctors to be required to take part in routine inquiries into deaths after surgery, maternal deaths, stillbirths, infant deaths and suicides
- doctors to be required to put their results in an audit of their specialty organised by their Royal College.

hostel: a *residential home* or provision which offers supervision and support to individuals who need somewhere to stay. Examples of people who might need hostel accommodation are:

- those coming out of prison
- young people leaving care
- *older people*
- those with *learning disabilities*
- those with psychological or *mental health disorders*
- women who need protection following *domestic violence*.

Houses of Parliament: consist of the House of Commons and the House of Lords. Parliament is responsible for determining law and social policy which affect the lives of the general public and the society in which they live. The government is formed from the ruling political party, the leader of which becomes Prime Minister.

housing is a collective term for places of shelter where people live. There are different regulations and legislation to ensure that suitable housing policies are being developed by *local authorities*. Housing and building legislation set standards to promote safe conditions.

housing benefit: see *benefits*.

human development can be seen in terms of developmental stages which include *infancy*, childhood, *adolescence* and *adulthood*.

Human Fertilisation and Embryology Act 2008: an Act of Parliament which makes it legal to assist reproduction. Key provisions of the Act with regard to fertilisation include:

- a ban on the selection of offspring for non-medical reasons. Selection of sex for medical reasons, e.g. to avoid a certain disease that affect only one sex, is allowed
- recognition of same sex couples as legal parents of children conceived through the use of donated sperm, eggs or embryos.

human growth and development: the way in which the body changes through the human life cycle. Growth and development includes:

- physical development – for example, the development of *bones* and *muscles* which affect body movement and co-ordination
- *social development* – the development of relationships through *socialisation* and self-management skills
- *intellectual development or cognitive development* – the development of learning, problem solving skills and reasoning; this includes *language development*
- emotional development – the development of emotional feelings including the bonding and attachment relationships between the newborn and his or her parents or primary care giver; this evolves later into the development of *self-esteem*
- cultural development – developing the person's cultural *identity* through reinforcing positive self-esteem
- spiritual development – the development of an individual's *belief* system.

In terms of human growth and development, consideration should be given to the individual's cultural and sexual identity. These aspects will develop and mature with the other changes within the life cycle.

Factors which can affect growth and development include low birth weight, lack of stimulation, accidents, illness, birth difficulties, inadequate diet, heredity and environment (see *nature–nurture*).

The study of human development is important to health and social care students because it helps them to understand and to clarify the needs of clients or service users. (See *development*, *learning theories*.)

human rights are the rights to which all human beings are entitled such as freedom of *choice*, rights to *confidentiality*, *dignity* and *autonomy*.

Human Rights Act 1998: an Act of Parliament which incorporates the rights and freedoms guaranteed under the *European Convention on Human Rights*. It also makes provision for certain judges to become judges in the *European Court of Human Rights*. The articles in the law include:

- the right to life, liberty and fair trial
- prohibition of torture, slavery, abuse of rights, forced labour and discrimination
- the right to education, security and no punishment without law
- the right to marry and respect for private and family life
- freedom of thought, conscience, religion, expression, assembly and association.

Huntington's disease: previously known as Huntington's chorea, this is a hereditary disorder of the *central nervous system*. In the United Kingdom over 20 000 people are affected directly or indirectly by the disease. Huntington's disease is caused by a faulty *gene*. In some way, which is not yet understood, the faulty gene leads to damage of the *nerve* cells in areas of the *brain*. This causes gradual physical, mental and emotional changes. Each person whose parent has Huntington's disease is born with a 50% chance of inheriting the faulty gene. Anyone who inherits the faulty gene will at some stage develop the disease. Its onset occurs in middle age. Recently tests have become available to inform young people whether or not they will develop the disease.

hydrocephalus is a condition which can be caused by an increase of *cerebrospinal fluid* in the cavities of the *brain*, leading to excessive pressure in the brain. An obvious outward sign that this is happening in infants is an accelerated increase in size of the head. If the excess pressure is caused by a blockage it can be relieved in order to minimise damage. This is usually done by inserting a valve or shunt which drains off the excess fluid into the abdominal or heart cavities. Many babies who are born with **spina bifida** have hydrocephalus but it also occurs independently at birth and later in life. Modern advances in treatment and therapy mean that many babies affected with this condition survive into adulthood.

hygiene: the procedures involved in maintaining cleanliness which also include *health and safety*. Personal hygiene *routines*, such as washing, bathing and changing clothes, are learnt at an early age. Children learn to wash their hands before meals and after going to the toilet and to wash their faces in the mornings. In addition, they learn to clean their teeth, wash their hair and bathe. Learning to dress and changing clothes develop as their manipulative skills emerge. Personal hygiene is an important part of caring. Retaining a person's *dignity* is a first priority in helping with washing and toileting. A clean and hygienic environment is essential in maintaining a service user's *health and well-being*. In order to maintain a high standard of hygiene in supporting care, carers are required to wash their hands at regular intervals, especially when moving from one service user to the next. Antibacterial scrubs can be used to enhance this process. (See *infection control*, *care environment and care context, food hygiene, food safety, MRSA* and *Clostridium difficile*.)

hypothalamus: the part of the brain situated above the *pituitary gland*. It provides the link between the *endocrine system* and the *nervous system*. Some of the functions of the hypothalamus are as follows:

- it controls the secretion of some *hormones*
- it controls some aspects of *homeostasis*
- it helps regulate the amount of fluid in the body; if the body requires fluids the hypothalamus gives rise to the feeling of thirst.

hypothermia: reduction of body *temperature* below the normal range. It is liable to occur in vulnerable clients such as *older people* and *babies*. It is important that babies and older people are kept warm and that their body heat is maintained as they can lose body heat very quickly. (See *care environment and care context*.)

hypothesis: a statement or research question which is identified at the beginning of an investigation or piece of research. It serves as a prediction or explanation of events. A hypothesis is an important aspect of research because it can be tested against reality (does the result indicate it is true, or not?) and can then be supported or rejected.

Aiming for a grade A*?

Don't forget to log on to **www.philipallan.co.uk/a-zonline** for advice.

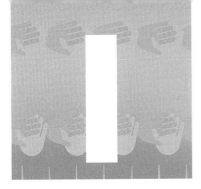

identity is a person's understanding of his/her self in relation to other people and society. It includes a person's view of themselves and develops in either a positive or negative way from early childhood. (See *self-concept, self-esteem*.)

ill health and disease can be classified as social, psychological, emotional or physical and can be defined as a breakdown in *health and well-being*. It can be due to:

- a deficiency of a chemical in the body, e.g. *diabetes*
- a physical disorder or dysfunction, e.g. *congenital* dislocation of the hip
- a *mental health disorder* or dysfunction, e.g. *depression*
- an *infection*, e.g. chicken pox
- an inherited disease, e.g. *haemophilia*
- a degenerative disease, e.g. *arthritis*.

Poor health has complex causes such as *ageing*, inadequate diet, lack of physical activity or the effects of sexual behaviour, *smoking, alcohol* and *drugs*. Social and economic issues play their part. These include *poverty, unemployment*, and *social exclusion*. Environmental factors such as air and water quality and *housing* also contribute to ill health.

image analysis: a *research method* used in *health promotion* which determines the audience or target group's attitudes towards the health topic being discussed.
A *questionnaire* is designed to collect evidence which can include:

- awareness of the topic discussed or presented
- attitudes
- practice.

imagination: using the creative faculty of the mind to form mental images. Developing imagination can be an effective way of improving a person's *communication skills*. A person can imagine what they might say in a certain situation or how they can be successful in what they do. Children use their imagination when they *play*. They use it in pretend or role-play. This can include playing shop with empty cartons and plastic money, dressing up and using face paints. (See *creative play*.)

imitation: copying another person's *behaviour*. Imitation is a powerful means of learning. Children in particular observe and imitate the actions of others. For example, a child might imitate what happens at home or in the home corner at *pre-school group* where the table is laid for a meal and different scenarios acted out.

immune response is the way in which the body's *immune system* responds when foreign *antigens* are introduced. *Antibodies* are produced which combine with these foreign antigens to inactivate them. This is the basic mechanism of *active immunity*. The main cells involved are *white blood cells* called lymphocytes. There are two main types:

- B-lymphocytes – these are manufactured in the *bone marrow* and then transported to the lymph nodes. When an antigen enters the lymph nodes, B-lymphocytes divide rapidly and

157

produce antibodies such as immunoglobulins which travel through the bloodstream. They provide the necessary protection against bacteria and viruses.

- T-lymphocytes – these also are manufactured in the bone marrow but they are matured in the thymus gland. They multiply and circulate around the bloodstream when an antigen enters the body. On contact with the cell containing the antigen they attack and destroy it.

immune system: this controls the way in which the body resists *pathogens*. The system consists of a number of structures and processes including:

- the skin, which provides a protective and waterproof covering to the body
- the production of immunoglobulins by bone marrow, spleen and all lymphoid tissue except the thymus
- the layers of mucous membrane which line the mouth, respiratory airways, alimentary canal and the vagina, they can produce antimicrobial enzymes as well as mucus which traps any particles
- the cilia in the respiratory tract which sweep particles away from the lungs
- the clotting of the blood which forms a protective barrier over cuts and wounds
- the secretion of acid in the stomach which destroys harmful organisms
- the enzyme lysozyme which is present in tears and destroys bacteria.

When foreign organisms enter the bloodstream, the body sets up an active response in order to eliminate those that may cause disease. This is called the *immune response*.

immunisation: a procedure which is used to combat many different diseases. Immunisation programmes are set up to give *vaccinations* to individuals or groups at appropriate intervals. Doctors and health visitors advise parents or carers about immunisations and discuss any worries they may have. (See *infection*.) This can also include immunisations used for travel reasons such as protection against cholera, malaria, tetanus, typhoid, hepatitis A and C and rabies.

Immunisation programmes

Age to immunise	Disease protected against	Method
2 months	Diphtheria, whooping cough, polio and Hib Pneumococcal infection	Injection
3 months	Diphtheria, whooping cough, polio and Hib Meningitis C	Injection
4 months	Diphtheria, whooping cough, polio and Hib Meningitis C Pneumococcal infection	Injection
Around 12 months	Hib Meningitis C	Injection
Around 13 months	Measles, mumps, rubella (MMR) Pneumococcal infection	Injection
3 years and 4 months or soon after	Diphtheria, whooping cough, polio and Hib Measles, mumps, rubella (MMR)	Injection
Girls aged 12 to 13 years	Cervical cancer caused by human papillomavirus types 16 and 18	3 injections over 6 months
13 to 18	Diphtheria, tetanus and polio	Injection

immunity is one of the ways in which a body resists the attack of disease and infection. The body deals with infection through the *immune response*. Immunity affects germs entering the body in different ways. There can be:

- total immunity – germs are destroyed
- partial immunity – there is not sufficient immunity to prevent the disease but there is enough to make the disease less severe
- no immunity – infection has developed and is fully evident.

There are various types of immunity which can apply to infections. They are:

- active immunity (acquired immunity) can be obtained when the body produces its own immunity or through vaccines
- passive immunity can be obtained through injection of a manufactured *antitoxin*
- foetal immunity is obtained by the foetus when antibodies cross the placenta from the mother's blood into the bloodstream of the *foetus*.

impairment: damage or loss of a physical function in the body. It can involve any part of the body. For instance a visual impairment limits the ability to see clearly as it affects the eyes.

in vitro fertilisation is a technique developed to fertilise the human egg using means outside the body. A woman is given *hormones* to increase the number of eggs she produces. Using a fine tube passed through the body wall, a doctor collects some of these eggs and places them in a dish containing a nutrient solution. Semen containing active sperm is added to the dish. *Fertilisation* of several eggs will occur. They are allowed to develop for three days before they are inserted back into the woman's uterus. In most cases at least one of these embryos develops into a baby. The technique is used in cases when a man and woman are unable to conceive naturally.

incidence: the number of new cases of an event occurring within a specified time period. This is a method of recording disease, crime rates and mortality rates from any type of disease.

inclusive practice describes the strategies used to ensure that all children are treated fairly and their rights and entitlements are met. This is underpinned by *anti-discriminatory practice*, ensuring that every child's individual needs are listened to and supported in their *early years provision*.

income: the amount of money which an individual or family receives from *employment*, investments and other sources to support their lifestyle. Income is described in terms of an amount per week, per month or per year. Income distribution describes the amount of money which is allocated throughout society. This is affected by:

- levels of employment/unemployment
- the cost of living
- lifestyle choices
- the use of credit, i.e. borrowing money to maintain levels of expenditure.

Unequal income distribution can lead to relative *poverty*.

income support: a method by which the government provides financial support to members of society who are unemployed or who receive less than a certain amount of money per week for the work they do. (See *benefits*.)

incubation period: the length of time which elapses from initial contact to the outward signs and symptoms of an *infection*. An example of this is rubella which takes 10–14 days for the first signs (rash, raised temperature and swollen neck glands) to reveal themselves.

independence: the ability to maintain activities which support an individual's *lifestyle* without the assistance of others. Independence is an important factor in care practice. Encouraging a child, teenager, adult, older person and those who are disabled to make choices, take decisions and carry out tasks themselves is an important dimension in *caring*. (See *activities of daily living, care value base*.)

independent living: a term which describes the way in which people with disabilities strive or aspire to live so that they have the most control, *choice* or *autonomy* over the manner in which they conduct their daily lives. (See *Disabled Living Foundation, aids and adaptations, activities of daily living, enablement, normalisation*.)

independent sector provides health and social care services which are independent from the state. These include:
- voluntary organisations – non-profit-making organisations whose management committees provide a service without receiving a salary. However, voluntary organisations do employ and pay administration staff to co-ordinate different programmes and schemes. They operate at national, local and regional levels
- private organisations provide a service at a cost. They charge for provision in order to make a profit for owners or shareholders
- not-for-profit organisations are set up as a charitable trust, where any surplus income is fed back into the trust. (See *charities*.)

individual need is based on the requirements of each service user, client or patient. These should be assessed and met by their carers. (See *basic needs, Maslow, additional needs, anti-discriminatory practice, effective communication, building a positive relationship* and *building confidence*.)

individual rights are the rights of an individual to *dignity* and *respect*, equal treatment, *access to treatment, anti-discriminatory care, safety* and protection, and to be able to communicate as desired with others using a preferred method or device.

individuality: a term which recognises that it is important to acknowledge that all people are distinct and vary one from another. These differences may include genetic make-up, *lifestyle, religion, culture, race*, life experiences and *intelligence*.

industrial tribunals are judicial bodies set up to support an individual who has been unfairly treated in their work or *employment* situation.

inequalities in health: an individual's well-being is affected by social and economic factors such as *poverty, unemployment* and *social exclusion*. In the Green Paper *Our Healthier Nation – A Contract for Health*, social and economic factors are confirmed as a link with ill health. Ill health is not spread evenly across society. In nearly every case the highest incidence of illness is experienced by the lowest social classes. Although death rates from lung cancer have been falling, mortality rates show that more people die from lung cancer in the North of England than in the South. The *National Contract for Health* is viewed as an opportunity to tackle such regional variations in health. (See *Black Report 1980, Acheson Report 1998*.)

inequality in society describes those inequalities which relate to *social and economic factors* and *disadvantage*.

infancy: the first stage of *human growth and development* following birth.

infant: a *newborn baby* completely dependent on the mother. This term is usually applied to a baby under the age of one year.

infant mortality is a measure of the death of babies under one year old. Infant deaths are measured by the number of babies who die under the age of one year per 1000 babies in the population. This infant mortality rate is used by statisticians as an indicator of child health in different countries.

infection: a condition which occurs as a result of contact with a disease-causing organism or *pathogen*, leading to signs and symptoms indicating that the individual is ill. The degree of infection and its effects will depend on the type of pathogen involved. The most common infections are colds and flu as well as chest, urinary and skin infections.

infection control: methods used to control infection particularly in a health and social care setting. Health and social care workers should be vigilant in their care in terms of:
- hand washing between contact with individual service users to reduce cross-infection
- maintaining their own personal hygiene such as daily washing and bathing
- ensuring personal safety by disposal of body fluids and solids in a safe way to a designated area
- making sure that *health and safety* regulations are in place in terms of food handling
- using protective clothing when attending service users such as when toileting or changing nappies. (See *hygiene*.)

infection control committee: a multi-disciplinary committee set up to formulate procedures to be implemented or carried out in hospitals or in the community in order to prevent and control *infection*. The committee consists of an *infection control nurse*, representatives from the different areas of nursing and community care, experts in food preparation and a microbiologist.

infection control nurse: a registered *nurse* who has specific responsibilities for the control of infection in *hospital*. He/she is specially trained and their knowledge and skills are used to help other nurses to carry out an *infection control* policy as part of their work. When a specific infection is evident, either in a ward or in an operating theatre, the infection control nurse investigates the source. In recent years the outbreak of *MRSA* and *Clostridium difficile* in hospitals has caused much concern. The nursing care of infected patients should be carefully monitored. The infection control nurse reports to the *infection control committee*.

infertility is the inability of an individual to conceive. Causes include:
- inactive sperm in the semen
- not enough sperm manufactured
- ovaries that are not producing eggs
- fallopian tubes that are blocked due to scarring or infection
- mucus lining in the cervix that has thickened to the extent that the sperm cannot enter
- the man being unable to have an erection ensuring full intercourse
- overproduction of prolactin by the *pituitary gland*, which leads to impotence in the male and infertility in the woman

- emotional and psychological pressures on both the man and the woman setting up a cycle of tension.

infestation: evidence of parasites, either on the skin, in the clothes or inside the body. These include scabies, head lice and threadworms.

inflammation is the body's response to any injury which causes damage to the tissue. The *signs and symptoms* of inflammation are:
- heat and redness – due to increased *blood* supply to the area
- swelling – when *tissues* develop oedema, which is the accumulation of excess fluid in the tissues surrounding the area of inflammation
- pain.

Inflammation may be caused by any injury such as a cut or bruise, exposure to ultraviolet light, *radiotherapy* treatment, intense *temperature* such as a burn, scald or frost bite, chemical burns, allergic reactions such as nettle rash, viruses and *bacteria*.

informal care is care which is given by family, friends and neighbours. According to the National Association of Carers:
- there are approximately six million unpaid and informal *carers* in Britain
- one in seven adults has a caring responsibility
- 1.4 million carers devote over 20 hours per week to caring
- one in five households contains a carer
- carers tend to be middle-aged women but can be men or even children
- one in five carers cares for someone who is not related to them
- most carers look after someone who is elderly
- many carers look after more than one person
- a quarter of carers receive no help from anyone inside or outside the family
- 50% of those caring for a spouse do so unaided.

information: knowledge which is acquired and transmitted from one person or organisation to another. In health and social care the way in which *i*nformation is acquired, given, selected and dealt with is a key requirement within the caring process. There are concerns about *confidentiality* and *access to information*. Some aspects may be protected by *legislation*. Carers handling information should be aware of the *rights and choices* of clients. Clients should be given as much information as possible. (See *Data Protection Acts 1984 and 1998*.)

informed choice is the ability to make a decision about care or treatment based on access to comprehensive and appropriate information. With this knowledge, service users are able to learn about the full range of options available to them and about any support which may be necessary and is available.

infringement of rights: an action or situation that interferes with someone's rights and the freedom to which they are entitled.

inhaler: a device which is used to introduce drugs to the body. Inhalers are most commonly used in the treatment of lung disorders. The patient breathes in a gas or vapour. The inhaler is designed so that the correct dose of inhalant drug is given. An inhaler is used particularly in the treatment of *asthma*.

inheritance of sex: the way in which the *chromosomes* determine the sex of an individual. Every *cell* in the human body contains 23 pairs of chromosomes. In 22 pairs of these chromosomes the two chromosomes look alike. The remaining 'pair' are the sex chromosomes. Females have two X chromosomes in the cell while males have one X and one Y chromosome. Eggs and sperm contain a single sex chromosome. In the egg the single sex chromosome is always an X. In the sperm the single sex chromosome can be either an X or a Y. When the sperm fertilises the egg there is an equal chance of uniting a sperm containing an X or Y chromosome – to produce XX (a girl) or XY (a boy). Therefore, the numbers of boys and girls born are more or less equal.

inherited disorders: any condition where a defective *gene* has been passed on to a child from either one of the parents. Examples of inherited disorders are *cystic fibrosis* and *haemophilia*.

inherited factors: see *genes*.

inoculation is the introduction of a substance, usually by the injection of vaccine, into the body as a means of protecting it against infectious diseases. (See *vaccination*, *immune system, immunisation*.)

inquiries are procedures set up to investigate the causes of tragic incidents or alleged malpractice. Such inquiries can range from informal, two-person panels to formal investigations which are legal proceedings involving a judge. The purpose of an inquiry is to ensure that there is justice for the victim and their family.

inspection: procedures which examine practice within an organisation. In health and social care this involves:

- inspection of premises with regard to suitability for client use, e.g. *residential homes, day care* provision, *pre-school groups* and *day nurseries*
- examination of procedures to ensure that legislation is implemented, e.g. *health and safety, equal opportunities*
- checking that staff practise quality care, e.g. adequate staff/client ratios, induction and in-service training.

institutionalisation can occur when people have been in hospital or residential care for a long time. They become accustomed to the same *routine* and are familiar with the daily tasks which are carried out for them. They find it difficult to carry out any new task for themselves and for this reason may be resistant to any change in their daily routine. Carers should ensure that they encourage clients to make decisions and to take part in personal tasks and activities.

insulin: a hormone produced by the cells of the islets of Langerhans in the *pancreas*. The amount of insulin secreted regulates the level of glucose in the bloodstream. When insulin is not produced the glucose level in blood rises, reducing the chemical breakdown of *carbohydrate* and increasing the breakdown of *fat* and *protein*. This is a condition called *diabetes mellitus*. (See *homeostasis, feedback systems*.)

integrated care is when health and social care services work together to provide a client, patient or service user with the individual care that they need. This is to ensure that, in the services they offer, health and social care workers have the:

- ability to work with individual service users in order to identify the whole range of their needs
- appropriate information on what else is available in the system and who else can help

- opportunity to work alongside other professional groups
- responsibility to supply the right care or service, when it is needed.

An example of integrated care includes nurses running care services in the community for patients with diabetes. Where necessary, they may need to refer a patient to a *chiropodist* for foot care and make decisions on what other health treatment or social care support is needed.

intellectual development or cognitive development is the development of the parts of the *brain* which are responsible for problem solving, reasoning, remembering and understanding. During childhood the brain grows rapidly. At the age of six years it has already reached 90% of its adult weight. In the first seven years of life a child learns rapidly about the world around them. (See *cognitive development, human growth and development*.)

intelligence: a term which describes a person's mental ability. This is tested to determine an individual's level of intelligence quotient (IQ). Intelligence is influenced by genetic inheritance which is called nature and by the opportunities provided in the child's environment which are called nurture (see *nature—nurture*).

interaction: communicating with others. People working in health and social care need to communicate with clients and with one another. They need to take part in one-to-one interactions with clients and other professionals, and in group interactions, such as case conferences, group work or staff meetings. These can be formal or informal. The purposes of these interactions are to:

- exchange *information*
- explain procedures, i.e. what takes place during treatment or the process involved in a care task
- promote *relationships* and client *well-being*
- assess client needs
- negotiate and liaise with clients, family members, colleagues and other professionals
- promote learning and support development
- promote group *social development*.

A typical plan for an interaction with a colleague or service user is to:
- determine the purpose for the interaction – for information exchange, brainstorming ideas, sharing opinions
- plan each stage – introduction, opportunity for discussion, explore the content
- evaluate the process – reflect on what has happened, analyse whether the interaction concluded with any decision making, evaluate if the result was to identify strengths, weaknesses and developing skills.

(See *active listening skills, effective communication, activities for health and well-being, activity-based interaction, interpersonal skills, strategies for effective communication, communication skills, conversational skills*.)

inter-agency co-operation: see *multi-agency working*.

intermediate care: services which are provided to promote independence. They are given to those people who could face long hospital stays, long-term residential care and continuing NHS care. It involves assessment of each individual's *care plan*. This takes the form of care designed to maximise independence and to enable patients and service users to return home. Intermediate care can last two to six weeks and involves support from a *multi-disciplinary team*.

International Classification of Diseases: a list of diseases which is published by the *World Health Organisation (WHO)* every ten years.

International Classification of Disorders is a classification system published by the *World Health Organisation (WHO)* relating to physical and psychological conditions. The WHO provides statistics from different countries on different disorders.

interpersonal skills: the skills that enable individuals to communicate with each other. Interpersonal skills are an integral part of the care process. Examples of such skills include using:
- verbal *communication*, using *language* and *conversation*
- *non-verbal communication*, body language, gestures, facial expressions and eye contact
- a safe and suitable environment for interaction to take place
- non-discriminatory policy and practice, respecting differences of race, language, culture, religion, sexuality, sexual orientation and political persuasion
- methods to promote the health and well-being of those being cared for and promoting a positive self-esteem
- non-judgemental attitudes to others and showing respect
- policies to maintain confidentiality and protect personal information about a client
- routines to encourage clients' autonomy and independence with regard to their rights and choices
- relevant and helpful information.

(See *care value base, strategies for effective communication, communication skills, building a positive relationship, building confidence, conversational skills*.)

intervention: a procedure which involves a carer taking action to improve the quality of an individual's life. This can include:
- *enabling* which encourages individuals to take control of their lives
- encouraging *coping* which allows individuals to come to terms with the presenting difficulties, disabilities or situations in their lives
- *caring* which gives a person support for their physical, social, intellectual and emotional needs.

intervertebral disc: a pad of fibrocartilage which is found between the bones (*vertebrae*) in the spine. The disc acts as a shock absorber protecting the *brain* and *spinal cord* from sudden impact caused by jumping, running and other body movements. (See *skeleton*.)

interview: a method used by researchers, health and social care professionals and others involving face-to-face contact with an individual. Interviews are a means of gaining detailed and descriptive information about a person. For the purpose of research there are different types of interviews, such as:
- structured interviews – the researcher collects information directly from the interviewee. A number of questions are compiled to ensure that the interview is carried out in exactly the same way with each interviewee. Such questions are called an interview schedule; it is similar to a questionnaire. This is a way of collecting *quantitative data* or evidence
- in-depth interviews – the researcher uses this technique to allow the interviewee to talk more freely and in an unstructured way. The researcher can provide guidance as the conversation progresses and the interviewee is encouraged to open up and provide as much detail as possible. In this way the researcher gathers the views and the beliefs of the interviewee. It is a valuable way of collecting *qualitative data* or evidence.

introversion is an aspect of the personality. It is characterised by a number of different traits such as the individual being passive, quiet and unsociable. In *Eysenck*'s personality inventory, introverted people try to avoid stimulation. An introvert may be characterised as a person who is interested in themselves rather than in the outside world. They tend to be self-conscious and find making friends difficult. (See *extroversion*.)

involuntary muscle is smooth *muscle* which works without the conscious control of the mind. For example, intestinal muscles work completely independently of conscious thought. Its microscopic structure is different from voluntary or striated muscle.

iodine: a *mineral* which is required in small amounts for healthy bodily growth and development. It is used by the *thyroid gland* in the production of thyroxine or thyroid hormone. A solution of iodine in potassium iodide solution can also be used in liquid form as an antiseptic.

A–Z Online

Log on to A–Z Online to search the database of terms, print revision lists and much more. Go to **www.philipallan.co.uk/a-zonline** to get started.

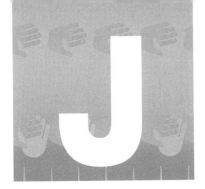

jobseekers' allowance: a financial *benefit* which was introduced in April 1996. The benefit is a combination of unemployment benefit and *income support*. It is available for claimants who have been unemployed for six months. During this time they have to prove that they have been actively seeking employment. If after six months they are not in work they receive *means-tested* payments in line with income support levels.

joint commissioning is a process where two or more agencies act together to co-ordinate their services and to take joint responsibility for *care* provision. It is often the way in which health and social care agencies work together to achieve:

- joint budgeting between agencies
- a clear assessment of population health needs as identified by the relevant agencies
- an agreed strategy of health and social care provision to meet local needs
- procedures for joint service planning, evaluation and monitoring of health and social care provision.

This way of working together is viewed as an efficient structure or framework which enables health and social care professionals to support the different and individual needs of their clients. (See *inter-agency co-operation, multi-disciplinary teams*.)

joint finance: a specific sum of money allocated each year via a joint consultative committee for innovative projects, e.g. community projects which support clients with *learning disabilities*.

joint planning: the process by which two or more agencies act together to plan service provision. It encourages the involvement of providers, users, carers, and the voluntary and community sectors.

joints are where the *bones* of the *skeleton* meet. Some are fixed allowing no movement, e.g. the sutures of the *skull*. Most joints, however, are movable and give the body movement and flexibility. The most common types of *synovial joints* are:

- hinge joints – those which work like any hinge, e.g. the knee joint. The movable part or bone can only move in one plane but in either of two opposing directions
- gliding joints, also called sliding joints – those in which flat surfaces glide over each other, e.g. those between the carpals which are the small bones in the hands. They are more flexible than hinge joints
- ball and socket joints – the most flexible joints, e.g. the hip joint. The movable bone has a rounded end which fits into a socket in the fixed bone. It can swivel in many directions.

justice: the legal right to fairness under the law. Justice is an ethic which is set in a framework of the court system within society.

key worker: usually a named person who co-ordinates the arrangements for a person's care. A key worker is frequently used in caring for children in a *day care* or residential setting. They are usually trained and experienced carers in their own particular area within health and social care. (See *named nurse*.)

keyhole surgery: a surgical procedure involving the use of a special instrument called a laparoscope or endoscope. A small cut is made in the skin. The underlying *tissue* and *muscle* is also cut. An instrument is inserted and surgery is carried out, e.g. removal of gall bladder or damaged cartilage in the knee joint. Such surgery is so-called because of the tiny size of the cut or incision. It also known as 'minimally invasive surgery' because of the limited side effects it can have on the patient. (See *trends in health care*.)

kidneys: the main organs of the urinary system. They are two bean-shaped *organs* situated one each side of the body in the lower back region. They contain:

- nephrons – tiny filtering units. There are about one million per kidney. Each consists of a renal corpuscle and a renal tubule
- renal corpuscles, or Malpighian corpuscles, which filter fluids out of the *blood*. Each consists of a glomerulus and a Bowman's capsule
- glomerulus – a circle of coiled-up *capillaries* at the centre of each renal corpuscle. The capillaries branch from an afferent arteriole entering the corpuscle and re-unite to leave the corpuscle as an efferent arteriole
- Bowman's capsule – the outer part of each renal corpuscle. It is a thin-walled sac around the glomerulus
- renal tubules – long tubes, each one leading from a Bowman's capsule. Each has three main parts – the proximal convoluted tubule, the loop of Henle and the distal convoluted tubule. These tubules have many capillaries wrapped around them. They are branches of the efferent arteriole and re-unite to form larger vessels carrying blood from the kidneys
- collecting tubule – a tubule which carries urine into the pelvis of a kidney.

The function of the kidneys is to separate waste products from the large amount of fluid which flows through them daily. Approximately 1.5 litres is excreted as *urine*.

King's Fund: a government 'think tank' which determines policy relating to *health care*. It was founded in 1897 by Edward VII to support London hospitals which, at that time, were being run by voluntary organisations. One of its most recent reports relates to transforming health care in London.

Krebs cycle: see *aerobic respiration*.

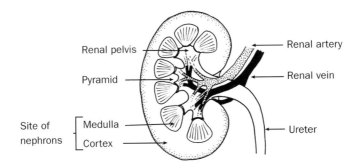

The kidney

Do you need revision help and advice?

Go to pages 292–304 for a range of revision appendices that include plenty of exam advice and tips.

K

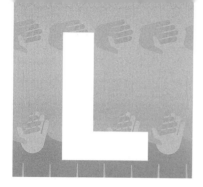

labelling identifies an individual as being of a certain type, belonging to a particular group whether they are members of that group or not. Labelling is the result of **attitudes** and **values** which become fixed and rigid through the process of **stereotyping**, e.g. labels which relate to people who are overweight inferring that they are lazy.

lactic acid is an acid naturally produced in the body as a result of the metabolism of glucose.

language: the development of communication, i.e. being able to communicate with others in a way that they can understand. This can involve using sounds, signs and symbols. (See *language acquisition*, *language development*, *sign language*, *Makaton*, *Bliss system*.)

language acquisition: a series of stages which relate to the achievement of language. These involve:

- prelinguistic – the stage before a child says their first meaningful words. At this stage the child will draw attention to objects and things by pointing, reaching out and touching
- holophrase – the stage where the child can identify objects and can communicate ideas using a single word. For example he may say 'duck' in the park because he wants to go and see the ducks
- telegraphic – the stage where more words are being spoken and the child is beginning to put two words together
- fully developed speech – the stage when the child constructs sentences and understands what he is saying and can make himself understood by others.

language development: the way in which a baby or a young child learns to communicate through noises and repetitive sounds. These gradually develop into words. The stages of language development are shown in the table opposite.

Children have an innate (inborn) ability to learn to speak. This ability is called a language acquisition device.

laser treatment: a treatment method involving a device which produces a very thin beam of light. The energy in the beam of light is very concentrated and therefore can be used to operate on a small body area with an abnormality such as in the treatment of gallstones. This method is also effective in dealing with certain conditions in the *eye*. Lasers can be used to unblock small *arteries* such as *coronary arteries*.

The stages of language development

Age	Language development
1–6 months	Cries when hungry or has discomfort. Turns face towards sounds and is startled by sudden noises. Makes cooing noises. Babbles and responds to the sound of voice.
6–9 months	Babbles and starts to imitate sounds. Babbling is now likely to be linked to language of familiar adults, parents or primary care givers. At this age the baby will shout, and make noises in order to be noticed.
9–12 months	Imitating word sounds and begins to string these sounds together. These word sounds have different tones like a conversation. This is called jargon. Understands simple instructions such as 'give it to me' and simple words such as 'cup', 'duck'. Can point to objects.
12–15 months	Continues to use jargon. Can use 2–6 words but understands many others.
15–18 months	Can say 6–20 words and points to pictures in a book or on the wall. Echoes words which are said by others. This is called 'echolalia'. At this stage they enjoy joining in songs and rhymes.
18 months–2 years	Can say about 50 words but understands many more. Can now put two words together and obey simple instructions.
2–3 years	Saying more words including plurals and pronouns. They can understand what is being said and join in simple conversations. Enjoys song and rhyme and stories.
3–4 years	Words and vocabulary are developing. Sometimes they have difficulty with pronunciation. Asks question 'Why' many times a day. Knows age and name.
4–5 years	More developed use of correct speech.

later adulthood: the last stages of life for those aged over 65 years. (See *older people*.)

learning is about the development of skills and knowledge. Learning starts at birth and continues throughout life. Learning can be either direct or indirect:

- direct learning is through the knowledge that the baby, child or individual experiences as they play and observe with the use of their different cognitive, physical and social skills
- indirect learning is through other people, and resources such as observing other children, teachers and through looking at books, television, internet and listening to sounds, music and the radio.

There are different strategies which develop learning including:

- experiential – through personal experience and discovery such as play or hobbies

- listening – through listening to others and learning from their knowledge and experience, listening to instructions, etc.
- visual – through looking at colour, displays, photographs and pictures in different media.

There are factors which can affect learning such as family relationships, lack of provision to play and limited access to education. Additionally, there is the environment and whether it is suitable for learning in terms of location and availability of resources.

learning and children: learning is a key aspect in a child's *development*. It is interlinked with different aspects of development such as physical, intellectual and cognitive, emotional and social. Children learn in a variety of ways:

- discovery or experiential learning
- modelling through observation
- reinforcement of learning through praise and encouragement
- research and reading, working with thematic activities such as transport and shopping
- reflection and analysis through thinking, reasoning and problem solving
- verbal instruction, learning through receiving and giving instructions. (See *learning techniques*.)

learning disabilities: a range of disabilities of mental capacity. Clients with learning disabilities may have a limited mental capacity but will generally be able to function to the full extent of such abilities. The causes of learning disabilities are as follows:

- genetic disorders, e.g. Down's syndrome
- intrauterine injury, injury to the growing *foetus* in the uterus such as an *infection* which causes damage to the *brain* and to parts of the *nervous system*, e.g. paralysis of a limb and loss of mental function
- *birth injuries*, any injury to the baby during birth affecting the brain and nervous system, e.g. *cerebral palsy*
- anatomical injuries to the brain or *spinal cord* such as *spina bifida* and *hydrocephalus*; there are different degrees of such disabilities which range from mild through moderate to severe or profound learning impairment.

In 2002, a government White Paper 'Valuing People – a New Strategy for Learning Disability for the 21st Century' was introduced with four underlying principles of rights, independence, choice and inclusion. It confirms the rights of all individuals in conjunction with the *Human Rights Act 1998* and *Disability Discrimination Act 1995 and 2005* which works for people with learning disabilities. (See *Protection of Vulnerable Adults*.)

learning techniques are methods used to promote learning. These include:

- allowing times for questions and questioning
- providing resources and materials to promote knowledge
- providing immediate feedback on performance
- using rewards and using encouraging comments such as giving praise
- providing prompts for learning such as making suggestions
- setting structured tasks with verbal instruction and opportunities to practise as a group or on an individual basis.

learning theories seek to explain how individuals achieve a permanent change in understanding and behaviour. Change usually occurs as a result of experience and is dependent on cognitive abilities such as *memory* and perception. There are two well-known levels of learning theory. They are:

- Classical conditioning or learning by association – this is involved in the *socialisation* of young children and also plays a part in the development of phobias. The principles of classical conditioning are seen in the treatment of phobias. For example, it is used in the treatment of alcoholics by creating a phobia. This is called aversion therapy. A special drug can be implanted under the skin so that it remains active in the body over a long period of time. If the alcoholic person has a drink during that time they are instantly sick. The taking of alcohol becomes linked with nausea and so the patient learns to avoid it.
- Operant conditioning – this relates to responses that bring about satisfaction or pleasure. When this happens such responses are likely to be repeated. This is termed positive reinforcement. Those reactions that bring about discomfort are not likely to be repeated and are termed negative reinforcement. *Behaviour* shaping or modification is associated with achieving the approved behaviour by rewarding the actions which produce the desired response. It is often used deliberately to generate socially acceptable behaviour. The control and management of misbehaving children at school is one example.

The management of behaviour can involve using:

- primary reinforcers – those which satisfy basic needs or drive, e.g. for food, water or praise
- secondary reinforcers – acquire their reinforcing properties through association with primary reinforcers, e.g. tokens, stars, money.

Carers may reward a client with signs of approval such as smiling. Praise is important in building self-esteem. (See *building confidence*, *behaviour modification*, *Pavlov*, *Skinner*, *Piaget*, *Vygotsky*, *behaviour theories* and *development theories*.)

legislation: the making of laws by Parliament. Legislation determines the policy framework and reflects the different statutory rights of organisations, groups and individuals. Laws result from:

- an awareness of issues which are evident and affecting the life of the nation
- the results of commissioned research
- recommendations from groups such as *pressure groups*
- government white and green papers, which are part of the stages of consultation before a law is made.

The various stages involved in making legislation are summarised in the diagram overleaf.

leisure is free time. People will have different ways of using their leisure time, such as watching television and videos, reading or sports activities. Individuals may also have hobbies, e.g. collecting antiques or stamps, DIY, shopping or gardening.

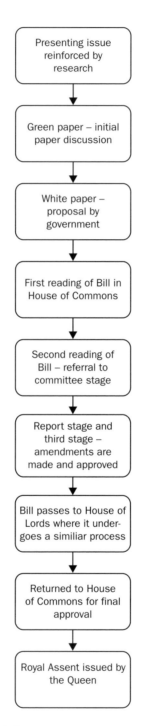

Stages involved in making legislation

lesbians/gays are those who form physical, sexual relationships with individuals from the same *gender* grouping. Females in a gender partnership are termed lesbians and males in such a partnership are gays or homosexuals.

life course is the sequence or pattern of different experiences and events that an individual goes through during a lifetime.

life events: events which an individual experiences during a lifetime. These can be predictable or unpredictable (See *change*.)

life expectancy is an estimate of lifespan. It enables comparisons between the ages and stages of life to be made across the population. It is affected by *mortality rates* including *infant mortality* rates.

life quality factors are factors which influence the quality of life of an individual in a psychological and physical way. These include approval, autonomy, choice, dignity, effective communication, exercise, balanced diet, safety, comfort, security, social contact and social support. (See *physical life quality factors* and *psychological life quality factors*.)

life skills training: the techniques used to support those with disabilities to lead more *independent* lives. (See *activities of daily living*, *aids and adaptations*.)

life stages are stages of growth and development that follow a sequence. The following ages and stages are approximate: *infancy* 0–3 years, childhood 4–9 years, *adolescence* 10–18 years, *adulthood* 18–45 years, middle adulthood 46–65 years, older adulthood 65 years plus.

lifestyle: the way in which a person chooses to live their life. Health educators believe that if a person has a healthy lifestyle then they will live longer. In order to maintain a healthy lifestyle a person is encouraged to:
- eat a healthy *diet*
- have plenty of *exercise*
- learn to manage *stress*
- take time out for *leisure* and recreation
- not to *smoke* cigarettes
- drink *alcohol* in moderation
- use *contraceptives* and not to have unprotected sex (i.e. use a condom)
- live in adequate *housing*.

However, it is important to add that not every person in society today has a choice in lifestyle. The more affluent the person the more choices they have as to the lifestyle which they adopt. Therefore, it is clear that *social and economic factors* affect lifestyle.

Lifting Operations and Lifting Equipment Regulations 1998 (LOLER): regulations set up to reduce the *health and safety* risk to employers, employees, contractors and others, when using or coming into contact with lifting equipment in the workplace.

ligament: a tough band of yellow elastic *connective tissue* which is found linking two *bones* together at a *joint*. Ligaments bind the articular surfaces together giving joints protection and strength. When the ends of one of the bones forming a joint is displaced it may interfere with the proper working movement of the joint. The ligament at the joint may be torn as a result of the displacement. This is the cause of a sprain.

lipids: see *fats*.

listening skills: the ability to listen to others in a way that conveys interest and positive regard. The person speaking then feels that what they are saying matters. Listening is an important aspect of the *caring* process and involves the following:

- sitting or standing in a position that enables the client or patient to feel that they are being listened to, keeping the 'open position', not folding arms or crossing legs
- making and maintaining eye contact demonstrating to the client that they are being listened to
- learning to control facial expressions so that whatever is being said can be seen to be important
- giving the client or patient time to express what they want to say; this is particularly important when the client has a speech impairment, or their use of English is limited.

(See also *active listening skills, communication, interpersonal skills, English as a second language, conversational skills*.)

literacy is the ability to read and write. In recent years the government has introduced strategies to develop literacy in children and young people. This involved using clearly designated teaching time to develop literacy skills, such as *listening skills* and speaking, reading and writing, and using fine *motor skills*.

liver: the largest internal organ of the body. It is situated beneath the *diaphragm* in the upper right side of the *abdomen*. It is protected by the ribs and weighs approximately 1–1.5 kg. It is dark brown in colour and has a smooth surface. The *blood* supply to the liver is provided by the hepatic artery, hepatic vein and hepatic portal vein. The hepatic vein takes blood from the liver.

The liver has many functions which include:

- regulation of glucose
- regulation of lipids
- regulation of proteins
- detoxification
- *bile* production
- breakdown of sex *hormones*
- formation of *red blood cells*
- breakdown of *haemoglobin*
- formation of plasma proteins
- storage of *vitamins*
- production of heat.

local authorities have statutory duties and powers with regard to the implementation of health and social care in their geographic area. Local authorities publish their services through their community care plans to ensure that health and care services meet the needs of local people. They have responsibility for various services such as:

- social service departments – supporting *personal social services* including care of children, clients with disabilities and elderly people; the registration for these services is also covered
- *housing* – council housing, residential and sheltered housing
- *community care* – elderly people, physical disability and sensory impairment, learning disabilities, mental health, drugs/alcohol, domestic violence, HIV/AIDS.

This involves care management, home care, day care services including palliative care and occupational therapists

- **benefits** and employment opportunities in their localities.

The areas of responsibility are outlined in Local Government Acts, the **Children Act 1989**, the **NHS and Community Care Act 1990, The New NHS – Modern, Dependable, Our Healthier Nation – a Contract for Health** and the Local Government Act 2000.

Local Safeguarding Children's Boards: the system of safeguarding and protecting children which has responsibility for overseeing inter-agency working in England, Wales and Northern Ireland.

lone-parent families: families consisting of a dependent child or children living with only one parent. This is usually the mother but may be the father. Over the last three decades, partly as the result of changing **family structures**, there has been a substantial increase in the number of lone parents.

loss is the separation from something or somebody on a permanent basis. There is a process of coping with loss as the person comes to terms with what has been lost. (See **grief**.)

LSD (lysergic acid diethylamide) is a hallucinogenic or psychedelic **drug** which causes disturbances in understanding and a changed state of consciousness and awareness. It is taken in small tablets and can make a person behave in an erratic and unpredictable way. For example, a person on an 'LSD trip' may climb to the top of a building and 'try to fly'.

lung volume is the amount of air taken in by the **lung**. The capacity of the lungs can be measured in various ways as follows:

- tidal volume – the amount of air taken in and out during one breath
- pulmonary ventilation – the amount of air taken in during one minute
- vital capacity – the amount of air which is breathed out (exhaled) after a maximum amount of air has been taken in (inhaled)
- residual volume – the amount of air which is left behind in the lungs after forceful exhalation.

lungs are the main organs of respiration. There is a right and a left lung. They fill the thoracic cavity and are situated on either side of the heart. (See **respiratory system**.)

lymph: see **lymphatic system**.

lymphatic system: a system of lymph vessels, lymph nodes and small organs of lymphoid tissue which are important in the recycling of those body fluids which help the body in the fight against disease. It produces lymphocytes which are disease-fighting **white blood cells**. The vessels of the lymphatic system transport a fluid called lymph around the body and return it into the **veins** and the lymphoid organs as a means of fighting infection. Vessels carry lymph from all body areas towards the left side of the chest. Lymph vessels are lined with endothelial tissue and have valves in order to prevent backflow. The thinnest vessels are called lymph capillaries. The **capillaries** join to form larger vessels called the lymphatics, which eventually unite to form two main branches which empty into the blood via the right subclavian vein via the right lymphatic duct and the left subclavian vein via the thoracic duct. Lymphoid organs connected by the lymphatic system include the **spleen**, tonsils and **thymus** gland.

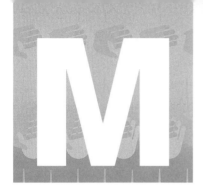

MMR: a triple vaccine given to protect a child against the diseases measles, mumps and rubella (German measles). (See *immunisation*.)

MRSA: see *methicillin-resistant Staphylococcus aureus*.

magnetic resonance imaging: (MRI) a technique used to produce images on a monitor of the soft tissues of the body such as the brain and spinal cord. The MRI scan has all the benefits of a *computed axial tomography* scan but without exposure to radiation. It is a method used to diagnose diseases such as cancer and multiple sclerosis.

mainstream schools are those which offer compulsory education for children from the age of 5 to 16 years. These schools follow the *national curriculum* from key stage 1 to key stage 4.

Makaton: a system of *communication*. It uses speech, signs and symbols to help people with learning difficulties to develop *language* skills. This can involve using some language, i.e. a word and a sign using hands or their bodies to communicate. This system contains a large range of signs and symbols.

male reproductive system: responsible for the male role in sexual reproduction. It is made up of primary *organs*, or *gonads*, which consist of two testes, and a number of additional organs. *Cells* in the gonads also act as *endocrine glands* secreting many important *hormones*.

- Testes – contain tube-like canals called seminiferous tubules which manufacture sperm. They are situated in the scrotum which hangs below the *abdomen*. The optimum temperature for sperm production is slightly lower than normal body temperature. (See *testicular self-examination*.)
- Penis – the organ through which sperm are ejected via the urethra during intercourse. It is made of soft, sponge-like erectile tissue, which has many spaces or blood sinuses, blood vessels and nerve endings called receptors. When a man is sexually excited, the sinuses and blood vessels fill with blood and this makes the penis stiff and straight. This is called an erection.

malnutrition: a disorder brought about by an inadequate *diet* or lack of *food*. Children and adults in countries where there is famine and war often suffer from severe malnutrition, sometimes leading to *death*. Once malnutrition occurs a person's physical condition

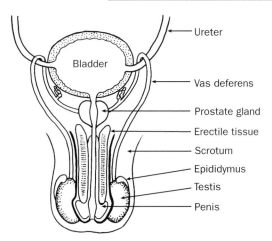

The male reproductive system

deteriorates. Research shows a rise in the number of people in *residential care* or in *hospitals* in the United Kingdom who are also suffering from malnutrition. *Age Concern* in a report in 2006 believed that insufficient attention has so far been given to the needs of *older people* in hospital. Consequently, there are problems in a number of areas which contribute to the prevalence of malnutrition in hospital. These include:

- suitability of the food on offer
- help with eating food
- monitoring of patients for signs of malnutrition
- involvement of patients, relatives and carers
- knowing how and who to raise concerns with. (See *balanced diet*.)

mammography: a special screening test of the *breast* employing low dosage *X-rays* which are used to detect the presence of cysts or *tumours*. (See also *breast self-examination*.)

Management of Health and Safety at Work Regulations 1999 are legal requirements for employers to assess all *health and safety* risks to their employees and others in the workplace. All procedures and practices should be carried out to minimise the likelihood of any risks.

Manual Handling Operations Regulations 1992 revised 1998 and updated in 2004 (MHOR): legal requirements for both employers and employees to reduce the *risk* to *health and safety* from manual handling operations. These include transporting or carrying a load which involves pushing, pulling, carrying or moving, lifting and lowering. Employers are required to carry out risk assessments with regard to risk of injury from lifting. Policies and procedures are set out to ensure that employees know what to do when they are lifting and what steps to take to ensure they are safe from risk. They should check that the equipment they are using is safe and make sure that they report any hazardous handling activities. (See *risk assessment*.)

marginalisation: the action taken by individuals or groups to isolate or to exclude someone else from society. This can lead to an individual or group being disadvantaged and oppressed. Individuals or groups may be discriminated against on the basis of age, social class, gender, race and ability.

Marie Curie Cancer Care: the UK's largest *cancer* care charity which provides nursing care for people with cancer through 11 in-patient Marie Curie centres. Over 6000 Marie Curie nurses nationwide are also available to look after patients in their own homes. All services to patients are free of charge. Marie Curie Cancer Care runs its own research institute and education department which provides training courses and conferences for health professionals on cancer and related topics.

marks of safety are labels which are put on potentially hazardous appliances to warn users of danger. The safety marks should be included in manufacturers' instructions which should also include warnings. The most regularly occurring marks of safety are:

- British Standard kite mark – this symbol means that the product has been examined and is deemed to be safe. The kite mark can be found on:
  - domestic appliances
  - children's equipment such as highchairs, prams and pushchairs
  - oil heaters
- fire resistant mark – which ensures that the equipment and goods purchased are fire resistant and meet appropriate regulations
- British Gas seal of service – which is found on all gas appliances which have been tested for safety
- British Electrotechnical Approval Board mark of safety – which ensures that all electrical goods and equipment have met government safety regulations.

Kite mark

Maslow, Abraham (1908–1970): a psychologist who is well known for his hierarchy of needs theory. This was based on layers of different human need. He suggested that each level of need had to be met before the next level could be reached. Those needs at the lowest level related to meeting basic physical requirements such as food, shelter, warmth and clothing, whilst at the top of the hierarchy was the idea of self-actualisation, i.e. the belief that an individual could reach their full potential.

mass media refers to the different forms of communication designed to meet the needs of a mass of individuals. Examples are television, radio, newspapers and the internet.

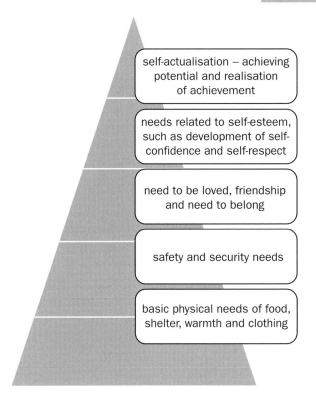

Maslow's hierarchy of needs

massage therapy: a *complementary therapy* which involves the gentle manipulation of the soft tissues of the body. Usually the hands are used as touch is an integral part of massage therapy, but sometimes other parts of the body such as the forearms, elbows and feet can be utilised. Massage can be an important part of a person's health and fitness programme. The functions of massage are to:

- reduce *muscle* tension
- improve *blood* and *lymph* circulation
- increase mobility and the range of movement in the *joints*
- relieve acute and chronic muscular pain
- encourage relaxation and reduce *stress*
- stimulate and soothe the *nervous system*.

maternal deprivation is the way in which a child reacts when separated for extended periods of time from their mother or primary care giver. Some children become anxious and stressed when separated from their mother. (See *separation, attachment, bonding*.)

maturation: the process of natural development in an individual. (See *human growth and development, ageing*.)

meals on wheels: a home care service which enables *older people* to have a meal delivered to them in their homes. There is a standard charge for the service. The delivery of this service varies from one area of the country to another. The meals are provided by social services departments and are sometimes delivered by the *Women's Royal Voluntary Service*.

means-testing: a system used to determine whether individuals are eligible to receive certain *benefits*. Means-testing is a way of delivering benefits to clients who are most 'in need', i.e. the system allows benefits to be targeted to those with the least financial resources.

mechanism of breathing is made up of inspiration (breathing in) and expiration (breathing out). Both actions are normally automatic, controlled by nerves from the respiratory centre in the medulla of the *brain*. The medulla is particularly sensitive to changes in the concentration of *carbon dioxide* in the *blood*. A slight increase in carbon dioxide causes deeper, faster breathing. Mechanisms of breathing therefore include:

- inspiration or inhalation; the act of breathing in. The intercostal muscles between the ribs contract, pulling the ribs up and outward and widening the cavity. The *diaphragm* also contracts and flattens, lengthening the chest cavity. The overall expansion lowers air pressure in the *lungs*, and air rushes in to fill them (i.e. to equalise internal and external pressure)
- expiration or exhalation; the act of breathing out. The intercostal muscles and diaphragm relax, and air is forced out of the lungs as the chest cavity becomes smaller.

(See also *respiratory system*.)

Medic Alert is a registered charity. Medic Alert provides internationally recognised medical identification emblems in the form of bracelets and necklets for people with hidden medical conditions, e.g. *diabetes*, *asthma*, *epilepsy* and heart conditions. These emblems are engraved with a personal identification number, medical condition and/or prescribed medication, plus a 24-hour emergency telephone number.

meeting individual needs involves the process whereby each individual need of a service user is identified and met. (See *assessment*, *care management, holistic care*.)

meiosis: cell division which takes place in the sex *organs* to produce the gametes. The gametes produced contain half the number of *chromosomes* present in the parent *cell*. Each gamete therefore contains 23 chromosomes rather than 23 pairs of chromosomes, as in other cells.

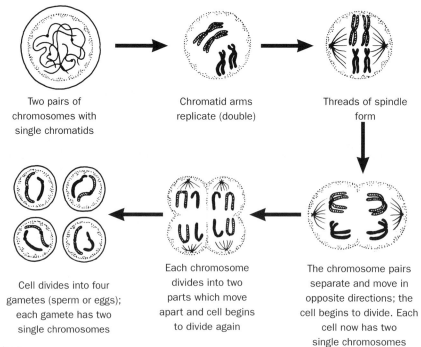

Two pairs of chromosomes with single chromatids

Chromatid arms replicate (double)

Threads of spindle form

Cell divides into four gametes (sperm or eggs); each gamete has two single chromosomes

Each chromosome divides into two parts which move apart and cell begins to divide again

The chromosome pairs separate and move in opposite directions; the cell begins to divide. Each cell now has two single chromosomes

melanocyte-stimulating hormone: a hormone manufactured in the anterior lobe of the *pituitary gland* and responsible for controlling the production of the pigment in the *skin*. The hormone acts on the melanocytes which produce melanin or skin pigment.

memory is the individual's ability to retain *information* about life, events and situations. The information is then stored and retrieved when the individual wishes to remember the incident and when it happened. Long-term and short-term memory may be affected by the *ageing* process. For example *older people* often find it easier to remember incidents from the distant past. Events which occurred only a day or a week before are harder to remember.

Mencap is a registered *charity* and voluntary organisation which supports clients with *mental health disorders.* It provides various services such as day care, respite care and residential care as well as *campaigning* for the rights of those with mental health disorders.

meningitis is the inflammation of the meninges in the lining of the *brain*. There are two main forms of meningitis:
- viral meningitis which is caused by a *virus*
- bacterial meningitis, caused by several different types of *bacteria*; meningococcal and pneumococcal meningitis are the most prevalent.

The bacteria that cause meningitis live in the back of the *throat* or nose of about 10% of the population and in up to 25% of young adults. They rarely give rise to illness but, when they do, infection progresses very rapidly and is fatal in one in ten cases.

Most cases of meningitis are seen in young children under five years of age with the greatest risk at around six months. The next highest incidence is among teenagers between 15 and 19 years and recent figures have shown an increase in cases of young people under the age of 25 years.

Antibiotics should be given immediately if bacterial meningitis is suspected. Oral antibiotics are recommended for close household or family contacts to prevent further spread. Early diagnosis is vital and most doctors now carry appropriate medication at all times.

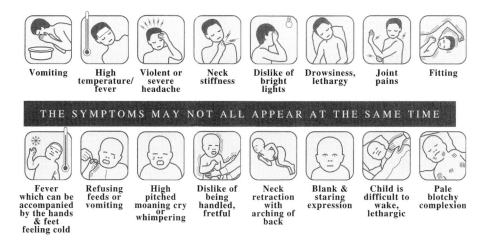

| Vomiting | High temperature/ fever | Violent or severe headache | Neck stiffness | Dislike of bright lights | Drowsiness, lethargy | Joint pains | Fitting |

THE SYMPTOMS MAY NOT ALL APPEAR AT THE SAME TIME

| Fever which can be accompanied by the hands & feet feeling cold | Refusing feeds or vomiting | High pitched moaning cry or whimpering | Dislike of being handled, fretful | Neck retraction with arching of back | Blank & staring expression | Child is difficult to wake, lethargic | Pale blotchy complexion |

Some symptoms of meningitis in adults and young people (above) and babies (below)

menopause: the cessation of *menstruation*, usually occurring naturally in women between 45 and 55 years of age. It marks the end of a woman's capacity for sexual reproduction.

183

The menopause is associated with changes in the balance of **hormones** in the body, particularly a reduction of the level of oestrogen. Women going through the menopause may experience signs and symptoms such as:

- hot flushes – at certain times the woman may feel unbearably hot and become red in the face
- night sweats
- instability, mood swings, **depression**
- loss of elasticity in the **skin**
- reduction in vaginal secretions
- reduced oestrogen weakens the bones which may lead to **osteoporosis**.

Some women going through the menopause may be prescribed **hormone replacement therapy (HRT)**.

menstruation: the process in a woman's body which leads to a discharge of blood every four weeks. It occurs in women of child-bearing age. The period during which blood is discharged may vary from three to seven days. Menstruation starts at about **puberty**. Young girls in their senior years of junior school are encouraged to learn about menstruation. Personal **hygiene** during the times of 'a period' is discussed. Menstruation is a series of changes which form the menstrual cycle. The cycle is controlled by **hormones** secreted by the **hypothalamus**, ovaries and **pituitary gland**. These hormones cause changes in the **uterus** lining or endometrium. After ovulation the empty follicle undergoes changes and becomes the corpus luteum. If the egg is not fertilised the corpus luteum persists, in the ovary, for about 14 days and then degenerates. The unfertilised egg disintegrates and the thickened wall of the uterus breaks down. The discarding of this tissue together with the loss of blood constitutes menstruation. If **fertilisation** does occur the lining gradually develops a new inner layer rich in blood vessels. Each menstrual cycle lasts about 28 days and occurs continuously from puberty to **menopause** (usually between the ages of 45 and 55), when ovum production ceases. The events of the menstrual cycle work in conjunction with the ovarian cycle, where the regular maturation of an ovum in Graafian follicles is followed by ovulation, i.e. the release of the ovum into a fallopian tube.

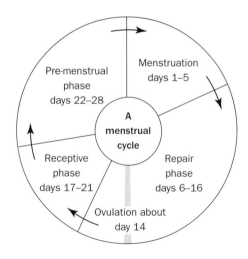

The menstrual cycle

Mental Capacity Act 2005: an Act of Parliament which provides the legal framework to protect and empower vulnerable adults (aged 16 +) who are unable to make decisions for themselves. The Act is supported by the Mental Capacity Act Code of Practice.

The five main principles are the right of:

- every adult to make his or her own decisions unless capacity to do so is proved insufficient
- individuals to be given help to make their own decisions
- individuals to make decisions that may by viewed as eccentric or unwise
- everything that is carried out for, or on behalf of, people without capacity to be in their best interest
- everything that is carried out for, or on behalf of, people without capacity to be the least restrictive to their *human rights*.

(See *advocacy, Mental Health Act 1983, Mental Health Act 2007, vulnerable people, Protection of Vulnerable Adults*.)

mental health: a person's ability to organise their thoughts in a coherent pattern and to act accordingly. Mental health is closely linked with a person's social and emotional state.

Mental Health Act 1983: an Act of Parliament which reinforces the rights of people with mental disorders and confirms the necessary procedures required to give them the appropriate care. A new legal framework is currently under review. This is being updated in the form of the Mental Health Order Act. (See *approved social worker, mental health disorder*.)

Mental Health Act 2007: an Act of Parliament which amends the *Mental Health Act 1983*, and the *Mental Capacity Act 2005*. It also extends the rights of victims by amending the *Domestic Violence, Crime and Victims Act 2004.* The main changes as a result of the Act are:

- amendments to the definition of *mental health disorder*, so that a single definition is applied throughout the Act
- criteria for detention, i.e. when an individual is sectioned and taken into compulsory care
- inclusion of civil partners as nearest relative as a means of contact (See *Civil Partnership Act 2004.*)
- new safeguards for patients with regard to electroconvulsive therapy, i.e. putting electrical charges into the brain
- age-appropriate services, i.e. that will care for individuals according to their age.

Mental Health (Care and Treatment) (Scotland) Act 2003: an Act of Parliament in Scotland which is based on a set of principles protecting individuals who are liable to have action taken against them because of the Act. These principles include non-discriminatory care, equality, respect for diversity, informal care, respect for carers, least restrictive alternatives, child welfare and benefits.

mental health disorder is a term used to describe mental health problems, personality disorders and *learning disabilities*. These can include:

- affective or mood disorders related to how a person feels and their moods, e.g. *depression*, phobias, bipolar disorder (extremes of low moods and elation)
- behavioural disorders related to how a person behaves which can affect their mental state, e.g. *alcohol* and *drug dependence*

M

- cognitive disorders related to thinking processes such as memory, information processing, attention including the ability to rationalise situations and experiences, e.g. *schizophrenia*
- personality disorders which relate to the character and *behaviour* of an individual. This can involve different areas of the personality and the resulting behaviour can cause personal and social disruption.

Mental health disorders are caused by:

- biochemical factors which include the activity of nerves, neurotransmitters and chemical reactions, levels such as that of serotonin and inadequate nutrition and the misuse of drugs
- genetics – the presence of predisposing genes
- *life events* such as *separation* through death, divorce and maternal deprivation
- physical influences such as postnatal depression
- socio-economic influences such as unemployment and inadequate housing.

The effects of a mental health disorder include:

- physical, and psychological, responses to situations which can be increased or reduced, e.g. no motivation to move out of the way of another pedestrian on the pavement, causing obstruction to others. This may be regarded as *anti-social behaviour*
- social and emotional health in the form of moods which can also affect others. This may result in the inability to maintain relationships
- inability to cope with daily living and *lifestyle* as well as being unable to deal with *harassment*, *discrimination* and *labelling*.

There are various methods and techniques which are used to treat mental health disorders. These include drug treatment, electroconvulsive therapy (putting electrical charges through the brain), *behaviour therapy*, cognitive therapy, psychoanalytic therapy such as *counselling*, family therapy (working with the family, giving opportunities for support, discussion, sharing and discussing *coping* strategies). Support is available through different networks such as community psychiatric nurses, general practitioners, advocates, counsellors and charities. (See *MIND*.)

Mental Health (Patients in the Community) Act 1995: an Act of Parliament which makes provision for patients with mental health disorders in England and Wales to receive care under supervision after leaving hospital. The Act also includes setting up community care orders.

Mental Health (Scotland) Act 1984: an Act of Parliament which reinforces the role of those in Scotland who work with, and manage, clients suffering from *mental health disorders*.

mental health tribunals are forums which have been set up to support service users of the mental health system. Their function is to hear cases related to *mental health disorders*. Each tribunal consists of a legally qualified person, a doctor and another person who could be a carer or service user. They were set up in Scotland, following the *Mental Health (Care and Treatment) (Scotland) Act 2003*.

mental health trusts are organisations which have been set up to provide health and social care services for people with mental health disorders. Many of these trusts work closely with local authorities and voluntary organisations to provide both short- and long-term care.

metabolism relates to the total number of chemical processes which take place in the human body. (See *basal metabolic rate (BMR)*.)

methadone is a manufactured synthetic opiate which is much longer acting than *heroin*. It is addictive and is used in clinics as a prescription for people undergoing withdrawal from heroin addiction. (See *drugs*.)

methicillin-resistant *Staphylococcus aureus* (MRSA) is a bacterium which is resistant to most antibiotics. MRSA is not a risk to healthy people, but to those whose resistance is low and who are vulnerable to *infection*. Examples are those being treated for *cancer* using *chemotherapy*. They can easily become infected with MRSA, because their *white blood cell* count is low. *Signs and symptoms* usually include high temperature or fever and the patient feels unwell. When MRSA has occurred the *infection control nurse* is informed and methods to prevent the infection being transmitted to others are implemented. The patient may be isolated from others and visiting may be restricted. All those in contact with the patient may be required to wear gloves, plastic aprons or overclothing as preventive measures. (See *hygiene.*)

micro-organisms are those organisms which are too small to be seen with the human eye but can be identified under a *microscope*, for example, *bacteria* and some algae.

microbiology is the science and study of micro-organisms. In medicine it is mainly directed at the isolation and identification of organisms which cause *disease*.

microscope: an instrument used to examine *cells* and *tissue* specimens. Microscopic examination is an essential part of detecting *disease*.

midwife: a qualified professional who works with women before, during and after they give *birth* to their *babies*. The midwife's role is to:
- give care and advice to women during pregnancy
- work alongside the mother during labour
- deliver the baby
- support and visit the mother immediately following the birth of her baby.

Midwives can either qualify through a three-year direct entry midwifery qualification or take an 18-month course following general nurse training.

milestones: see *developmental norms or milestones*.

MIND: a registered charity and voluntary organisation which supports the needs of the mentally ill. It actively campaigns for their rights, e.g. on such issues as the care of mentally ill people in the community.

minimum wage: see *national minimum wage*.

minerals: inorganic substances many of which are essential for general *health*. (See table on page 188.)

Minerals

Mineral	Source	Function	Deficiency
Iron	Liver, eggs, chocolate, meat	Forms haemoglobin in red blood cells which carry oxygen around the body.	Anaemia, pallor, breathlessness, lack of energy.
Calcium	Milk, cheese, butter, bread, flour	Builds strong bones and teeth. Aids clotting of blood when injured. Aids normal working of muscles.	Rickets (bones fail to harden), dental cavities, delayed blood clotting, cramp in muscles.
Phosphorus	Milk, cheese, fish, oatmeal	Helps to build strong bones and teeth, needed for the formation of enzymes and all body tissue.	
Iodine	Seafoods, water supply, vegetables, may be added to salt	Used by the thyroid gland to make thyroxine which regulates use of food in body.	Adult – goitre (enlarged thyroid gland). Baby – causes cretinism (retarded development).
Sodium chloride (salt)	Added to food kippers, bacon	Needed to maintain salt balance concentration of blood.	Cramp in muscles.
Fluoride	Water supply; may be present naturally or added artificially	Combines with calcium in teeth, so making enamel more resistant to decay.	Dental cavities.
Zinc	Meat and dairy products, breast milk, infant formula milks	Needed for growth and healing wounds. Helps activity of enzymes.	Mild – poor growth; poor healing. Severe – skin rashes, disturbances in the brain, gut and immune system.
Potassium	Cereals, some fruits	Needed for growth and healthy cardiac muscle.	Muscle weakness, tiredness.

miscarriage is the spontaneous loss of a *foetus* from the *uterus* in the early stages of *pregnancy*. This is very distressing for a woman and she will need sensitive support to enable her to grieve for her lost baby.

The Miscarriage Association provides information and support for those who have suffered the loss of a child through miscarriage. (See also *abortion*.)

mission statement: a formal statement of an organisation's aims and objectives with regard to the service, care and support it seeks to offer to the service user.

mitochondria: spherical or cylindrical bodies within the *cell* cytoplasm, which are the sites of internal respiration.

mitosis: *cell* division which takes place when new cells are produced for growth and to replace worn out, mature or damaged cells. The cells produced through mitosis contain the same number (46 in humans) of **chromosomes** as the parent cell and are genetically identical.

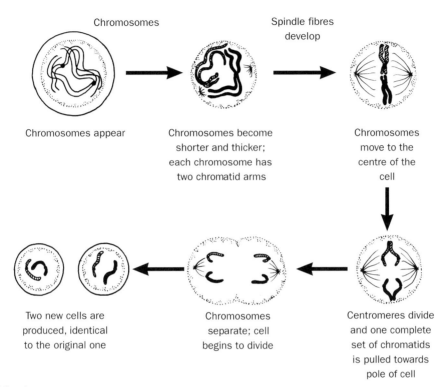

Chromosomes   Spindle fibres develop

Chromosomes appear

Chromosomes become shorter and thicker; each chromosome has two chromatid arms

Chromosomes move to the centre of the cell

Two new cells are produced, identical to the original one

Chromosomes separate; cell begins to divide

Centromeres divide and one complete set of chromatids is pulled towards pole of cell

Mitosis

mixed economy of care: the way in which community and social services are provided through different organisations in the statutory, independent and voluntary sectors, e.g. respite care may be offered through a local voluntary group such as **Mencap**.

mobility: the ability that a person has to walk, run and use the range of movements necessary for daily living. A service user's **mobility** is assessed as part of their **care plan**. (See **activities of daily living, aids and adaptations, calliper, Zimmer frame**.)

models of abuse are theories which have been created to provide some explanation or reason for **abuse**. The theoretical models are the:

- feminist model – explores the power relationships between men and women within a family and society. It does infer that most abusers are men but it is accepted that women can also be abusers
- medical model – explores the argument that abuse should be viewed as a **disease** with signs and symptoms which can be treated. However, it does not explore some of the more complex areas of abuse such as the different predisposing factors, including family breakdown and **stress**
- sociological model – explores the changes which take place in society and family life such as the effect of socio-economic issues. This includes inadequate housing, **poverty** and

unemployment which are seen to contribute to abuse. However, abuse happens across all areas of race, class and gender

- psychological model – explores the issues of how individuals in the family relate to each other. It examines dysfunction in families where communication has broken down and believes that supporting family relationships and improving communication will deter abuse from occurring in the future.

molecules are formed when atoms are chemically bonded together. For example, a molecule of water is represented as H_2O because it consists of one atom of oxygen with two hydrogen atoms bonded to it.

mongolian blue spot: a bluish patch on the skin present at birth. It looks rather like a *bruise*. It usually affects children of Afro-Caribbean origin.

monitoring health and fitness: requirements which identify the level of fitness in an individual. These include:
- standard height and weight charts
- body mass index
- measurements of pulse rate before, during and after exercise
- circumference of waist
- rate of perceived exertion, e.g. a scale of measured exercises used to predict perceived future exercise potential.

monosaccharides contain one simple *sugar* unit. In digestion all *carbohydrates* are broken down to simple sugars. Examples include:
- glucose – found in honey
- fructose – found in sweet fruits
- galactose – forms milk sugar or lactose.

morals: principles which determine the difference between right and wrong. Moral development is part of the *socialisation* process whereby a child will learn about right and wrong and how to behave accordingly. As a result of moral development individuals acquire a conscience, i.e. an internal set of moral principles that each person learns to live by.

moral development relates to the way in which young children develop a sense of right and wrong. From an early age, children can understand what pleases and what upsets others. With the support of family, teachers and other carers, children can learn to be loving and kind and to be instilled with a sense of fairness. As they grow older they find it much easier to view situations from the perspective of others.

morbidity data is the information which is collected with regard to illness, its type, nature and extent within the population. It is usually measured by the number of hospital admissions and doctor/patient consultations. Statistics relating to time off work as a result of sickness and self-reported illness data are gathered from health surveys.

morphine is a narcotic derived from opium. It is used as a powerful painkiller or analgesic drug, administered particularly to those who are suffering from severe pain. It is given to patients with *cancer*, for example. It can be addictive and is therefore registered under the Misuse of Drugs Act 1971.

mortality rates: the number of *deaths* per thousand of the population during a year. These rates are often split into the following groups: age, class, race, gender, children and infants. (See *infant mortality, mortality rate, standard mortality ratio*.)

motivation is the way in which a person uses their thought processes to encourage themselves to carry out tasks and activities. It is often related to a person's **self-esteem** and their belief in their ability to perform.

motor development is the development of the large and fine **muscles** which are found in the body. (See **motor skills**.)

motor neurone disease: a progressive **degenerative disease** which affects the motor neurones in the nervous system. It occurs in middle age and leads to increased muscle weakness. The Motor Neurone Disease Association assists sufferers and their families.

motor skills: aspects of **physical growth and development** which can be grouped together as the following:
- fine motor skills – manipulative skills using small movements of the hand, wrist and fingers and which involve some **hand–eye co-ordination** such as screwing and unscrewing a lid
- gross motor skills – involving large muscles and large limb movements such as running, walking, skipping and dancing.

mouth: composed of the upper and lower lip, teeth, hard palate and soft palate (which forms the roof of the mouth), tongue, tonsils and uvula, which is a projection from the soft palate. The mouth has important functions. The mouth:
- is the point of entry to the body for **food** and drink
- chews food and mixes it with **saliva** to help with swallowing
- enables food to be tasted
- is an **air passage** to the **lungs**
- makes speech possible.

multi-agency working is the way in which different agencies within health and social care liaise and work together in the care of clients. (See **multi-disciplinary teams, joint commissioning**.)

multi-disciplinary teams: health and social care professionals, each with different skills, who work together to meet the individual needs of a client. This is also known as **multi-agency working**.

multiple sclerosis: a disease affecting the nervous system which is characterised by the formation of patchy degenerative change in areas of the **brain, spinal cord** and the optic nerves. The signs and symptoms include numbness, weakness and unsteadiness in the legs, and **eye** problems such as double vision. The disease goes through cycles of relapse and remission.

muscles may be voluntary muscles, i.e. able to be controlled by conscious action, or involuntary muscles, i.e. those not under conscious control.
- Voluntary muscles – contractions of voluntary muscles are brought about as a result of nerve impulses reaching the muscle. Voluntary muscles are made up of voluntary muscle tissue. All voluntary muscles, except some of the muscles of the **tongue**, are attached to the **skeleton** by means of **tendons**. They cause movement of the skeleton by contraction of the muscle fibres. Skeletal muscles work in pairs. Flexor muscles cause bending at a joint and extensor muscles cause straightening. Skeletal muscles are usually arranged in antagonistic or opposing pairs. (See **antagonistic muscles**.)
- Involuntary muscles – are present in the wall of the gut, in blood vessels and in the dermis of the **skin**. These muscles are under involuntary control. Involuntary muscles usually open and close tubes or cavities.
- Cardiac muscle is found only in the **heart**.

muscular dystrophy: disorder which affects the *muscles* and the *nerve* supply to the muscles. There are several different types of the condition, which are all progressive, hereditary and result in muscle weakness.

The progressive breakdown of the muscle fibres over several years leads to the destruction of the muscle tissues. During this time the damaged fibres attempt to regenerate but are replaced by fibrous *tissue* and *fat*. The resulting muscle weakness and loss of muscle bulk cause difficulty in walking and affect the use of arms and legs, reducing mobility.

muscular tissue is a type of *tissue* which is contractile. There are three different types of muscle tissue.

Striated or striped muscle – voluntary muscle tissue which makes up skeletal muscles. It consists of long cells called muscle fibres grouped together in bundles called fasiculi. Each fibre has a striped or striated appearance and is made of many smaller cylinders, called fibrils or myofibrils. Fibrils contract when a fibre is stimulated by a nerve.

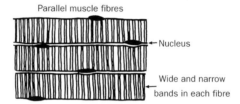

A section of striated muscle to show
actomyosin banding within the fibre

Parallel muscle fibres

← Nucleus

Wide and narrow
bands in each fibre

Cardiac muscle – involuntary muscle tissue, which makes up cardiac muscle in the heart. It is a special kind of striated muscle. Its constant rhythmical contractions are caused by stimulation from special areas of the tissue itself, which produce their own electrical impulses.

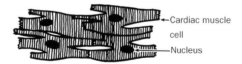

A surface view of cardiac muscle

←Cardiac muscle
cell

Nucleus

Smooth muscle or visceral muscle – involuntary muscle tissue which makes up the visceral muscles supporting the organs of the body. It consists of spindle-shaped cells, much shorter than the complex fibres of striated muscle.

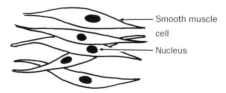

A surface view of smooth muscle

Smooth muscle
cell

Nucleus

musculoskeletal system includes the *muscles* and the *skeleton* of the body. Its function is to:

- assist movement
- support the body
- protect vital organs.

Dysfunctions of the system cause *arthritis*, *osteoporosis* and *fractures*.

music and singing are activities which help to develop different skills in young children. They can be used to:

- teach different sounds and noises
- develop vocal and singing skills
- give a child the opportunity to learn an instrument
- develop *memory*.

Just as music and singing are satisfying experiences for young children, they can be beneficial in other age groups, particularly the elderly. A regular 'sing song' round the piano helps older people to retain their memories. It gives them a creative experience which promotes happiness and satisfaction. *Reminiscence* using songs and music from the past is an excellent way of communicating with older people.

music therapy: the use of music to help individuals cope with stress and aggression in their lives. Music can be soothing and relaxing. The ability to make music and create sound can be a satisfying experience.

myalgic encephalomyelitis: (ME) a disorder or disease which is characterised by extreme fatigue. Other symptoms include poor circulation, pain in the *joints* and *muscles*, dizziness, general tiredness and a feeling of being unwell or malaise. The cause is unknown, but it often occurs after a *virus* or *infection* and, therefore, can be referred to as post-viral fatigue. Treatment involves rest and medication until the patient begins to feel better. In some cases ME can be a prolonged and debilitating disorder.

myocardial infarction: see *heart attack*.

M

Do you need revision help and advice?

Go to pages 292–304 for a range of revision appendices that include plenty of exam advice and tips.

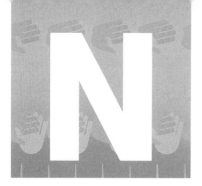

named nurse: the nurse, midwife or community nurse who is responsible for a patient's care. Whenever a client, patient or service user requires treatment or care then they should be told the name of the qualified nurse, community carer or midwife who is looking after them. (See *charters, key worker*.)

nannies are employed privately by parents to look after children in the family home. Nannies are exempt from registration if they look after the children of only one or two families, but must be registered with *OFSTED* if they care for the children of three or more families. Nannies can also work as au pairs which means they are employed for a limited period of time and can work in foreign countries. They may or may not be qualified as *nursery nurses*. Au pairs may be expected to carry out some housework and usually 'live in' with the host family.

National Advisory Committee on Nutrition Education: (NACNE) a government committee which issues nutritional guidelines for *health education* in Britain. A report was produced in 1993 which dealt with health-related issues such as body weight, carbohydrate and fat intake, *coronary heart disease*, salt and *blood pressure* and the effects of *alcohol*. The report concluded that being overweight increased a person's health risk. It made the following recommendations:

- *fats* – total fat intake should be reduced and ways of increasing the ratio of *polyunsaturated fatty acids* to saturated fatty acids should be considered. It provided evidence that a diet with a high proportion of polyunsaturated fatty acids could reduce the incidence of cardiovascular disease
- *carbohydrates* – sucrose (sugar) intake should be reduced and that of complex carbohydrates and fibre should be increased. A reduction in sugar is part of a strategy to reduce the overweight proportion of the population. They also identified a link between sugar intake and tooth decay
- fibre – to increase intake by 50%. The report suggested that low levels of dietary fibre were associated with large bowel disease, including irritable bowel syndrome, constipation, diverticulosis and colon cancer
- salt – to reduce the salt intake. The report indicated that high intakes of sodium chloride led to high blood pressure (hypertension).

The NACNE report looked particularly at the health education aspects of nutrition and how these related to *lifestyle*. Therefore, the targets set were those which would lead to a beneficial change in people's attitudes to nutrition and diet. (See *Committee on Medical Aspects of Food Policy*.)

national child care strategy: a government initiative to provide child care places for under fives. As part of the initiative each local authority has set up an early years and child care partnership. These partnerships are made up of a group of professionals from the private, voluntary and statutory sectors who work with young children and their families and representatives from social services, employment and training organisations. Working parents may be able to claim some money for child care costs through the tax system.

National Children's Bureau: a registered charity which identifies and promotes the interests of children and young people. It is a multi-disciplinary organisation and its aim is to promote co-ordination and co-operation amongst all those agencies serving children and young people.

national contracts for health: a government initiative set up to improve health in four priority areas, namely *heart disease and strokes, accidents, cancer* and *mental health*.

A contract for health

Government and national players can	Local and community players can	People can
Provide national co-ordination and leadership.	Provide leadership for local health strategies by developing and implementing health improvement programmes.	Take responsibility for their own health and make healthier choices about lifestyle.
Ensure that policy making across government takes full account of health and is well informed by research and the best expertise available.	Work in partnerships to improve the health of local people and tackle root causes of ill health.	Ensure their own actions do not harm the health of others.
Work with other countries for international co-operation to improve health.		
Assess risks and communicate those risks clearly to the public.	Plan and provide high-quality services for everyone who needs them.	Take opportunities to better their own and their families' lives, through education, training and employment.
Ensure that the public and others have the information they need to improve their health.		
Regulate and legislate where necessary.		
Tackle the root causes of ill health.		

(Source: *Our Healthier Nation – A Contract for Health* (1998) HMSO.)

National Council for Voluntary Organisations: the main umbrella body for the voluntary sector. It acts as:

- a focal point for formal and informal debate
- an information centre

- a focal point for networking
- an influence with regard to policy
- a campaigner for the voluntary sector
- a promoter of voluntary sector interests.

National Curriculum: a government reform introduced in 1988 as part of the Education Reform Act. Education is compulsory for all children between the ages of five and 16 in state *schools*, including special schools. The National Curriculum is divided into four key stage areas. There are regular and *standard assessment tests* (SATS) at the end of each key stage. The stages are:

- key stage 1 – children aged 5–7 years
- key stage 2 – children aged 7–11 years
- key stage 3 – children aged 12–14 years
- key stage 4 – children aged 14–16 years.

National Disability Advisory Council: provides advice on disability-related issues. It encourages consultation between members of the Commonwealth, the government, carers and service providers within the disability sector.

national food survey is a continuous social survey which monitors diet and food consumption in the United Kingdom. It is carried out by the Social Survey Division. They produce their findings for the Department of the Environment, Food and Rural Affairs.

National Health Service: see *NHS (National Health Service)*.

National Health Service and Community Care Act 1990: see *NHS and Community Care Act 1990*.

national health targets: set by the government in four priority areas. These are: *heart disease and strokes*, *accidents, cancer* and *mental health*. (See also *health education, Our Healthier Nation – A Contract for Health*.)

National Institute for Clinical Excellence: (NICE) an organisation set up under the recent government reforms for the NHS. The Institute's membership is drawn from individuals in the health professions, NHS academics, health economists and those representing patients' interests. It gives coherence and prominence to information about care and clinical treatment and its cost effectiveness.

national insurance: see *benefits*.

national minimum standards: requirements set up by the government to ensure that services provided within health and social care organisations meet minimum standards of practice. (See *Care Homes for Old People National Minimum Standards 2003*).

national minimum wage: a wage per hour set at a level decided by the Low Pay Commission. No employee should be paid less than this agreed sum.

National Service Frameworks: (NSFs) long-term strategies set up by the government to improve specific areas of care. They include conditions such as cancer, coronary heart disease, mental health disorders and diabetes. They also cover patient groups such as children and older people.

National Society for Prevention of Cruelty to Children: (NSPCC) a voluntary organisation with *statutory* powers to act in the care of children and their families. It has the authority to take legal action on behalf of a child and to obtain access to records such as the register of children at risk. To carry out this work it employs qualified *social workers* and

operates closely with the statutory **personal social services** and **police officers**.
A child may be referred to the NSPCC which investigates the case and works with the family.
If there is a need for the child to be taken into care, then the case may be taken to court by
the NSPCC or passed over to the local authority social services department. The emphasis
of the organisation is on protecting children, working with families and seeking to prevent
their break-up.

National Statistics Socio-economic Classification: (NS-SEC) an occupation-based
classification that is used for all official statistics and surveys. Although it is based on occupation,
it has been altered to ensure that the categories cover most of the adult population.

NS-SEC analytic classes are:
1   Higher managerial and professional occupations
    1.1   Large employers and higher managerial occupations
    1.2   Higher professional occupations
2   Lower managerial occupations
3   Intermediate occupations
4   Small employers and own account workers
5   Lower supervisory and technical occupations
6   Semi-routine occupations
7   Routine occupations
8   Never worked and long-term unemployed.

For complete coverage, the three categories: Students; Occupations not stated or
inadequately described; and Not classifiable for other reasons, are added as 'not
classified'. (Source: Office for National Statistics.)

National Vocational Qualifications (NVQs) are those qualifications which provide
proof of competence in the workplace. The holder of the award has met the requirements
of the relevant national occupational standards. There are a variety of awards including
community work, care, hospital operating department support, caring for children and young
people, **early years** care and education.

nature–nurture: a debate which discusses the factors influencing the way in which
children grow and develop, comparing the impact of home environment (nurture) and
inherited traits (nature). (See **socialisation**.)

needs: the requirements necessary for maintaining life at a certain standard. There are
basic needs such as warmth, fresh air and sunlight, healthy **diet**, affection, good health,
independence, good **hygiene**, a sense of belonging, social contact, **play** (to be occupied in
work or involved in a hobby), protection from harm, and **safety. Care** involves providing the
relevant support to meet all of these, within the context of a client's physical, intellectual,
emotional, cultural and religious needs. (See **Maslow, basic needs**.)

negative behaviour: the **behaviour** of an individual which may be interpreted as
antisocial. This includes **tantrums**, screaming, shouting and swearing. This form of behaviour
needs firm but sensitive handling. (See **challenging behaviour, anti-social behaviour**.)

neglect is the failure to provide a child or person with the basic necessities of life such as
food, warmth, clothing, housing and the security of being cared for. Carers who neglect their
clients may:
- leave them alone for long periods
- not make adequate provision for their clothing and hygiene needs

- not consider their dietary needs and routine of regular feeding
- isolate them by not giving them love and companionship.

(See also *abuse*.)

nerve impulses are messages carried or conducted along the various *nerve* fibres in the body. For example, sound, light, touch and heat stimulate the sense *organs* to send impulses along a nerve *cell* or neurone to the brain and to any part of the body. Neurones are linked to each other and form a body network connecting with the *brain* and *spinal cord*. However, the neurones are not joined directly together. There is a small gap or synapse between adjoining neurones. When an impulse is conducted along a nerve, a release of chemicals at the synapse enables the message/impulse to be conducted to another nerve cell. Neurones are nerve cells which carry messages to and from the *brain* via the *spinal cord* and the peripheral nervous system. They vary in size and shape but are classified in groups according to their different functions, which include:

- sensory neurones – carry messages or relay impulses from the sensory organs to the central nervous system
- motor neurones – carry messages or relay impulses from the central nervous system to *muscles* and *glands*
- intermediate neurones – relay messages between the different neurones.

nerves are bundles of fibres which are responsible for carrying messages or relaying impulses to and from the *brain* via the *spinal cord* and the peripheral nervous system to all parts of the body. There are 43 pairs of nerves situated in the *central nervous system*. These consist of:

- 12 pairs of cranial nerves which connect the brain to all parts of the body
- 31 pairs of spinal nerves which connect the parts of the body to the brain.

Each nerve contains bundles of fibres which vary in thickness and number. Some nerves consist of one or two fibres and are thin threads while others are thicker with many more fibres. Nerves continually branch off and therefore penetrate all parts of the body. Such fibres may be sensory or motor nerves; which they are determines the type of action they initiate.

nervous system: this provides the fastest method of communication within the body. There are two parts of the nervous system: the *central nervous system* (CNS) and the peripheral nervous system. It is a network of nerve cells called neurones which carry messages to and from the *brain* via the *spinal cord* and peripheral nervous system to all parts of the body. The central nervous system consists of the brain and spinal cord. The peripheral nervous system consists of bundles of motor and sensory fibres which take messages to and from different parts of the body. Dysfunctions of the nervous system cause *Parkinson's disease* and *multiple sclerosis*.

nervous tissue is composed of *cells* which conduct messages or impulses to and from the *brain* and other parts of the body. The nerve cells are also called neurones.

network: the formation of a number of friends, colleagues or people who group together to offer *support* in the following ways:

- *counselling*
- sharing *information*
- sharing expertise
- fundraising for local self-help projects

- publicising a service
- setting up localised training sessions.

Networks are links made between different **groups** of people. Networks are important because they perform a number of functions:

- sharing of information
- giving emotional and practical support
- giving individuals a sense of belonging and included within a group situation.

(See **support groups**.)

network analysis is a method of evaluating the effectiveness of how **groups** function within a network.

newborn baby (neonate): the **baby** in the first month of its life. When babies are born they are curled up in the foetal position (arms and legs are bent inwards towards the body). After **birth** the newborn begins to adopt different positions such as:

- prone – the baby lies on its front with its head turned to one side. The bottom is raised and the knees are curled up under the tummy. The arms are bent at the elbows and tucked under the chest. The fists are clenched
- supine – the baby lies on its back. The arms are turned inward and bent towards the body. The knees are also bent towards the body. The baby exhibits jerky kicking movements in the legs
- ventral suspension – when held horizontally under the tummy the baby's head and legs fall below the level of their back and the baby's body forms a downwards curve
- sitting – when the baby is pulled into the sitting position its head falls back. This is called head lag. As the baby's body comes up its head flops on to its chest.

(See **reflex actions of the newborn**.)

NHS and Community Care Act 1990: an Act of Parliament following the white paper 'Caring for People' 1988 which introduced reforms into NHS and social care services. The principal areas covered by the Act included:

- local authority community care plans
- assessment and care management
- purchasing, providing of health and social care services
- GP fund-holding
- community care reforms
- NHS reforms.

The most recent government reforms in the NHS have amended or replaced some of these recommendations.

NHS Direct: a 24-hour telephone **advice** line staffed by **nurses** to deal with enquiries from the general public.

NHS (National Health Service): a free, comprehensive and state-provided health system. The NHS was set up in 1948 following the Act of Parliament, the NHS Act 1946. The shape of the NHS in 1948 consisted of three distinct and separately managed areas. These were **hospitals**, run by management committees, primary care (**GPs**, **dentists**, **opticians** and **pharmacists**), run by executive councils, and **community health services** (district nursing, ambulances), run by **local authorities**. The NHS was reformed in 1974 when there were major changes to its structure and to that of local government. A new three-tier system of managing the NHS was introduced, i.e. regional health authorities, area health authorities and district health authorities. The aim was to separate responsibilities to the different levels, and to improve management and resource allocation. There was further major reform following the **NHS and Community Care Act 1990**. The aim this time was to create a more efficient NHS by making it more business-like through the setting up of an 'internal market'. It divided the service into '**purchasers**' and '**providers**' of health care. Purchasers – such as district health authorities and GP fund-holders – would draw up contracts with providers such as **NHS trusts** to deliver health care. This introduced an element of competition into the system which was designed to improve efficiency and reduce costs (see **economy, efficiency and effectiveness**). Another reform was to introduce care in the community. This was a means whereby mental health and learning disability care was provided in the community. Social services were to be responsible for assessing the 'package of care' and then for organising the delivery of that care for the client (see **community care**). Following the White Paper in December 1997, '**The New NHS – Modern, Dependable**', further changes were implemented. These changes included:

- fair access to high standards of care
- **national service frameworks** – ending two-tier GP fund-holding and giving all GPs the same level of influence
- **primary care trusts** – involving all GPs, other primary care professionals and Social Service input, i.e. shape services in line with local needs
- more responsibility inside **NHS trusts** for their clinical staff
- health authorities to monitor a **health improvement programme** with a legal duty of partnership which includes stronger links with local authorities
- national bodies such as the **National Institute for Clinical Excellence** which leads on clinical and cost effectiveness and local commitments to **quality assurance**.

NHS restructuring in April 2002 led to 95 health authorities being replaced by 80 strategic health authorities making primary care trusts the main NHS organisations with responsibility for assessing need planning and securing all health services and improving health in their localities. Further restructuring has led to the modification of the NHS authorities and trusts.

NHS plan: this was published in 2001. It set out initiatives such as:

- new working arrangements in the form of joint health and social care trusts
- enabling social care to be carried out in new settings such as GP surgeries and health centres
- defining **nursing care** as all services carried out by a registered nurse, and defining other care carried out by health care assistants as **personal care**.

NHS resources: **funding** which applies to the NHS. The NHS is financed through general taxation. The **Department of Health** is responsible for allocating **funding** to the **primary care trusts.**

NHS trusts: organisations which provide **patient** services in **hospitals** and in the community. Trusts are responsible for providing health and community care for millions of people in the United Kingdom. NHS Trusts include **acute trusts, foundation trusts**, **ambulance trusts, care trusts, primary care trusts**, **mental health trusts, strategic health authorities**, and **special health authorities**.

NICE: see *National Institute for Clinical Excellence*.

non-accidental injury: the act of deliberately physically hurting a child, causing injury. Physical injuries can take the form of:

- *bruises* – marks which may be caused by beatings with belts, shoes and sticks
- burns – such as cigarette burns
- *fractures* – caused by hitting, or dropping on the floor
- head injuries – hitting or shaking a child which may cause *brain* damage
- *poisoning* – feeding a child harmful substances such as *alcohol*.

(See *abuse*.)

non-profit-making organisations are health and social care services which provide care for clients on either a voluntary basis or for a minimum cost, e.g. Dial a Ride, a transport service for the disabled and the elderly. (See *voluntary sector organisations*.)

non-verbal communication: ways of communicating with others using body language such as:

- the *eyes* – using eyes to make contact and build rapport can indicate interest. However, in some cultures a sustained eye contact with another would be viewed as showing a lack of *respect*
- facial expressions – the face can show whether the person is happy, bored, irritated or concerned
- gestures and body posture – how a person uses their body can send out strong messages to others
- physical proximity – how close a person is in proximity to another person is very important. Moving too close can often be viewed as an intrusion of body space
- tone of voice.

(See also *communication*, *barriers to communication*, *building confidence*, *personal space*, *interaction*, *effective communication*.)

norms: patterns of *behaviour* that are expected to be followed by members of a particular group. Different groups have their own sets of norms to which members are expected to conform. (See *peer groups*.)

normalisation is a theoretical model which describes how people with disabilities integrate into society. They should be given opportunities to develop their skills and abilities so that they can play a fuller role. (See *enablement*.)

Northern Ireland Act 1998: an Act of Parliament which places a legal responsibility on public authorities in respect of the promotion of equality of opportunity in Northern Ireland. It covers relationships between:

- persons of different religious belief, political opinion, racial group, age, marital status or sexual orientation
- men and women
- persons with a disability and those without
- persons with dependants and those without.

Northern Ireland health provision: health and social care services in Northern Ireland are managed through health and social care service boards. On 1 April 2009 the Health and Social Care Board (HSCB) replaced the previous four HSS Boards. The focus of the HSCB is on *commissioning*, *resourcing of services*, performance management and improvement.

notifiable diseases: a list of diseases including *diphtheria*, hepatitis, *food poisoning*, tetanus and *HIV*. When they occur they must be reported to the relevant authority. Notifiable procedures are a means whereby:

- *records* of diseases or infections are maintained as they occur
- adequate provision is made for available *hospital* beds
- research is kept up to date
- local *doctors* are regularly informed of any outbreak of disease in their area.

(See *Reporting of Injuries, Diseases and Dangerous Occurrences Regulations 1995*.)

numeracy is the ability to think and reason with numbers. It is a skill which is developed and learned from an early age through cognitive thinking and reasoning. This leads to number recognition, working with numbers by adding, subtracting, multiplication and division. As basic numeracy skills are understood then this progresses into more complex problem solving and number working. There are strategies in place in schools to develop children's learning with regard to numeracy.

nurse: a professional qualified to care for people in a variety of settings. Nursing involves training for three years. Half way through this training, nurses specialise in one of the four main branches, adult, *mental health*, *learning disability* and children's nursing. The professional qualification in nursing can enable a person to develop their skills in other career directions, such as *health visiting*, oncology or caring for *cancer* patients. Nurses may now qualify at diploma or degree level.

nursery nurse: a trained professional person who works with children from newborn babies to children of different ages and stages in a variety of childcare settings. Nursery nurses promote the physical, emotional, social, intellectual, cognitive and cultural development of children. They work in nurseries, infant or special schools, hospitals, family homes, as holiday play representatives and play scheme workers. Nursery nurse training can take up to two years leading to a Diploma in Child Care and Education or to a BTEC Diploma in Children's Care, Learning and Development. Other qualifications such as *National Vocational Qualifications (NVQs)* may be completed over a shorter period of time. A nursery nurse may be called a childcare and education worker or early years worker. (See also *nannies, human growth and development*.)

Nursing and Midwifery Council: the regulatory body for nurses and midwives set up in 2002.

nursing care is assessed in terms of a client's individual needs and requirements. Care in residential homes is categorised as:

- personal care – dressing, undressing, bathing, feeding and other tasks which influence the *health and well-being* of *service users*
- nursing care – carried out by trained nurses – dressing a wound, treating ulcers and pressure sores. This care is free of charge.

Residents in care homes receive some state funding which varies from region to region. In Scotland, personal and nursing care is free. Wales is the same as England in that clients pay for personal care but nursing care is free.

nursing home: residential accommodation which provides professional *nursing care*. They are registered and inspected by the *Care Quality Commission*.

nutrients are the essential components of *food* which provide the individual with the necessary requirements for bodily functions. They are essential in the composition of a healthy diet. They comprise:

- *carbohydrates*, *fats* and *proteins*. These are also known as macro-nutrients because they are present in larger amounts
- *vitamins* and *minerals*. These are also known as micro-nutrients because they are present in smaller amounts.

nutrition: the study of the food process in terms of the way that it is received and utilised by the body to promote healthy growth and development. The science of nutrition explores aspects of different diets, and of diseases caused by dietary deficiency. (See *balanced diet, minerals, vitamins*.)

Nutrition Standards for School Lunches and Other School Food 2006: regulations introduced by the government which cover how food should be nutritious and should promote healthy eating in children. Food requirements are dependent on sufficient portions of vegetables and fruit, fish and the serving of red meat twice a week. It is a strategy to reduce the amount of 'junk food' and processed foods being eaten by school children.

nutritional health is about eating a *diet* which supports good health. There are various influences affecting nutritional health:

- dietary habits – meals, snacking, bingeing
- *lifestyles* – eating out, eating at home and frequency of take-aways
- socio-economic and cultural variations – cost of food and food availability
- *health education* – educating people to eat more healthily
- relevant *legislation*.

(See *balanced diet, healthy eating plate, Five-A-Day campaign*.)

Are you studying other subjects?

The *A–Z Handbooks (digital editions)* are available in 14 different subjects. Browse the range and order other handbooks at **www.philipallan.co.uk/a-zonline**.

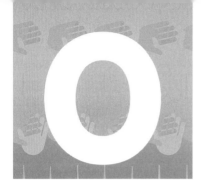

obesity: the excessive deposit of fatty *tissue* in the subcutaneous region around the body. Obesity is caused by the consumption of an excessive amount of calories taken in the form of food and drink. Obesity is measured by body weight against body height, which calculates the *body mass index* (BMI).

observation: a procedure in which one person watches or studies another person or a group of people. There are different types of observation:

- direct observation – the researcher remains detached from the subjects he or she is observing. Subjects can be watched as they go about their daily lives. Both *qualitative data* and *quantitative data* can be collected. Observers can count participants in terms of race, class, gender and age and any other characteristic. They can also record qualitative data such as how individuals behave towards each other. Direct observations are the only way to monitor some groups. Observation of clients as a means of assessment involves noting the general appearance of the client, their colour, dress, mobility, facial expressions, body posture, gestures and the way they speak
- participant observation – means that the researcher becomes part of the group being studied. Some researchers have spent years living and working with their subjects, while at the same time recording data about them
- naturalistic observation – observing people in their natural setting, e.g. watching children interact with their mother or primary care giver.

Recording an observation can be simple, e.g. writing what is being observed in a note book. In some cases a video camera may be used or photographs may be taken, if permission is given beforehand. Permission is sought from the client, carer and in some cases the care manager if necessary, so that the individual rights of the client are protected. Observations may be recorded:

- for a defined period and with a specific aim in mind, e.g. a childcare student may wish to observe an aspect of a child's development, such as their physical co-ordination, as they play
- at regular intervals in order to collect evidence for a project, e.g. a student may observe others in the college refectory every lunch time for a week in order to note the eating habits of students
- on a chart, e.g. quantitative readings such as temperature, pulse and respiration.

observational skills are skills which are developed through assessing, monitoring and recording the *behaviour* of others.

occupational diseases result from particular types of employment, usually as a result of long-term exposure to a specific substance, environment or a repetitive physical act. Examples are conditions caused by:

- dust, e.g. asbestosis is caused by breathing in asbestos dust which results in damage to the *lungs*
- *chemical poisoning,* such as lead compound poisoning which results in **bone marrow** damage
- working with continuous loud noise which can result in damage to hearing
- being exposed to radiation which can result in some *cancers*
- repeated movements of parts of the body which can result in repetitive strain injury
- the constant glare of a computer screen which can result in visual disturbance.

occupational health nurses are registered *nurses* who work with people in their place of employment. They promote physical and mental health and carry out **risk assessment** with regard to any physical hazard which may result in employees contracting work-related *diseases*. They are often involved in **health screening**, record keeping, environmental monitoring, accident prevention, **health education**, **rehabilitation** and any follow-up treatment. They also deal with minor accidents.

occupational health service: the department within an organisation which looks after the health needs of employees.

occupational therapists are trained professionals who treat patients, clients and service users with temporary or permanent physical or learning disability or mental disorder. Occupational therapists work in a number of different settings supporting clients from a variety of backgrounds. These settings can include general and specialist *hospitals*, health centres, local authority social services, **residential homes** and *day centres*, children's and mental health services, in people's own homes and in industry and commerce. An occupational therapist has to combine knowledge and skills when working with people of all ages. They support clients with different problems, such as psychological or physical illness, accident recovery or ageing. Fundamentally their role is to encourage individuals to take action for themselves. They assist clients to improve the quality of their own lives and enable them to remain independent and autonomous for as long as possible. This may involve visiting a client's home and assessing their need for necessary **aids and adaptations**. Registered occupational therapists qualify after a three-year course at university.

Office for Standards in Education: (OFSTED) an organisation which inspects, monitors, and reports on the performance of *schools* and *early years provisions*. Visits to schools are carried out by teams of inspectors which include lay members (people who do not have a background in education). It is intended that services are inspected on a regular basis. Summaries of the reports must be published, and distributed to the appropriate people.

Office of Population Censuses and Surveys: an organisation which collects data to be published in national, local and medical population tables. The results recorded include *morbidity data, mortality rates, employment* statistics, marriage and *divorce* rates.

OFSTED: see *Office for Standards in Education*.

older people: a term given to people who are aged 65 years and over. They form one group of service users or clients and patients who use the health and social care services. Services provided for older people include health care, social care, **domiciliary services**, **day care**, private and voluntary care. There are other terms for older people such as senior citizens, old age pensioners, elders and elderly people. Older people form a high proportion of the population in the United Kingdom. In recent years there has been an increasing number of older people and, therefore, this has put pressure on the demand for health and social care services. (See **frail and elderly, caring for older people**.)

The rights and needs of older people

Needs of older people	Rights of older people
Affection	To feel cared for and valued as an individual
Communication	To be able to relate to others independent of disability or impairment; to be given the appropriate equipment to promote communication, e.g. hearing aids, Bliss boards
Dignity and self-respect	To be respected for their individual beliefs; to be encouraged to participate in activities which support their personal identity and promote positive self-esteem
Exercise and mobility	To be able to take regular exercise; to be encouraged to be as mobile as possible and, if appropriate, for suitable aids and equipment to be supplied
Healthy diet	To be supported with a diet which meets their dietary needs. Support should be given if required with shopping, cooking, or provided by meals on wheels
Independence	To be able to make decisions about their daily lives; to live in a place of their own choice, preferably their own home whenever possible; to receive relevant support so that they can be as independent as possible
Relationships	To meet others with similar interests; to build rapport and share experiences with others, e.g. reminiscence
Rest and a sense of safety in a secure environment	To be able to feel safe and protected and free from harm; to live in a safe environment, whenever possible, an older people's environment should be assessed as being safe and healthy
Routines, e.g. hygiene, washing, showering, housework	To be able to maintain relevant routines necessary to support daily living; to receive assistance as and when required
Stimulation	To be able to continue with lifelong learning if they wish; and to meet with others for recreation and hobbies, e.g. keep fit, card games, etc.

older people – abuse: a deliberate act to hurt or harm an older client, patient or service user. This can take the form of:

- verbal *abuse*, such as calling a client names, or shouting at them when they need help or they cannot move fast enough
- physical abuse, such as hitting them with a hand or piece of equipment such as a hairbrush or coat hanger; often, the abuser will injure a client in a place which is covered with clothing so that it cannot be seen

- neglect: for example the client might be left alone without being washed, dressed or bathed. Toileting might be carried out infrequently and the client might wet or soil themselves. This may make a client more vulnerable to other forms of abuse
- emotional abuse, for example where the elderly client is put on the toilet and the door is left open or they are strip washed in front of others. They are not given any involvement in decisions about their care. There is no sense of kindness and compassion in the caring that they receive and they can easily feel unloved, unwanted, isolated and alone
- sexual abuse, such as touching, fondling and intimidating behaviour.

Caring for older people can be demanding as they may need a great deal of attention, concern and *holistic care.* Every aspect of their different and individual needs should be considered and met.

ombudsman: an appointed person whose role is to help improve public services. They do this by investigating complaints from individuals about the way they have been treated by UK government departments and by the NHS in England.

opinion poll: a survey method to collect data with regard to public opinion on different issues. *Quota sampling* and street *interviews* are methods often used to test public opinion.

ophthalmic optician: see *optometrists*.

ophthalmologists are qualified *doctors* who have specialised in the treatment of the *eyes* and visual impairments. They also detect, diagnose and treat eye infections. They care for the visually impaired and look at strategies for preventing loss of sight or blindness.

opticians are professionals trained to examine and test the eyesight of clients and customers. They can detect *eye* disorders and prescribe the appropriate lenses to be fitted into spectacles or glasses. Opticians usually charge for eye tests. However, there are certain individuals who are exempt from this charge, such as *older people* and the disabled. (See *optometrists, ophthalmologists*.)

optometrists are professionals involved in testing eyesight to detect and measure any visual disorder or impairment. They may prescribe lenses to correct such defects. They are also able to detect any disease or dysfunction of the *eye*. They either work in private practice or within the *NHS (National Health Service)*.

oral presentation: see *giving a talk*.

organ: a structure consisting of different *tissue* types carrying out a particular function or functions; an example is the *heart* which is made up of *muscle tissue* called cardiac muscle, and nervous tissue, supported and bound by *connective tissue* and *epithelial tissue*. When different *organs* work together they form an organ system, e.g. the circulatory system which includes the heart, lungs, arteries, veins and capillaries.

organ transplant: see *transplantation*.

organisations are bodies of people set up to achieve specific aims. They are characterised by a structure and a culture. Organisations are often placed where there are decision-making processes and information exchange. Those in health and social care have been established to meet the health and social care needs of society, at both local and national level. They will usually be managed by a senior group who will direct different teams working with various client groups (see *hospitals*, *social services*). However, there are also much smaller organisations such as playgroups and day centres. In such examples there is usually just one senior leader of a team which works together in the care of their clients. Organisations should have policies in place to ensure that a positive care environment is maintained and promoted. These polices include:

- a **mission statement** – as an intent towards good practice
- **equal opportunities** – to ensure anti-discriminatory practice
- **codes of practice** which describe working practices such as food hygiene, food safety, health and safety, recruitment, training and staff selection
- availability and access to services especially for those with disabilities.

Organisations in health and social care include:

- statutory, voluntary, private or independent organisations
- formal and informal organisations (see **caring**)
- social services
- strategic health authorities, primary care trusts, NHS trusts, mental health trusts and children's trusts (see **health and social care organisations, statutory organisations, voluntary sector organisations**).

organisational culture is a network of strategies which create either a positive or a negative atmosphere within an organisation, e.g. target setting where meeting targets can dominate and undermine the individual care of service users. (See **barriers to organisational culture**.)

orthopaedic specialist: a qualified **doctor** who specialises in detecting, diagnosing and treating diseases, disorders and dysfunctions of the **bones** and **joints**.

orthoptists are professionally trained people who work with individuals, usually children, who have any visual defect or disorder, abnormal **eye** movement or any other correctable eye condition. Their role is to prescribe eye exercises and to monitor the patient's progress during the course of treatment. Most orthoptists work in **hospitals** but some operate in the community providing vision screening in **schools**, mobile units and health clinics. (See **optometrists, opticians**.)

osmosis is the process by which solvents pass through a semi-permeable membrane under osmotic pressure. The solvent molecules, e.g. water, pass from an area of lower solute concentration to an area of higher solute concentration until the concentration of solutions on both sides of the semi-permeable membrane is equal.

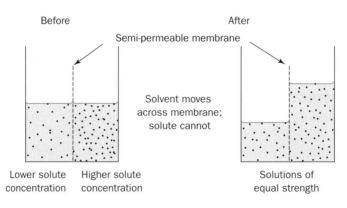

Osmosis

osteopathy: a *complementary therapy* which focuses on dysfunctions or disorders of the *muscles* and the skeletal system. A method of manipulation is used to help the body to heal itself. The basic principles applied in osteopathy are:

- the body has self-healing mechanisms which can be identified by the osteopath and put to work
- the body is made up of units and parts which inter-relate with each other and can work together to maintain *health and well-being*; this indicates the *holistic* nature of the treatment
- the structure and functions of the body link and inter-relate with each other, for example sore and painful muscles may lead to poor circulation so by diagnosing the different causes of pain and releasing the *blood flow*, the healing process is facilitated.

Qualifying to be an osteopath takes four years. For qualified *doctors* it takes thirteen months.

osteoporosis is a disorder which affects the *bones*, causing thinning or reduction in the mass of bone present in the body. It is frequently to be found in older people. Lack of physical activity can promote generalised osteoporosis. *Fractures* and *disability* are linked with this disease, because of its effect on the bones. It affects women more than men due to the reduction of oestrogen (female sex hormone) following the *menopause*. *Hormone replacement therapy (HRT)* is sometimes given to reduce or slow down the process of osteoporosis. Taking sufficient calcium as part of a woman's daily diet may help to prevent osteoporosis in later life.

Our Healthier Nation – A Contract for Health: a Government Green Paper which sets out ways to improve the health of the population by increasing the length of people's lives and the number of years that people spend free of illness. It also explores strategies which seek to improve the *health* of the worse-off in society and to narrow the health gap. The report considers issues such as:

- *inequalities in health*
- the causes of *ill health*
- setting up national contracts for health
- setting national targets for health – *heart disease and strokes, accidents, cancer* and *mental health*.

outdoor play: a type of play which children enjoy outside, in the open air. Outdoor play, when weather permits, is an integrated part of a child's school day. Opportunities to run, skip, hop, play ball, chase, and play *games* are encouraged. *Physical play* gives a child's *muscles* the exercise needed to develop body co-ordination and movement.

out-of-school care is the provision available to children before and after school. They are now required to register all supervised provision for children up to the age of eight with the *Office for Standards in Education (OFSTED)*. For those children of school age this includes provision in out-of-school clubs, play centres, adventure playgrounds and holiday play schemes. Children are delivered to, and collected from school, during term time by club workers they know and trust. Once at the club, children are registered, given food and offered play opportunities until collected by a parent at a later time. Some clubs operate all day throughout school holidays. There are different types of provision for children of this age, including facilities run by *local authorities*, *voluntary sector organisations*, the *private sector* and those that are employer sponsored. Parents usually make a contribution towards costs. Other clubs may operate only during term time, or for certain parts of the year. (See *after-school clubs*.)

ovulation: the release of an egg or ovum from one of the ovaries occurring about every 28 days. The egg is moved along the Fallopian tube towards the *uterus* by muscular movements called *peristalsis*. In addition to this the lining of Fallopian tubes has ciliated epithelium, which helps the movement of the ovum. The journey from the ovary to the uterus usually takes about seven days. (See *menstrual cycle*.)

oxygen: a colourless, odourless gas that makes up 21% of the earth's atmosphere. It is vital for life. It supports combustion, dissolves in water to form a neutral solution and is a very reactive oxidising agent (e.g. it oxidises iron to iron oxide). Oxygen is essential for some of the chemical processes in the body, and it is breathed in via the *lungs* and taken to different parts of the body. It is used in cell respiration. (See *gaseous exchange, mechanism of breathing*.)

oxytocin is a *hormone* produced in the posterior lobe of the *pituitary gland*. It causes the uterus to contract during labour. Oxytocin also controls the release of milk during the suckling period.

Aiming for a grade A*?

Don't forget to log on to **www.philipallan.co.uk/a-zonline** for advice.

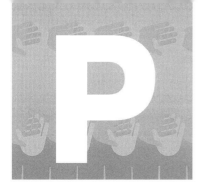

paediatrician: a qualified *doctor* who specialises in treating children. Paediatricians usually work in *hospitals* and have a specialist knowledge of the disorders, disease and dysfunctions which affect children. Children are referred to a paediatrician by their *general practitioner (GP)*.

palliative care: care which is given to a *patient* who is suffering from *terminal illness*. 'It affirms life and regards *death* as a normal process, neither hastens nor postpones death, provides relief from pain and other distressing symptoms, integrates the psychological and spiritual aspects of patient care and offers a support system to help the family cope during a patient's illness and in their bereavement' (*Health Provision* (1984) WHO).

This type of provision involves home and day care, and in-patient hospital care, *bereavement* support and voluntary support. (See *Cancer Relief Macmillan Fund, Marie Curie Cancer Care, Mencap, holistic care*.)

pancreas: a large *gland* situated in the first loop of the duodenum at the back of the *abdomen* behind the lower part of the *stomach*. It is a large whitish *organ*. The pancreatic duct links the pancreas to the duodenum. During *digestion* the pancreas secretes digestive juices which are poured onto food as it passes into the duodenum. These digestive juices are alkaline, to provide optimum conditions for the pancreatic enzymes to work. The functions of the pancreas are as follows:

- it produces pancreatic juice containing the *enzymes* lipase which digests *fat*, amylase which digests starch, and trypsin which digests *protein*
- it produces insulin from special pancreatic cells called the islets of Langerhans. Insulin reduces the level of glucose in the *blood* ensuring that the glucose level is kept constant. Excess glucose enters the cells of *muscles* and the *liver* for storage as glycogen
- it produces glucagon in the islets of Langerhans. This raises the level of glucose in the blood by causing the release of glycogen in the liver.

paralysis: loss of nervous function to part of the body. This may be due to damage to the sensory or motor nerves or to both. There are many different causes of paralysis, which can either be temporary or permanent. It may be due to:

- pressure on *nerves* blocking off any nerve reactions, e.g. tumour
- disease of the *spinal cord*, e.g. *multiple sclerosis*
- *brain* damage, e.g. *cerebral palsy*
- injury to the spinal cord or peripheral nerves, e.g. injury in a car accident.

paramountcy principle: the concept that the welfare of the child is the paramount consideration in proceedings concerning children. (See *Children Act 1989, Working Together to Safeguard Children 1999, Working Together to Safeguard Children 2007*).

paraplegia is *paralysis* of a person from the waist down.

parasympathetic nervous system: part of the *autonomic nervous system* which slows the heartbeat rate, lowers blood pressure and promotes digestion. There are two important nerves which form part of the parasympathetic *nervous system*. They are:

- the vagus nerve which extends from the base of the spine networking to all parts of the body
- the pelvic nerve which extends from the lower part of the spine networking to the lower parts of the body.

It works in opposition to the *sympathetic nervous system*.

parathyroid glands: there are four such *glands* embedded in the *thyroid gland*, two in each lobe. They secrete a *hormone* called the parathyroid hormone. This hormone controls the level of calcium in the blood. (See *endocrine system*.)

parent and toddler groups are small informal groups which offer *play* opportunities for children. The children are usually under the age of three years and attend the group with their parents or carers such as *childminders*. These groups may be linked with other forms of provision, such as *schools, pre-school groups* and *clinics*.

parental responsibility defines the duties of parents or primary care givers according to the relevant legislation with regard to children. This involves their rights and responsibilities as well as the necessary statutory powers to care for children. Parental responsibility can be given to a person who is not the biological parent and can be shared amongst a number of people. It may be acquired through an agreement or court order. (See *adoption*.)

Parentline: a national voluntary organisation offering telephone support, guidance and counselling services to any parent or carer of children. It provides help for parents under stress and facilitates and maximises a family's capacity to care for its children. It helps to break the cycle of family unhappiness by enabling those who are parenting to share with others the difficulties of bringing up children. Parents can telephone when they are in a crisis or when they just feel the need to talk.

Parkinson's disease: a slowly progressive, degenerative *disorder* of the *central nervous system*. The cause of Parkinson's disease is not known but it is believed to be associated with one small group of nerve cells in the *brain* (the basal ganglia) failing to function normally. This affects the production of dopamine, a chemical substance involved in the transmission of messages between *nerves* and the *muscles* they supply, causing the muscles to stiffen and respond slowly or not at all. Once established, the symptoms may be mild, but they can increase gradually over the years, although there may be a period of time when they seem to remain static. *Intelligence* is not affected and life expectancy is normal. There are three main symptoms which are usually present to some degree in each case of the disease.

- Tremor is not always present but, if it is, this slight shaking begins in one hand or one arm. It generally decreases when active or asleep.
- Rigidity or stiffness in the muscles is an early sign, and everyday tasks become difficult.
- Slowness of movement plus a difficulty in initiating movement are characteristic. Walking becomes an effort and voluntary movement may be interrupted.

participant observation: see *observation*.

partnership with parents: the practice of working closely with parents or other carers to ensure that the needs of individual children are met. This involves:
- building mutual trust and respect through the sharing of information which is relevant to the care of each child
- ensuring that there are communication systems in place so that parents have access to relevant information
- making sure that record keeping is regularly updated in consultation with the parent and kept confidential and secure. This would include an up-to-date record of any particular issues. (See *working in partnership*.)

passive immunity is the process by which antibodies produced in one individual are passed into the body of another to reduce the risk of specific disease. Passive *immunity* can take the form of:
- injection of *antibodies* from another mammal – when these are injected in the form of a serum, they are absorbed into the bloodstream and the individual gains immunity, e.g. treatment of diphtheria and *tetanus*
- immunity transfer between mother and *newborn baby* – antibodies cross the placenta from the mother's blood. Therefore the baby has the same protection against the same diseases as the mother. When the baby is *breast* fed, the baby receives antibodies in the breast milk. These antibodies also provide some immunity for the first few months of a baby's life.

pathogen: any micro-organism which causes a *disease*.

pathologist: a trained professional who is responsible for examining specimens of body *tissue* and detecting any disease, degeneration or dysfunction. (See *histology*.)

pathology: the study of *disease* and how it progresses. Pathology also explores the causes of disease and its other aspects. Specimens of *tissues* and *cells* and other samples from the body are sent to the pathology laboratory. Here they are examined using a variety of methods such as microscopy. The presence of any disease, disorder, *degenerative disease* or *dysfunction* is detected and a report written. This is a good example of indirect care as the laboratory technicians have little or no contact with their patients.

patient: a person who is receiving medical treatment and nursing care.

patient and public involvement forums were set up in 2004 to monitor services within *primary care trusts* and *NHS trusts*. They are made up of *patients* and members of the general public, and represent as wide a range of views as possible.

patient's survey: national *surveys* which provide *information*, gained from *patients* and *service users*, on their experience of health care. The results of these surveys can then be used to make improvements to services.

Pavlov, Ivan (1849–1936): a psychologist who developed a learning theory called classical conditioning. In an experiment known as 'Pavlov's dogs', Pavlov taught some dogs to salivate when they heard a bell ringing. The dogs learned to associate the noise with food. This learning by association is called 'conditioning'.

peak flow is the maximum speed at which air can be forced out of the *lungs*. A peak flow meter records the maximum speed at which the air is forced out from the lungs. It is used to assess the width of the trachea and bronchi. If the trachea and bronchi are narrowed, the air rushes out more slowly. This happens when a person is suffering from *asthma*.

peer assessment: the process of being observed and monitored by others in a group. It involves receiving verbal and written feedback in the form of constructive criticism from members of the group.

peer group: a collection of people who share common characteristics or circumstances. Peer groups have an important function in the *socialisation* process. Through peer group membership, individuals learn different roles and identify with the *norms* and *values* of the group. A set of friends of the same age in a class at school represents a kind of peer group.

pelvis: the bony structure situated in the lower part of the trunk. The pelvis consists of the ilium, ischium and pubis. These units form the two innominate bones. This framework supports the *bladder*, rectum and reproductive organs. (See *skeleton*.)

percentiles are the 100 sections on a *centile* chart which indicate, for example, the range of weight of boys and girls. The 50th percentile is called a median and represents the middle of the range. Children move from one percentile to another if their weight increases or decreases more or less than the 'average' for their peer group. The percentile positions are calculated from a typical sample of 100 children. (See *centile charts*.)

peristalsis is the rhythmic contraction and relaxation of the longitudinal and circular layers of smooth *muscles*. This muscular action moves objects in a particular direction. It is the process whereby *food* is passed through the oesophagus into the *stomach* and by which it is pushed along the *alimentary canal*.

personal care: the *care* which meets the personal needs of a client such as:
- personal *hygiene* – washing and bathing
- continence management – toileting
- nutrition – feeding and special diets
- supporting *mobility* – walking using mobility aids, e.g. *Zimmer frames*
- assisting with medication
- personal assistance – dressing, undressing, getting up and going to bed
- *counselling* and support.

(See *nursing care*.)

person-centred care places the *service user* at the centre of decision making with regard to their care. This ensures that the individual needs of the service user are met and that they are given the individual care that they require. (See *individual needs*.)

personal preferences identify the preferred *choices* of the *service user* which are appropriate to their needs.

personal social services provide care for vulnerable people including *client* groups with *special needs* such as older people, children and the disabled. *Local authorities* have statutory responsibilities to provide care for these clients. For example, *social workers*, home helps, *residential homes* for older people.

personal space: the physical separation between one person and another which is both culturally and individually determined. It is an important aspect of *communication*. When a person stands too close to another while they are in conversation, it may be viewed as intimidating, especially if the conversation is between two people who do not know each other well. Personal space and positive communication practice rely on:
- the distance between people; too close is viewed as intimidating, too far can be viewed as the person being disinterested or 'stand-offish'

- the different culture patterns of **behaviour**
- body language and **gestures** used
- how well people know each other.

Learning what is acceptable in terms of personal space is an important aspect of working with people and is a skill which should be developed. Students should spend time observing communication in different settings. They should also evaluate what they feel is an invasion of their own personal space. (See **observation, non-verbal communication, interaction**.)

personality: the characteristics or traits of an individual that underline consistencies in the way that they behave over time and in different situations. (See **introversion, extroversion, Eysenck**).

pH scale: this indicates the degree of acidity or alkalinity of a solution. It is particularly important for **carers** and **nurses** when they are testing the pH of a patient's **urine** as the results can contribute to a clinical picture of a patient's medical condition. It is a simple test to perform. It involves using a small plastic strip with pH-sensitive areas which is dipped into the patient's urine sample and left for the time specified. The resulting colour change gives the pH of the urine and provides an indication of how the **kidneys** are functioning. The kidneys play a vital part in regulating acid levels.

phagocytosis: the process used by **white blood cells** to engulf the micro-organisms which attack the body.

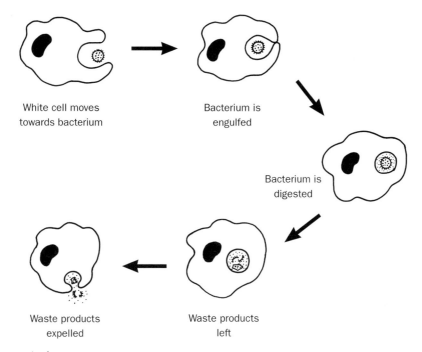

White cell moves towards bacterium

Bacterium is engulfed

Bacterium is digested

Waste products expelled

Waste products left

Phagocytosis

pharmacists are professionals qualified in the field of **drugs** and medication. They are trained to dispense doctors' prescriptions and may also sell medicines for minor ailments. People often ask a pharmacist for advice with regard to mild medical ailments. In order to carry out their roles and responsibilities pharmacists have an indepth knowledge of drugs and their impact on the body, as well as any adverse reactions that drugs may cause. There are three different categories of medicines which the pharmacist will manage:

- prescription-only medicines – as their name implies, these medicines are only available on a prescription written by a doctor and are dispensed by a pharmacist from approved premises
- pharmacy medicines – only available for sale from a pharmacy under the supervision of the pharmacist
- general sales list medicines – these are freely available from pharmacies and other retail outlets, such as supermarkets.

physical disability: a disorder, *disease* or *dysfunction* which affects or restricts movement and co-ordination of one or more parts of the body. Physical disabilities can be:

- congenital – present at birth, e.g. congenital dislocation of the hip
- *genetic* – passed through the generations, e.g. *Huntington's disease*
- acquired – through accident, disease or a disorder which occurs at any time in a person's life, e.g. *multiple sclerosis*.

physical growth and development: the way in which the body increases in size, e.g. height and weight, and its ability to perform tasks and activities. As a child's *bones* and *muscles* grow and develop, his or her muscular co-ordination will also increase. Growth and development are rapid during the first year of life and then steady throughout the childhood years. During *puberty*, there is a sharp increase in the growth of secondary sexual characteristics. Following late teens and early adult life, growth begins to slow down. Progress should be monitored from the day that a baby is born. A child's height and weight may be regularly checked by the local *primary health care team*. (See *centile chart, motor skills, sensory skills*.)

physical life quality factors are requirements which enhance the physical *well-being* of a *service user*. They include *exercise*, a *balanced diet*, a safe environment, freedom from pain and physical discomfort. It is important to add that these factors will differ in detail between service users.

physical play: a type of activity which stimulates a child's physical growth and *muscle* control. Physical play encourages co-ordination and movement which develops gross motor skills. Gross motor skills involve limb movements which use the large *muscles* of the body. Such movements include running, walking, skipping and jumping. There are various groups which promote physical play and related activities, such as Tumble Tots and Jungle Gyms. (See *play, outdoor play*.)

physical skills: see *motor skills*.

Physically Handicapped and Able Bodied (PHAB) is a voluntary organisation which integrates people with and without *physical disabilities*. Their aim is to promote and encourage everyone, whether they have physical disabilities or not, to share activities together. One of the functions of the organisation is to arrange holidays. They view this as an excellent example of bringing disabled and able-bodied people together on equal terms.

physiology: the science which is the study of the functions of the various parts of the body. (See *anatomy*.)

physiotherapist: a qualified professional who treats disorders with physical means. These include methods such as the application of heat, *ultrasound*, electro-therapy, massage and manipulation to help individuals maintain and develop movement and *mobility*.

Such methods can assist in rehabilitating patients. Physiotherapists may work in the **NHS (National Health Service)**, or in the **independent sector**. They train for three years to achieve qualified status.

Piaget's theory of cognitive development supports the view that **play** can be used to reinforce a child's cognitive or learning experience. Early sensori–motor co-ordination may help children to understand the **symbolic** world in which they live, thus encouraging co-operation, and co-operative play. At each stage of Piaget's theory, **imagination** is to be encouraged by parents, teachers and others. Toys and **games** should develop problem-solving skills, muscle development and **hand–eye co-ordination**. Play develops and enhances a child's learning.

Piaget's three stages

Stage	Age	Development
Stage 1 Sensori-motor stage	0–2 years	The developing child uses their senses to discover the world around him/her. Senses such as sight, hearing, touch, taste and smell. As an example, a baby will often put objects in its mouth.
Stage 2 Pre-operational stage	2–7 years	During this stage the child is developing different skills such as hand–eye co-ordination and problem solving. Children learn through their imagination and 'let's pretend play'. Language development enhances this stage.
Stage 3 Concrete operations stage	7 years and over	The child develops skills which involve working with rules, sharing responsibilities with others and taking turns.

pictogram: a method of presenting data collected from **research**. The results are illustrated using a **bar chart** with the length of the bar modified to show a line of pictures or images.

Pictogram: the number of children who went to see Santa Claus in various department stores on December 22

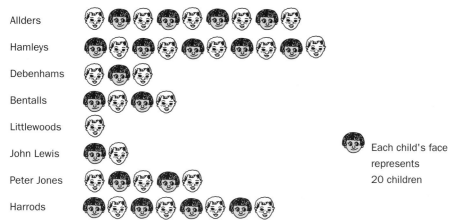

A pictogram

P.I.E.S. refers to the physical, intellectual, emotional and social development of individuals through their **life stages**.

pie chart: a method of presenting data collected from research. A full circle is drawn. The relative quantities of different data alternatives are represented as sectors of the circle. The sectors vary in size according to the frequency of the results. By this means the results of *quantitative research* can be shown in an easily understandable way.

pituitary gland is a small *gland* situated at the base of the *brain*. It is attached to the hypothalamus by a short stem. It is called the 'master gland' because its secretions affect the functions of all the other endocrine glands. It has two lobes which are the:
- anterior lobe – produces growth hormone, prolactin, follicle-stimulating hormone, thyroid-stimulating hormone, and adrenocorticotropic hormone, ACTH (see *endocrine system*)
- posterior lobe – produces antidiuretic hormone and oxytocin.

placenta: the mass of *tissue* which develops within the *uterus* of a *pregnant* woman. It contains *blood* vessels. *Oxygen* and nutrients are passed from the mother into the developing foetus. Waste products and *carbon dioxide* are passed from the foetus into the mother's blood supply to be excreted. The blood supply from the mother runs alongside the blood supply from the foetus, i.e. maternal and foetal blood supplies are different.

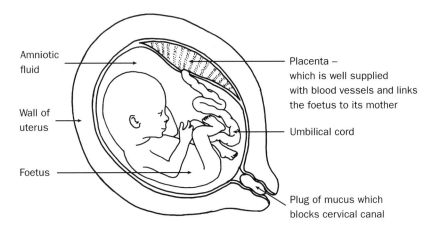

A developing foetus and placenta

placement: see *work experience*.

Placing Assessment and Counselling Teams (PACTs) are teams set up to help people with disabilities to find a job and to go to work as part of the access to work scheme. This scheme is available in job centres but it is the PACT that support applications and give advice.

plasma is a straw-coloured fluid in the blood which contains 90% water. Plasma also contains the following:
- proteins such as fibrinogen (aids *blood clotting*), serum albumin (absorbs materials in the blood) and serum globulin (antibodies)
- prothrombin which is an enzyme which aids blood clotting
- inorganic materials such as chlorides and phosphates
- digested food in the form of glucose and *amino acids*
- nitrogenous wastes as a result of metabolism in the tissues.

platelets are tiny structures found in blood *plasma*. They are irregularly shaped and colourless. They are produced in the red *bone marrow* and have an important function in *blood clotting*. There are approximately 250,000 per cubic millimetre of *blood*.

play is the activity through which children discover the world around them. It occupies an important part in a child's life. It stimulates physical, intellectual, emotional, social and cultural development. It promotes a child's ability to learn and develop different skills, such as *hand–eye co-ordination*. Play helps a child relate to other children through talking, sharing and taking turns. Making and building objects gives a child a sense of achievement and therefore helps them to develop a positive *self-esteem*.

There are several types of play which include:
- *physical play*
- play with different natural materials such as sand, water, dough, clay and wood
- construction play with blocks, building bricks and kits
- *creative play* such as painting and collage
- imaginative play, involving drama, acting out and role modelling
- *music and singing* and *storytelling*.

Play has different stages such as:
- solitary play – a baby will play on its own
- parallel play – the small child sits or stands next to another child. Children will play alongside, but do not interact with each other
- co-operative play – the child seeks out the company of other children. They play various games and carry out activities together
- *games* with rules – the children work within the guidelines or rules making games more complicated. (See *Piaget's theory of cognitive development*.)

Benefits of play include creating a sense of satisfaction and positive *self-esteem*, discovering the world around them, diverting inappropriate *behaviour*, encouraging development skills, preventing boredom and reducing *stress*. (See *symbolic play*.)

play therapy: the way in which *play* is utilised as a form of treatment in order to support a child. This may take different forms such as:
- supporting treatment for a child with a physical disorder – gentle physical *exercise* may be the ideal follow-up treatment following a leg operation, for example playing a stretching *game* can be a means whereby a child has fun during their exercises
- relief of pain – providing different and stimulating activities can help support a child who is in pain either from their condition or following an operation
- a method of diagnosing a child's *behaviour* problem – a child may display what they are secretly worried about; this is frequently used when *child abuse* is suspected when the child is given different toys to play with, including anatomically correct dolls
- a form of treatment – when a child has a lot of frustrated or pent-up feelings; play can be a satisfactory way of releasing these feelings.

playgroups: see *pre-school groups*.

playworkers are individuals who are either trained or experienced in the area of children's *play*. They form part of a team which provides opportunities for children's play in different childcare settings. They work closely with youth workers but are usually associated with the age group of children from 3 to 15 years of age. They are based mainly in adventure playgrounds, play centres, community projects, children's wards in hospitals, **after-school clubs** and holiday play schemes. Play work involves creating a safe and happy **environment** which supports children's **creative, imaginative** and social development.

poisoning occurs when a dangerous **chemical** or substance has been taken into the body causing physical distress and harm. Poisons can enter the body in a number of ways which include:
- eating and swallowing contaminated **foods**, **drugs** or chemicals
- inhaling, breathing in poisons from the atmosphere, or through vapours and **solvents**
- absorbing poisons such as garden fungicides, through the **skin**
- poison injected into the skin such as from snake bites
- poison produced in the body, i.e. the body has an allergic response to 'toxins' which it produces itself.

police officers are responsible for maintaining law and order and ensuring that the public and their property are protected. They investigate **crimes** and are concerned with crime prevention. They work with other professionals to maintain the **criminal justice system** within the United Kingdom.

policies are statements which are written to describe how an organisation intends to function in terms of good practice. Some policies such as **equal opportunities policies** are underpinned by **legislation**. Other policies include **confidentiality**, on **harassment** and anti-**bullying**. Policies are implemented by raising staff awareness through recruitment, induction training and during subsequent employment. Policies should be implemented, monitored, evaluated and reviewed in order to ensure that they are fostering positive attitudes between staff and service users. Policies influence national and local care by:
- improving practice
- encouraging joined-up thinking, i.e. professionals working together in terms of the direction of care practice
- changing and adapting the level and pattern of provision
- using funding to target national priorities.

polio (poliomyelitis): an infectious **disease** formerly called infantile paralysis, which is caused by a **virus**. After initial flu-like symptoms, the virus can attack the **spinal cord**, causing **muscle** paralysis which can affect any part of the body. Polio can be prevented by **vaccination** followed by a booster vaccination.

pollution: the release of poisonous substances, fluids and vapours into the environment. These can have harmful effects on the soil upsetting natural processes, the atmosphere, rivers and oceans. Substances causing such problems are known as pollutants. Examples of pollution include the accidental release of chemicals as a result of an industrial process.

polysaccharides: **carbohydrates** consisting of many sugar units which are chemically linked or bonded together in long chains. Examples are starch and glycogen. Starch is found in most human **diets. Foods** containing starch include bread, potatoes, rice and pasta.

polyunsaturated fats: molecules of **fat** which occur in plant and animal cells. High levels are found in nuts, nut oil and fish. **Diets** containing high proportions of such fats have been linked with low blood **cholesterol** levels in some populations.

portage is a home teaching programme for children with **special needs** and their parents. Set up in America in the 1960s, it involves a specially trained portage worker who supports the family by:

- carefully explaining developmental areas such as **language**, motor skills, **cognitive** skills, stimulation, self-help and **socialisation**
- working in partnership with parents to produce a learning programme for a child with a number of tasks to be achieved
- helping a child to achieve the tasks set in a learning programme by breaking them down into smaller and more manageable actions, for example, the task of doing up a button will be broken down into several smaller movements, and over a period of time the child works towards achieving each of these until eventually the task can be completed as a whole. All effort is accompanied by a lot of encouragement and positive reinforcement
- ensuring that tasks are realistic for the child concerned, i.e. that they are not too difficult nor too easy
- encouraging the parent to reinforce the task at different times in the week when there is opportunity to sit quietly with the child and work together.

All successes are carefully recorded and enjoyed by all those involved. The portage scheme can be used with children with a variety of **disabilities**. (See **children with disabilities**.)

positive care environment is one which provides the appropriate care for its **service users**. It maintains this by:

- implementing the **care value base**
- using **effective communication** between service users and their carers (see **strategies for effective communication**)
- fostering positive relationships and **building confidence** and trust
- challenging **discrimination**
- ensuring the appropriate **policies** and procedures are in place
- training staff and updating their knowledge
- ensuring that records are accurate and securely stored, and monitoring the sharing of **information**.

(See **care environment and care context**.)

post-natal care: care given to a mother and her baby following birth. The **primary health care team** will monitor the progress of the mother and baby.

post-natal depression: a psychological disorder characterised by a new mother feeling sad, worthless and overwhelmed by motherhood. Mothers with post-natal depression need medical supervision, support and practical help.

post-traumatic stress disorder: an **anxiety** disorder arising from a situation which has occurred in the life of the victim. This can be the result of:

- an accident such as a car or train accident
- a frightening event such as a fire or bombing
- being involved in a war or a disaster involving many casualties.

The **victim** suffers persistent recurrence of images, mind pictures and nightmares. This can lead to insomnia, feelings of isolation, loss of concentration and guilt. Victims need support and *counselling* to help them come to terms with these incidents. (See *victim support*.)

posture is the position in which the *muscles* of the body support the *skeleton* when standing, sitting, walking or working. In every muscle there are fibres which are continually contracted to create muscle tension, or muscle tone. Muscle tone is responsible for keeping the muscles ready for immediate contraction and keeping the body in an upright position without conscious thought. Upright posture is maintained by the contraction of both the flexor and extensor muscles holding *bones* and *joints* in position. When the body is held upright with the minimum of muscular effort, the distribution of body weight on the hips and leg bones keeps the body balanced. This is regarded as good posture. Posture can be affected by weight, a poor working environment, inadequate seating or shoes and clothes which do not fit properly. Posture is maintained through *exercise*, *balanced diet* and a healthy *lifestyle*.

poverty: a state of being with little or no money or other resources. It can be applied to an individual, group or country. Two types of poverty can be distinguished:

- absolute poverty – where there is not enough money to pay for food, water and any form of shelter. This type of poverty exists in some developing countries
- relative poverty – where there is not enough money to support a certain standard of living. This person may have an income which is much lower than others in the population. People may not be able to pay for an adequate diet and housing. Relative poverty is often closely linked to unemployment.

poverty trap is the way in which people on low incomes may become even worse off financially. This is due to the fact that a small increase in wages or salary begins to affect their eligibility for *means-tested* benefit that they previously received, so trapping them in relative *poverty*.

practice nurses are qualified *nurses* who are based at a GP's surgery. Their role includes supporting:

- *older people* with *chronic* health problems such as leg ulcers
- patients requiring holiday vaccination programmes
- *health promotion*, e.g. asthma clinics
- routine health checks and *immunisations*
- well man and well woman clinics.

pre-coding is a method used to analyse answers provided in a *questionnaire*.

pre-conceptional education is advice to a woman who is preparing to conceive. This involves ensuring that the woman knows about:

- eating a balanced and healthy *diet*
- taking a folic acid supplement
- giving up *smoking* cigarettes and not drinking *alcohol*
- not taking any *drugs* or medicines which could harm a developing *embryo*.

pregnancy: the period of time, normally 40 weeks, extending from *conception* and the date of the last menstrual period to a baby's *birth*.

pre-judgement: see *assumption*.

prejudice: preconceived ideas about a person based on attitudes and *beliefs* which lead to discriminatory behaviour and practice. (See *attitudes, discrimination*.)

pre-menstrual syndrome: a number of signs and symptoms which may affect a woman about 7–10 days before a period. These include:

- feeling irritable and tense
- feeling nervous and anxious
- feeling bloated, especially around the abdomen
- headaches
- increased tiredness and lethargy.

Treatment may involve taking oil of evening primrose and vitamin supplements.

pre-natal development is growth of the unborn baby which takes place in the mother's *womb*. The three stages of prenatal development are as follows:

Stage	Pre-natal development
1 Germinal	Following fertilisation, there is rapid cell division
2 Embryonic	The major body systems and organs begin to develop and take shape
3 Foetal	The bone cells appear with rapid growth and changes in body form

pre-school groups offer care and early education to children under five years on a sessional or full day basis. They can be run privately as small businesses or as registered charities. Pre-school groups follow the *Early Years Curriculum* and are inspected on a regular basis by the *Office for Standards in Education* (OFSTED). Most pre-school groups can cater for children with *special education needs*.

pressure groups are groups who 'lobby' parliament or local government on different issues or areas of concern in society. They are set up to:

- highlight the needs of individuals and groups in society
- investigate ways in which legislation can be introduced to support those whom they represent
- explore ways of improving services.

Example of pressure groups are *Age Concern, Child Poverty Action Group*.

pressure points are points in the body where an *artery* crosses a *bone* (see diagram overleaf). In cases of severe bleeding from a limb, indirect pressure can be applied to a pressure point above a bleeding artery. For example, in severe bleeding from a wound in the lower arm, indirect pressure can be applied to the brachial pressure point (source: St John Ambulance 1997). (See *pulse*.)

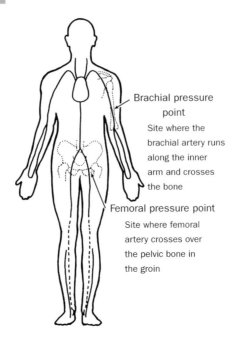

Brachial pressure
point
Site where the
brachial artery runs
along the inner
arm and crosses
the bone

Femoral pressure point
Site where femoral
artery crosses over
the pelvic bone in
the groin

Pressure points

preventive care: strategies which are in place to prevent the need for future medical care, e.g. *immunisation*.

primary care trusts are groups of professional carers such as GPs and nurses working together in a locality. These were set up under NHS reforms in 1997. The functions of primary care trusts are to:

- contribute to the health authority's *health improvement programmes* on health and healthcare, helping to ensure that they reflect the needs of the local community and the experience of patients
- promote the health of the local population
- commission health services in their area from the relevant *NHS trust* within the framework of the health improvement programmes
- develop primary care by means of joint working across practices, skills sharing and deployment of resources.

In April 2002, PCTs were made responsible for control of local health care.

primary health care team: the health professionals who care for individuals in the community. They usually include GPs, health visitors, community nurses, midwives, dentists, pharmacists, optometrists and ophthalmic medical practitioners.

privacy: one of the principal needs of a *patient* or *client* who is being looked after by health or social care workers. Clients may occasionally need to be alone and to have some time to sort out their affairs. Some clients wish to retain some *information* which is private to them. Patients and clients often need privacy when they are being toileted. If it is impossible for the client to be left alone, then *carers* should make sure that the client is covered and that the toilet door is closed. Carers should be sensitive to the fact that privacy is a way in which clients can retain some of their own personal *identity*.

private sector: consists of organisations set up to provide health, education and social care services 'at a price'. They are income-generating and profit-making services and can include:

- public and independent *schools*
- health insurance companies
- some *hospitals*
- childcare providers
- private care homes and hostels
- *complementary and alternative medicine*
- some *screening* services.

(See *independent sector.*)

prognosis: a prediction of how a *disease* may take its course from beginning to end. It allows for the fact that it will differ between *patients* because of factors such as:

- impact of the disease on the body
- progression of the disease
- changes to care strategies.

prostate cancer: this is a *cancer* of the prostate gland, which is to be found at the base of the male *bladder*.

Protection of Vulnerable Adults (POVA) is a *policy* which has been introduced by the government to ensure that vulnerable adults are protected from possible harm. It does this by raising the quality of care through the *National Service Frameworks* and by regulating providers of care so that the care which service users are given meets *national minimum standards*. The policy applies to adult placement schemes, care agencies, registered service providers of care and employment agencies, as well as businesses who supply workers to these providers. Providers are required, as part of the *Criminal Record Bureau* application process, to check that potential workers are not on the POVA list which contains the names of people who are unsuitable to work with vulnerable adults. Care providers are also required to refer care workers who have harmed vulnerable adults in their care for inclusion on the list. All care providers must ensure that a copy of the relevant guidance is available to staff and that staff are advised accordingly. (See *Safeguarding Vulnerable Groups Act 2006.*)

proteins: important substances required by the body to support almost all its functions. Proteins contain the elements *carbon, hydrogen, oxygen*, nitrogen, phosphorus and sulphur. The units from which protein molecules are built are called amino acids. There are 21 different *amino acids* present in the human body. The amino acids are linked together by peptide bonds to form long chain molecules. The shape of the chain and the sequence in which the amino acids are linked together determines the function of the protein. Protein is an essential part of a healthy diet and is used to promote growth and to replace and repair body cells and tissues. The main source of protein is found in meat, dairy produce, fish, nuts and in smaller quantities, vegetables (particularly some cereals and beans).

providers are any organisations which provide health and social care services. This could be, for example, *NHS trusts*, *GPs*, *voluntary* and *private sector* organisations and some parts of *personal social services*.

psychiatric service: a branch of the health service which specialises in the detection, diagnosis and treatment of *mental health disorders*.

psychiatrist: a qualified *doctor* who has chosen to specialise in the area of *mental health*. Psychiatrists work with people suffering from *mental health disorders* and those with *learning disabilities*. They often work in a team of other professionals including *psychologists* and *occupational therapists*.

psychological life quality factors are requirements which enhance the psychological well-being of a service user. These include *effective communication*, *choice*, *dignity*, *privacy*, *autonomy*, *social support networks*, *trust*, *confidentiality* and *affection*.

psychologist: a professional trained to observe and interpret both normal and abnormal human behaviour. A psychologist has specialist training following the completion of a psychology degree. They can work as:
- clinical psychologists – dealing with *patients* in the treatment of *mental health disorders*
- *educational psychologists* – supporting the emotional needs and problems of children and young people up to the age of 19 years
- occupational psychologists – advising organisations on the different job training needs of service users
- criminological and legal psychologists – in prisons, special *hospitals*, youth custody centres and secure units.

puberty: changes which occur in the body during the teenage years. Young people develop secondary sexual characteristics due to the release of certain *hormones* into the bloodstream. (See *adolescence*.)

Secondary sexual characteristics which develop in males and females during puberty

Males	Females
Growth spurt	Growth spurt
Hair growth on chest, in the axilla and on the pubic areas	Hair growth in the axilla and on the pubic areas
Shoulders broaden and hips narrow	Development of breasts. Hips broaden and body curves occur
Enlargement of penis, scrotum and testes	Menstruation or periods commence
Can perform an erection of the penis and ejaculation of sperm	

public health: the maintenance of *health* in society. This involves a number of regulations relating to social, political, economic and environmental hazards. Public health is monitored by *environmental health officers* and the *Health and Safety Executive*. Different legislation supports its requirements and procedures. Each *strategic health authority* has a public health department responsible for monitoring the well-being of the local population. Public health policy and practice is concerned with:
- controlling communicable disease
- developing programmes to reduce risk and screen for early disease
- developing *policies* which promote the health of the population
- identifying the health needs of the population

- monitoring the health status of the community
- planning and evaluating the national provision of health and social care.

Factors relating to public health include:

- links between social change, *lifestyle* choices and emerging public health topics such as increasing *obesity,* the occurrence of certain *cancers*, *drug misuse*, *mental health disorders* and *sexually transmitted diseases*
- patterns and inequalities of health and illness experience within the population in the United Kingdom
- possible causes and explanations for patterns of health as well as recent changes in the public health status of the population of the United Kingdom.

Public Health (Control of Disease) Act 1984 and the Public Health (Infectious Diseases) Regulations 1988: a legal requirement for doctors to report any *notifiable diseases* to the *Department of Health*.

public health strategies are methods used to implement public health policies. Strategies used in the United Kingdom include measures that:

- aim to reduce the environmental harm of industrial, household and biological waste products through water, sewage and air treatment processes
- aim to protect the population from infectious diseases (*notifiable diseases*) through *disease surveillance*, *immunisation* and *screening programmes* and to reduce *inequalities of health*
- are taken by local authorities and central government with regard to action on recycling and waste
- highlight *food safety*
- support and protect the national environment
- are taken by environment protection agencies, environmental health officers and public health staff in monitoring and implementing public and environmental health policies and legislation
- are taken by pressure groups such as Greenpeace, and international governmental organisations such as the World Health Organisation, to monitor and respond to global environmental and public health issues.

pulse: rhythm produced by the regular pumping of *blood* by the *heart*. The pulse can be taken by placing a finger on the spots where an artery crosses the bone (see *pressure points*), for instance in the wrist, the groin and the neck. The normal pulse rate for an adult is approximately 70–80 beats per minute. It is faster in a baby or child, usually between 100 and 120 beats per minute. The pulse is usually recorded at the wrist (the radial pulse) or at the neck (the carotid pulse) when an emergency arises.

purchasers are organisations with the responsibility to buy health and social care services from health and social care providers.

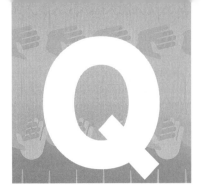

qualitative data: information which cannot be recorded in numerical form. The *data* collected relates to the views, *attitudes* and *values* of the respondent. Qualitative data is usually collected through *interviews*. It can also be gathered in other ways, e.g. from secondary sources of information, such as textbooks or research documents.

quality assurance: a framework of standards set up by organisations to maintain a professional service in health and social care. It includes the management and monitoring of a service through:

- auditing and identifying poor service provision
- dealing with and responding to complaints
- detailing individual roles and responsibilities of workers and managers
- listening to service users
- responding and giving feedback to service users.

quality assurance mechanisms are systems set up by organisations to ensure that they have *quality assurance* measures in place. These include:

- developing *complaints procedures*
- evaluating the quality of services through surveys by service users, e.g. patient *surveys*
- improving information and consultation with service users, e.g. 'Your guide to the NHS'
- implementing quality service standards, e.g. *national service frameworks*
- improving registration and inspection procedures, e.g. *OFSTED*
- rewarding good practice, e.g. *Charter Mark*
- using performance ratings, e.g. *star ratings*.

quality of life: the daily way of living which is created by the client, patient and service users and their carers. It relates to the physical, psychological, social, spiritual and emotional *health and well-being* of the individual. Carers have a vital role to play in ensuring the quality of life for their clients in terms of physical care, emotional support, social contact and the provision of interesting and stimulating activities to promote *cognitive development*. (See *life quality factors*.)

quantitative data: information which can be collated in numerical form. The *data* is recorded in the form of graphs and *charts*.

quarantine is the separation from others of people who have an infectious disease (*notifiable disease*). Patients are isolated for a few days longer than the incubation period of the disease.

(See *methicillin-resistant Staphylococcus aureus*.)

questioning: a procedure which involves asking people questions on a specific topic or subject. Its aim is to ensure that the questions asked are suitable to obtain objective answers and to provide the researcher or carer with the required *information*. There are different types of questions which can be asked. They include:

- opinion or attitude questions – those which ask about the respondent's beliefs, values and attitudes
- closed questions – those which have a single or a fixed set of answers
- open questions – those which, when asked, enable the respondents to answer in their own words, the questions reflect views and opinions and can be a means whereby qualitative research is collected
- probes – a form of questioning designed to extract more detailed information from the respondent; they can be used to deal with response problems and can be used to clarify an answer
- prompts – a statement which aids questioning techniques; the researcher may repeat questions in order to reinforce the respondent's understanding of the information being sought in the answer.

Questioning is used in many different aspects of *caring*, e.g. as part of the *care planning* process. (See *listening skills*.)

questionnaire: a list of questions which is used to collect data. Questions in a questionnaire should:

- be structured in such a way that the researcher gains the information required
- be ordered so that they reflect the breadth of the research
- be short and to the point
- be reviewed to ensure that there is limited or no bias in the wording
- not be embarrassing or intrusive.

The questions used can be open or closed. Questionnaires can take a number of forms:

- self-completion in a given situation. The questionnaire is completed and returned immediately
- postal questionnaires. The returns on these are often slow, making it an inefficient way of achieving results
- part of a simplified interview technique where the researcher ticks off answers for the respondent.

Questionnaires are a means whereby large numbers of individuals can be given an opportunity to participate in a research project.

quota sampling: a *sampling* method where a specific selection of people in the population is chosen for use in a research project. This ensures that targeted groups of people are involved in the research representing appropriate categories by age, race, class and gender. Interviewers are given lists of people to interview from each category.

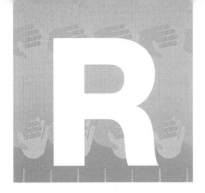

race is a broad term given to individuals and groups who are identified by their *culture* and ethnic grouping. This may include sharing similar biological features such as *skin* colour and hair type. These days, ethnic grouping is a term which is also used. The focus for *ethnic groups* tends to be on cultural similarity rather than on a set of physical features.

Race Relations Acts 1976 and 2000: Acts of Parliament which makes it illegal to discriminate against anyone on the grounds of their colour, race, nationality or ethnic origin. The Acts are enforced in the following way:

- if a person is discriminated against on racial grounds they can go to a county court. If the alleged *discrimination* is in the field of employment then they can also go to an *industrial tribunal*.

In 2000, the Act was amended in England by placing a statutory general duty on local authorities and other public bodies to eliminate unlawful discrimination and to promote equal opportunities and good race relations. Then, in 2003, the Race Relations Act 1976 (Amendment) Regulations 2003 were brought in to strengthen the Race Relations Act 1976.

Race Relations Act (Northern Ireland) 1976 and 1997: legislation which acts against discrimination on grounds of colour, race, nationality or ethnic or national origin. The Irish Traveller community is specifically identified in the Order as a racial group against which racial discrimination is unlawful.

racism: *discrimination* and unfair treatment on the basis of *race*. It can take the form of:

- racist language where name calling can be upsetting and destructive to the *self-esteem* of the person concerned
- behaviour which involves ignoring another person; this can create embarrassment (see *discrimination*)
- rejection in terms of employment. For instance, individuals from certain racial groups may apply for advertised jobs and then be told that vacancies have been filled even though the potential employer continues to advertise.

radiographers: specially trained, but not medically qualified, professionals who work in *multi-disciplinary teams* led by radiologists. They mainly work in *hospitals* as:

- diagnostic radiographers – carrying out a range of procedures such as using *X-rays, computed axial tomography* (CAT) scans, *ultrasound* and *magnetic resonance imaging* (MRI)
- therapeutic radiographers – administering radiation treatment to patients as prescribed by the doctor.

Training as a radiographer usually involves three years of full-time study at degree level.

radiologist: a trained *doctor* who works in the radiology department of a *hospital*.

radiology: methods of detecting or treating *disease* using radiation. It can involve the use of *X-rays* for diagnosis such as radio diagnosis or diagnostic radiology, and treatment (radiotherapy) but also incorporates many other methods of diagnostic imaging and treatment. The two separate branches of the specialty are now called:

- clinical radiology – involves patients undergoing X-rays including CAT scans and other diagnostic procedures such as *ultrasound* and *magnetic resonance imaging* (MRI)
- clinical oncology – involves patients undergoing ionising radiation treatment mainly for *malignant* disease (i.e. X-rays, radium and other medical methods).

radiotherapy: a method of treating malignant *disease* such as *cancer* or *tumours* using radiation. *X-rays* are intensified and their beams are directed onto the area where *treatment* is required. In some diseases radium needles or rods are inserted into the tumour or the area of disease. Another treatment using radium involves the patient drinking radioactive liquid.

ranking: a method applied in research with regard to *data* collection. Ranking is used in the recording of the results of *questionnaires* when the researcher wants to measure the degree of the respondents' *attitudes*, views and *beliefs*.

rating scale: a method used to record answers to closed questions when collecting results for research. The respondents indicate their opinion by choosing the appropriate scale point.

rationale: the reason for any form of research or investigation. In health and social care there are many subjects which can be researched.

recommended dietary allowance: (RDA) the suggested average daily intake of a nutrient for healthy people in a population. (See *Committee on Medical Aspects of Food Policy*.)

records are the way in which information is maintained about individual patients, *clients* and *service users*. Any records which are kept may take the form of:

- hand-written notes – reports stored in a filing system
- computerised records – letters and reports written and stored on a hard disk, CD or data stick.

Whatever form of recording is used, access to information and confidentiality is protected by legislation (see *Data Protection Acts 1984 and 1998*). Records should be therefore maintained in a secure place; they are legal documents and can be used in court.

recovery position is the position in which a person is placed when they are unconscious. This position prevents the tongue from blocking the throat and, because the head is slightly lower than the rest of the body, it allows liquid to drain away from the mouth and reduces the risk of the casualty inhaling the stomach contents. The head, neck and back are kept aligned, while the bent limbs keep the body propped in a comfortable and secure position. Placing the unconscious person in the recovery position is usually carried out by a trained first aider. For health and social care students, learning about first aid is an important health and safety requirement which will enhance their care practice.

(Source: *First Aid Manual*.)

red blood cells (erythrocytes) are cells produced in the red *bone marrow* in the long *bones* and the ribs, vertebrae and the skull. The red pigment in the cells is called *haemoglobin*. Red cells remain functional for approximately 120 days. When they die they are broken down in the *spleen*. They are biconcave in shape and carry *oxygen* and some *carbon dioxide* in the haemoglobin. The average person has a million red cells per cubic millimetre of blood.

redress: see *systems of redress*.

referencing: a method of identifying sources of material used in *research* and assignment writing. It is important to reference all work that is not one's own. Place a list of all source material at the end of the research work or assignment, using the following system to reference books:

- author(s) or editors name(s) (year the book was published), *title of the book,* edition if not the first, town or city the book was published in, name of publisher; e.g. Richards J. (2003) *Complete A-Z Health & Social Care Handbook,* 2nd edition, Tonbridge, Hodder Arnold.

When referencing journal articles:

- author (year journal was published), title of article, *title of journal,* volume and issue numbers, page number(s); e.g. Jones D. (2007) *Journal of Health and Social Care*, 12(4), 45-46.

When referencing websites:

- title of website (year), *title of article* [online], HTML address [date accessed].

When referencing in the body of the assignment or research text:

- place quotation marks around the extract if taking words directly from the source, and then, in brackets, the author's surname, date of publication and page number.

referral to health care services: the means whereby a person has an appointment arranged for medical treatment or therapy. This can include:

- professional referral. Every person should be registered with a *general practitioner (GP)*. When there is a health need which requires hospital treatment, the GP refers the patient to a hospital consultant or specialist, e.g. a child with persistent earache and ear discharge will be passed on to a specialist for examination
- self-referral – the person refers him/herself, for example by making an appointment with the *dentist*
- compulsory referral – when a person's life is in danger, or they are a danger to others but refuse to accept treatment, they can be detained under legislation (*Mental Health Act 1983*)
- referral by others – the person is referred to the service by another person, e.g. a neighbour may be concerned about the way a child is being treated at home. If the neighbour contacts social services to report this, they have then referred the child to social services
- emergency referral – referral following an *accident*. If the patient is taken to *hospital* in an ambulance, the hospital staff will decide, when the patient reaches hospital, whether or not to admit the patient. Being taken to hospital in the ambulance is a way of referring the patient to the hospital service.

reflection: see *reflective practice*.

reflective practice: thinking about practice and looking for ways to improve and learn from experience so as to improve future practice. This can involve:

- reviewing one's own thoughts, *attitudes* and *beliefs*
- making an accurate analysis of practice, i.e. exploring relationships between colleagues and service users

- being able to evaluate practice, i.e. determining strengths and weaknesses and making changes
- reviewing all aspects of practice on a regular basis. This could involve writing a reflective log.

reflex action is a simple act of behaviour in which a stimulus provokes a response. The response is usually specific and short-lived.

reflex actions of the newborn: a number of automatic movements which are present in the first weeks of a baby's life. These movements include:

- sucking – when anything is placed in the baby's *mouth* it will immediately start sucking and swallowing
- grasp or palmar and plantar reflex – when an object is placed on the palm of the baby's hand its fingers will grip it firmly. Similarly, if an object is placed on the sole of the foot, the toes will curl around it
- moro or startle reflex – the way in which a baby will jerk in response to a sudden noise
- stepping reflex – when the baby is held upright on a flat surface, it will make stepping movements with its feet
- rooting reflex – when the side of the baby's cheek is stroked, it moves its head towards the movement as if searching for a nipple.

(See *newborn baby*.)

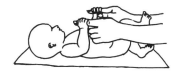

Sucking reflex

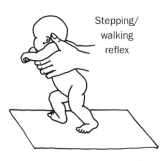

Stepping/ walking reflex

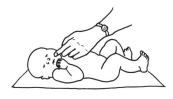

Grasp (palmar and plantar) reflex

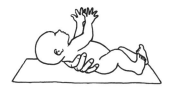

Moro/startle reflex

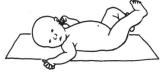

Rooting reflex

The reflex actions of the newborn

In addition, a newborn baby will communicate by crying, waving its arms and legs and turning its head from side to side.

After about three months these reflexes disappear and are replaced by more conscious and controlled movements. As a baby grows and develops, many different skills and responses have to be learned.

reflexes are the involuntary motor neurone responses to a stimulus, e.g. the act of sneezing in response to pollen or dust.

Stages involved in a reflex action

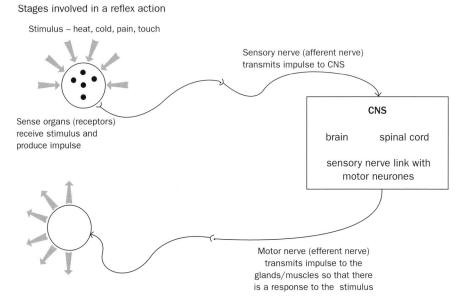

Reflexes

reflexology: a *complementary therapy* involving foot *massage* which can have a profound effect on the entire person. According to the principles of reflexology, the feet are a map of the body and dysfunction in any area of the body can be reflected there.

registered nurse: a trained professional who has completed a recognised training programme in nursing.

Regulations for Reporting of Injuries, Diseases and Dangerous Occurrences (RIDDOR) 1995 are regulations concerned with recording and reporting *accidents* and ill-health at work. When more than ten employees are based in the place of work, there must be an *accident book* to record:

- accidents
- sickness which may have been caused by work
- dangerous occurrences and 'near misses'.

Employers must report to the *Health and Safety Executive* or to the environmental health department of the local authority whenever the following events occur:

- fatal accidents
- a major injury or condition requiring medical treatment
- dangerous occurrences

- accidents causing incapacity for more than three days
- some work-related *diseases*
- gas incidents.

Many serious accidents and dangerous occurrences must be reported immediately, and a written report provided within seven days.

There are special forms which must be completed when diseases occur. There are 28 categories of reportable diseases including *poisoning, skin* and *lung* diseases.

Trade union safety representatives, if it is applicable, must have access to all information relating to all such problems in the workplace. The Employment Medical Advisory Service (EMAS), which is part of the Health and Safety Executive, gives *advice* and *information* on the reporting of diseases. In addition to these procedures, legislation exists designed to record and control diseases which are not necessarily linked to the place of work. Diagnosed cases of HIV and *AIDS* are reported in anonymous returns to the Centre of Communicable Diseases which is attached to the *Department of Health*. This centre is responsible for keeping statistics on HIV, AIDS and other diseases.

Regulatory Reform (Fire Safety) Order 2005: an Act of Parliament which ensures that those responsible for all workplaces carry out a specific fire *risk assessment* as part of their fire precautions.

rehabilitation: the development of procedures and a *care plan* which support *clients* or *patients* after any *accident*, surgery or any other form of medical treatment. Examples include:

- *physiotherapy* – if the person has suffered injury to a limb or part of the body in an accident, he/she will need physiotherapy and support in order to restore normal health and function. However, if full recovery is not possible, then they will be encouraged to organise their life to achieve as much independence as possible
- *occupational therapy* – when a person suffers from *depression*, for instance, they should be encouraged to pick up the threads of their life again. They may attend day centres, go shopping, learn to make decisions again and, if possible, return to *work*
- counselling therapy – following a disaster such as a fire, a person may need *counselling* to help them come to terms with what has happened.

Rehabilitation is an important part of any person's recovery as it is essential that the person learns to adapt and function again as an active member in society. This involves them being entitled to their own *rights and choices*. (See *activities of daily living*.)

RELATE: a confidential counselling service for people with relationship difficulties.

relationships: links and associations with others within the framework of society. These can include:

- Biological relationships – links with family, e.g. in family life they are important because they provide opportunities for individuals to learn about relating to others. It is where a child is loved and can learn to love in return. Family life should be a secure place for a child to develop physically, emotionally, socially, intellectually and culturally.
- Social relationships – links with friends and peers. The ability to build and maintain friendships is an important aspect of an individual's life. It provides opportunities to give and receive mutual support (see *network*).

- Formal working relationships within education and employment. The relationship between a manager and employee, or between a child and teacher, is not the same as that in a social or biological relationship. Learning and working together assists individuals to develop and mature.
- Sexual relationships – links involving a physical attraction for another person. Developing a close and intimate relationship should be a satisfying experience for those involved.
- Caring relationships **–** links supporting others either as a professional or *informal carer*.

Relationships are a major focus in the life of any individual. The ability to build positive relationships is closely linked to *self-esteem*. Every type has a code of *behaviour* attached. When this code is broken or violated, the relationship bonds are often broken and in some cases the damage is irreparable, for example, in some cases of child abuse. There are several organisations which offer support with regard to relationships.

relaxation techniques are used to reduce tension and *stress* in the body. There are a variety of methods such as:

- breathing *exercises*, creating even and controlled breathing which relaxes and calms the body
- forms of *muscle* relaxation exercises, such as tightening the muscles and then gently letting each muscle relax and extend
- lying in a candle-lit room on a comfortable bed, listening to quiet music
- using different lights and imagery to create a sense of peace and relaxation
- meditation or prayer
- yoga and specialised exercise programmes which are learned and practised
- different leisure pursuits
- a *massage* with soothing oils.

religion is regarded as a system of *beliefs*. Different religions have varying views on acts and displays of worship. Acknowledging an individual's personal beliefs and religious views is a key requirement in caring for people. (See *care value base*.)

reminiscence: sessions set up for *older people* which include discussion and information sharing. This usually involves sharing memorabilia from the past. In order to stimulate memory and discussion the group leader may produce a reminiscence box containing a number of items such as old pictures, coins and artefacts.

renal system: see *urinary system*.

reproductive system: see *male reproductive system* and *female reproductive system*.

research is a systematic investigation of a subject which involves gathering *data*, analysing results, drawing conclusions, writing reports and making recommendations. The purpose of research is to:

- review existing knowledge, exploring any changes in terms of additional analysis required to develop a deeper understanding of a subject
- describe a situation or problem, e.g. looking at specific needs in a population, community or group
- study a social science, psychology or scientific issue.

Research used in health and social care is valuable because it provides:

- epidemiological and census data which can be used in policy making and service planning
- experimental findings which can be invaluable in the development and testing of medical or other treatment interventions
- survey and interview research findings which can be used to assess **service user** satisfaction with local and national health and social care provisions.

Preparation for research involves:

- choosing a subject
- setting out a **hypothesis**, issue or research question
- writing aims and objectives
- selecting **research methods**
- considering ethical issues such as **confidentiality,** guaranteed **privacy, respect, trust,** written **consent**
- **record** keeping – references, sources and date and time of accessing internet sites
- checking that **data collection** of evidence is reliable, i.e. that it would produce the same results if repeated, valid, i.e. that it is a true picture of what is being researched, and unbiased, i.e. that the research is not carried out in a way that favours one group over another.

research methods: methods used to conduct research include:

- experiments
- questionnaires
- interviews
- observations.

research presentation: a suggested method by which research should be presented. The following outline could be used:

- presentation page with title
- abstract – brief summary
- introduction
- methodology – justifying choice of design including ethical issues
- presentation of data
- analysis of results
- conclusion and evaluation of research
- recommendations.

residential home: provides accommodation and personal care in a home for a range of client groups. There are usually no professional medical staff employed in the home but a GP or doctor is on call should the need arise. These homes are registered by the **local authority**. The care given in these homes is called residential care. (See **Home Life 1984, Better Home Life 1996.**)

resourcing of services: the methods used to ensure that adequate financial and human resources are available to the different health and social care services issues. Resourcing issues relate to:

- improving efficiency and effectiveness
- reviewing social welfare problems such as child care shortages, teenage pregnancies, and under-funding for older people, vulnerable people and those with mental health disorders.

respect is a caring quality in which a person is given and is seen to be given their rights. It includes:

- ensuring that the client has the *privacy* and space they need
- *listening* to the client, their requests, their conversation
- allowing the client the right to their personal beliefs
- retaining a client's right to **confidentiality**. (See **dignity**.)

Respect Task Force is a unit set up by the government to tackle **anti-social behaviour**. The task force works within the agenda of respect and helps communities, parents and young people to accept responsibility for their behaviour and supports appropriate and acceptable behaviour in society. The task force is supported by parents, children's services, police and teachers. It is hoped that this task force will encourage more responsible behaviour in young people and adults.

respiratory system: the system responsible for **breathing**. Respiration consists of two processes, external respiration and internal respiration.

External respiration (**gaseous exchange**) involves:

- taking air into the **lungs**. The **oxygen** from the air passes into the blood capillaries lining the lungs
- expelling **carbon dioxide** from the body. The carbon dioxide from the cells passes out of the blood capillaries lining the lungs and is breathed out.

Internal respiration involves:

- the release of energy through the breakdown of food. Oxygen is used in this process and carbon dioxide released.

The component parts of the human respiratory system are:

- larynx. The 'voice box' at the top of the trachea. It contains the vocal cords – two pieces of **tissue** folding inwards from the trachea lining and attached to plates of **cartilage**. The opening between the cords is called the glottis. During speech, **muscles** pull the cartilage plates (and the cords) together, and air passing out through the cords makes them vibrate, producing sounds
- trachea or windpipe. The main tube through which air passes on its way to and from the lungs
- bronchi (singular bronchus). The main tubes into which the trachea divides. The first two branches are the right and left primary bronchi. Each carries air into a lung, alongside a pulmonary artery bringing blood in. They then branch into secondary bronchi, tertiary bronchi and bronchioles, all accompanied by blood vessels, both branching from the pulmonary artery and merging to form pulmonary veins
- lungs. The two main breathing organs, inside which gases are exchanged. The lungs contain many tubes (bronchi and bronchioles) and air sacs (**alveoli**)
- bronchioles. The millions of tiny tubes in the lungs, all accompanied by blood vessels. They branch off tertiary bronchi and have smaller branches called terminal bronchioles, each one ending in a cluster of alveoli
- alveoli (singular alveolus). Millions of tiny sacs attached to terminal bronchioles. They are surrounded by **capillaries** (tiny blood vessels) whose blood is rich in carbon dioxide. The blood passes out through the capillary walls and in through the alveoli. The oxygen breathed into the alveoli passes into the capillaries, which then begin to merge together (eventually forming pulmonary veins) (see **mechanism of breathing**)

- pleura or pleural membrane. A layer of tissue surrounding each lung and lining the chest cavity (thorax). Between the two layers of pleura there is a space (pleural cavity) which contains fluid. The pleura and fluid-filled cavity make up a cushioning pleural sac
- *diaphragm*. A sheet of muscular tissue which separates the chest from the lower body, or *abdomen*. At rest, it lies in an arched position, forced up by the abdomen wall below it.

The respiratory rate is measured by watching and timing the chest rise and fall with inspiration and expiration. The normal rate is between 18 and 22 breaths a minute. Dysfunctions of the respiratory system cause bronchitis, pneumonia, *asthma*, colds and flu.

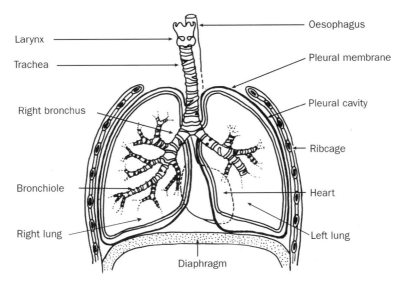

The respiratory system

respite care provides a service which offers regular breaks to *carers*. This is a valuable means of support for carers who are looking after relatives or friends on a long-term basis. Since the implementation of the *Carers (Recognition and Services) Act 1995* the value of respite care has been highlighted. It can take the form of:
- the client being cared for in a residential setting for one or two weeks so that the carer can take a holiday
- a professional or volunteer carer taking over for short periods so that the carer has some free time
- day centre care.

(See *caring for the carer, young carers*.)

respondent: the individual who participates in a project by answering questions in an interview or by filling in a questionnaire.

rest home: residential care which is available usually for older people who do not require nursing care. The home is registered with the local authority and the care is given by care assistants who are not necessarily qualified.

resuscitation: see *ABC of resuscitation*.

retirement: see *change*.

rhesus factor in blood describes a method of *blood grouping*. The rhesus factor is named after the rhesus monkey in which it was originally discovered. Approximately 85% of humans have rhesus factor in their blood. Such individuals are termed rhesus positive. The remaining 15% of humans do not have this factor and are rhesus negative. Rhesus negative patients cannot receive rhesus positive blood. Rhesus factor is inherited.

RIDDOR: see *Regulations for Reporting of Injuries, Diseases and Dangerous Occurrences (RIDDOR) 1995*.

rights are the expectations of an individual in their treatment and care. A service user has a right to be treated equally, to respect, to privacy, to protection and security, to be cared for in a way that meets their individual needs or additional needs.

rights and choices: the freedom that individual people in society have to choose their own preferences, *beliefs* and *lifestyles*. Within the context of health and social care provision, *clients* or *service users* have individual rights and choices which should be acknowledged, valued and supported.

rights and responsibilities of service users and providers: requirements which are necessary to meet the needs of both the service user and the provider. These include:
- appropriate knowledge of relevant legislation
- facilitation of rights of access to fair treatment and care
- implementation of care values in the care and treatment of service users by professionals involved in care provisions
- understanding the right to refuse treatment and to withhold or give *consent*.

risk: the way in which a client or carer can be exposed to harm from others or from their *care environment*.

risk assessment: the procedure which examines a care setting for potential risks and hazards to service users and their carers. Following this the areas of concern are recorded and addressed. This assessment has five stages:
- stage 1 – look for hazards
- stage 2 – assess who may be harmed
- stage 3 – consider the risk, are precautions adequate?
- stage 4 – record findings
- stage 5 – review risk and revise if necessary.

risks to health: see *alcohol*, *smoking* cigarettes, *drug misuse*, *obesity*.

risk management involves identifying health and safety hazards in order to implement strategies to eliminate and prevent such risks. Risk management involves:
- carrying out a formal risk assessment and making a written record
- reducing risk in different care settings by training, early warning systems, *health and safety* policies, warning and safety signs, safety equipment in place and personal protective equipment being available
- ensuring fire precautions are in place
- providing security in early years provisions and other vulnerable people's settings to prevent unwanted visitors, intrusion and to ensure the safe collection of children.

role: the behaviour adopted by individuals when they are interacting in social situations. People learn their roles through the *socialisation* process and may play many different roles throughout their lives. Examples include *nurse*, father, *police officer*.

role model: an individual whose behaviour may be copied or aspired to. Young individuals in particular model their *behaviour* on the adults around them. When working with children, adults should develop their *communication* and *interpersonal skills* in such a way as to show their concern and respect for others, irrespective of different racial or ethnic background. Also they should demonstrate sensitivity to different needs, and should develop their listening skills, as a way of helping young children to learn to listen. A positive, encouraging, interested and stimulating adult role model can be a key person in a child's personal development.

role-play: a learning method used by students in *education* or training. It involves the student taking a part and acting it out in a given situation. Other students observe the role-play and give feedback in the session. Role-play is also used by children in different ways as they develop their imagination.

roles and responsibilities: the function of the *care practitioner* in their job role and the different requirements attached to it, e.g. *person-centred care* and supporting the *care value base.*

Rogers, Carl (1902–1987): an American psychologist who believed in the humanistic approach to psychology. His main theories related to the *person-centred* approach. He believed that individuals could achieve *self-actualisation* or achievement of their potential.

routines are periods of time or methods of working which ensure that the overall care of clients, patients or service users is fully catered for. They will involve:
- times for getting up and going to bed
- meal times including food preparation, service and feeding
- personal hygiene, changing clothes, bathing, washing, toileting times
- recreation and leisure activities.

Routines are part of care practice because they can create a sense of security. Also if several workers are involved in caring for a large number of clients, each carer will have roles and responsibilities to maintain a routine.

Royal Association for Disability and Rehabilitation: (RADAR) a national voluntary organisation which is run by, and works with, the physically disabled. It acts as a *pressure group* to improve the environment for disabled people, campaigning for their rights and needs, and challenging negative attitudes and stereotypes. RADAR is particularly involved with issues surrounding civil rights, social services, social security, employment, education, *housing* and *mobility*. (See *disability*.)

Royal Commission for Long-term Care: a government committee set up in 1998 to look at:
- establishing *values* with regard to the system of long-term care
- reviewing aspects of care in *residential homes*
- reviewing hospital care and *rehabilitation*
- devising a fair system of paying for care. (See *nursing care*.)

Royal National Institute for the Blind: a voluntary organisation which provides national services for blind and partially sighted people. This includes people with sight problems such as older people with cataracts. The RNIB offers an information service in all matters relating to eye health and blindness.

Royal National Institute for the Deaf is concerned with the needs and problems of people of all ages suffering varying degrees of hearing loss.

Royal School for the Blind: see *SeeABILITY.*

Royal Society for the Prevention of Accidents: (RoSPA) a professional *organisation* and registered *charity.* Its basic aim is helping to save lives and reducing the number of injuries from *accidents* of all kinds. Accidents have been identified as a *national health target* in the latest government health initiatives. RoSPA's accident prevention activities include safety on the road, at work, in the home, at leisure, on and in the water and safety education for the young.

A–Z Online

Log on to A–Z Online to search the database of terms, print revision lists and much more. Go to **www.philipallan.co.uk/a-zonline** to get started.

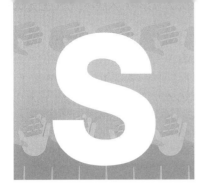

safety: procedures which are taken into account to protect clients, patients and service users from harm. It is one of the most important issues for carers working in health and social care. Clients need to feel physically safe and secure in their care settings. Safety procedures are strategies for providing and maintaining a safe environment. If procedures are to be effective, all workers, managers and clients should be aware of them and understand how they work. They should be written down so that there is no misunderstanding about what is expected. Carers, other workers and clients need to be informed when they are changed. There are a variety of working procedures which can be developed in the range of **care settings**. These are closely related to the **health and safety** of both clients and the workers involved. Examples of such procedures include:

- checking the care setting and carrying out a **risk assessment.** Once a setting is deemed safe, then procedures are put in place to ensure regular monitoring and maintenance with regard to health and safety
- checking that any equipment or toys which are being used have been manufactured and installed safely
- maintaining records with regard to staff, clients, equipment and the different resources used in the care setting
- supervising activities and staff–client ratios
- ensuring **fire drills**, evacuation procedures and **first aid** are regularly practised
- transporting clients in vehicles, travel arrangements and outings
- ensuring that all procedures comply with health and safety regulations written into legislation such as the **Health and Safety at Work Act 1974**.

safety marks: see **marks of safety**.

safeguarding: systems in place to protect service users from **abuse** and harm. They are a key method of promoting and protecting the rights of service users.

safeguarding children: a term used to describe the systems that are in place to protect children from abuse. These include the role of:

- relevant legislation and policies such as **Working Together to Safeguard Children 1999, Working Together to Safeguard Children 2007, Children Act 1989, Children Act 2004, Every Child Matters**, Protection of Children Act 2004 (Scotland), Protection of Children and Vulnerable Adults (2003) Northern Ireland
- local authorities in supporting children at risk
- **Local Safeguarding Children's Boards** set up in the **Children Act 2004**. These have a **statutory** responsibility for inter-agency working to safeguard children
- different agencies working together to meet the needs of children and their families. (See **child protection**.)

S

Safeguarding Vulnerable Groups Act 2006: an Act of Parliament which legally requires changes to be made with regard to the way that individuals work with vulnerable groups (children and vulnerable adults). These changes include:

- setting up the Independent Safeguarding Authority (ISA) which will make all decisions with regard to POVA, i.e. the **Protection of Vulnerable Adults**
- maintaining records of those banned from working as teachers or in children's services and keeping a separate record of those working with vulnerable adults (see **Vetting and Barring Scheme – Every Child Matters**).

salivary glands are responsible for secreting saliva into the **mouth**. Saliva prepares food for **digestion**. Whenever **food** is smelled or tasted then saliva is poured into the mouth. It is mixed with the food and aids digestion. It contains about 95% **water**. It also contains lubricating mucus and the enzyme salivary amylase, which changes cooked starch into maltose (a disaccharide sugar).

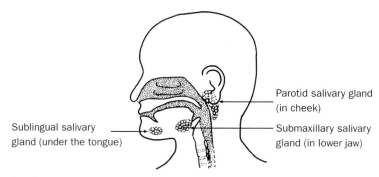

Sublingual salivary gland (under the tongue)

Parotid salivary gland (in cheek)

Submaxillary salivary gland (in lower jaw)

Salivary glands

salmonella: a group of **bacteria** which causes certain types of **food poisoning**. Salmonella bacteria are found in raw meat and are destroyed by cooking. Salmonella infection can be caused by:

- meat, especially poultry, not being thoroughly defrosted. When cooked the temperature inside the meat is not high enough to kill off bacteria and the meat (if eaten) may cause food poisoning. Bacterial toxins reach the intestines of the person eating the contaminated meat and a fever accompanied by vomiting and diarrhoea develops
- unwashed hands. Salmonella bacteria on the hands can be transferred to food by the person handling and preparing the food not having washed their hands thoroughly
- unhygienic food preparation, e.g. cooking surfaces which are not regularly cleaned allow bacteria to be transferred to cooked meat.

Careful attention to hygiene, food preparation and food storage are an essential requirement to prevent salmonella infection. (See **food safety**.)

salts are ionic compounds containing at least one cation and one anion. The properties of salts are that they:

- are often soluble in water
- have high melting and boiling points
- dissociate into ions in solution and so are electrolytes.

Sodium chloride (NaCl) is the best-known salt. Salts have many industrial and domestic uses.

Samaritans: a voluntary organisation which offers a listening and befriending service by telephone. It provides support to those who are suicidal or in despair at any hour of the day or night. This service is available to any member of the general public who wishes to talk about their problems. (See *counselling*.) It is supported by specially trained *volunteers*.

sample: a group of individuals who are assumed to be representative of the population from which they have been drawn. In research it is not always possible to study the whole population at once and, therefore, a sample is used.

sampling is a process which involves choosing a representative proportion of the population to be studied. It is a widely used procedure in many different types of research. The aim of sampling is to make the chosen group of individuals as representative as possible of the entire population but still manageable in terms of the numbers involved. The conclusions and recommendations drawn from such research can then be applied to the population as a whole. The results are then said to have been 'generalised'. (See *sampling frame, sampling methods*.)

sampling frame: usually a list of people (survey population) from which the sample is drawn. These lists can be drawn from club membership or school rolls, for example.

sampling methods are ways in which representative samples are selected. There are a variety of methods, such as:

- random sample – each member of the population being studied stands an equal chance of being selected, e.g. the National Lottery
- stratified sample – the composition of the sample reflects the composition of the population, e.g. 48% males and 52% females in the population determines that the sample should itself contain a selection of 48% males and 52% females
- quota sample – the researcher chooses a selection of people roughly in proportion to their occurrence in the population, e.g. quota of different age groups
- opportunity sample – selecting whoever is available at the time of research.
  (See *data collection*.)

scattergram: a graphical representation of the correlation between two sets of measurements. These measurements are called variables and the relationship between two variables can be plotted graphically. The more the points on the scattergram are clustered around some definite pattern, the stronger the correlation. In a linear correlation, the points fit along a line. A direction of bottom left to top right represents a positive correlation, while a direction from top left to bottom right indicates a negative correlation.

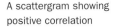

A scattergram showing positive correlation

A scattergram showing negative correlation

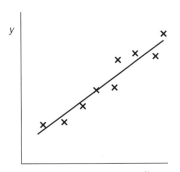

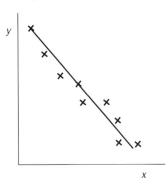

schizophrenia: a severe mental disorder. It affects one in a hundred people worldwide. The symptoms can be divided into two groups:

- 'positive symptoms' which include delusions, for instance, when a person believes that they are someone else and suffers hallucinations such as hearing voices and seeing, feeling, tasting or smelling things which are not there
- 'negative symptoms' such as withdrawal, difficulties in communicating and in expressing emotions.

schools: it is a statutory requirement in Britain for all children between the ages of 5 and 16 years to attend full-time education.

SCOPE: a *charity* and voluntary organisation which provides a range of services for people with *cerebral palsy* and their families and *carers*, including *schools, residential care, information* and careers advice. They also offer *counselling*. The monthly newspaper 'Disability Now' provides information relevant to all forms of the disability. A network of local teams provides contact with SCOPE social workers and over 200 local affiliated groups.

Scotland and its Parliament: Scotland controls its own affairs through the Scottish Parliament. Following the White Paper 'Scotland's Parliament', the Scottish Parliament and executive have responsibilities for various areas such as:

- *health* including the *NHS (National Health Service)*, public and mental health in Scotland
- *education* and training including pre-5, primary, secondary, further and higher education
- local government, social work and housing
- the law and home affairs, including most civil and criminal law and the criminal justice system.

screening programmes: procedures which are carried out on people in order to look for a specified disease. For example, a woman may attend a *GP*'s surgery for a *cervical smear*, when a sample of *cells* is removed from the cervix and sent to a laboratory to be examined for pre-cancerous cells. For a screening programme to succeed the *disease* must exhibit specific characteristics. It must:

- have a high risk of occurrence in the population
- be treatable if detected
- be dangerous if undetected
- be reasonably easy and inexpensive to diagnose at an early stage.

(See also *breast self-examination, cervical smear, testicular self-examination*.)

seamless services are the way in which health and social care providers work together in order to meet the care requirements of clients or service users. (See *continuum of care*.)

Secretary of State for Health: the government minister who is responsible for the provision of health and social care services. The Secretaries of State for Northern Ireland, Scotland and Wales are responsible for health in their own areas of the UK.

Sector Skills Councils (SSCs) provide opportunities for employers to target skills gaps and shortages in order to improve opportunities in the work force. They also seek to develop learning through apprenticeships, higher education and national occupational standards. Within the health and social care sector, the Sector Skills Councils have developed the skills for health. They are designed to:

246

- deliver more skilled *health and social care workers* who will improve health and *care practice*
- influence the training and development of workers and therefore enhance their skills
- identify where there are shortages of skills.

SeeABILITY: (formerly known as the Royal School for the Blind) a charity which supports individuals with *visual impairments* and assists with their education and learning. It is estimated that in Britain today there are over 30,000 people who are blind, visually impaired or have some other visual disability – only 1% of these people are receiving adequate care.

self-actualisation: an inner drive to grow and develop or a *belief* that an individual can work towards recognising and developing their potential and, as a result, achieve self-fulfilment. *Carl Rogers* recognised this as part of his client-centred approach to counselling. *Abraham Maslow*, in his hierarchy of needs, stated that self-actualisation was the final psychological level that was met when all the *basic physical needs*, including love and affection, had been achieved.

self-advocacy is the process by which a service user speaks on their own behalf. This should be encouraged amongst clients and service users, particularly those who have *special needs*.

self-assessment: the ability to monitor and evaluate one's own performance through the process of developing *self-awareness*.

self-awareness: the state of knowing oneself. Achieving self-awareness involves individuals learning about their own feelings, attitudes and values. It works on the idea that if a person knows themselves better, they are able to relate more effectively to others.

self-concept: the way we see ourselves. The self-concept can be explored in order to understand ourselves. (See also *self-awareness* and *self-esteem*.)

self-confidence: an individual's belief in his or her own ability to achieve something or to cope with a situation. Self-confidence may influence and be influenced by *self-esteem*.

self-disclosure: the way in which individuals reveal intimate *information* about their lives as they build relationships with others. As the client/carer relationship is built up, the client may reveal certain details about themselves. It is important for the carer to ascertain whether details given in this way are *confidential*.

self-efficacy is the way in which an individual believes in their own ability to carry out tasks and activities, or their belief in their own competence. This is closely linked to a person's thinking or cognitive ability, motivation and response to life's challenges.

self-empowerment: a process of helping individuals to obtain a higher degree of control over themselves in terms of motivation, ability and achieving potential.

self-esteem is the view that an individual has of themselves, their own worth and their own identity. Having a positive self-esteem means that an individual is able to identify their strengths and weaknesses and 'feels good about themselves'. Building a positive self-esteem in others is an important requirement in the caring process, and includes:
- *effective communication* skills
- giving praise and encouragement where necessary
- helping individuals to identify their strengths or what they can achieve.

Helping an individual build their self-esteem takes time and is often achieved by building a constructive relationship with the person or child concerned. (See *building* confidence, building a positive relationship, interpersonal skills, strategies for effective communication, listening skills and active listening.)

self-fulfilling prophecy: when what a person predicts will happen does indeed come to pass. A person's thought processes are activated so that they begin to behave in the predicted way. The prophecy comes to pass because of behaviour which is unconsciously designed to bring it about. Self-fulfilling prophecy can often be built on negative behaviour, producing negative reactions which reinforce the behaviour.

self-help: the way in which individuals and groups are encouraged to deal with their feelings and to solve their own problems. This can be achieved through a range of activities such as:

- *counselling* on a one-to-one basis
- co-counselling which involves partnering with another person and sharing experiences
- joining a group, each of whom has been through or is going through a similar process or experience (see *bereavement, support agencies*)
- joining an organisation and working as a *volunteer*.

Self-help is closely related to *empowerment*.

self-image: the view that an individual has of herself or of himself.

self-perception is the way in which an individual observes their own *behaviour* and makes decisions as a result of that behaviour.

self-referral: a means whereby clients can refer themselves for treatment or therapy. (See *referral to health care services*.)

SENCO: *special needs* co-ordinator. (See *statementing*.)

sense organs: parts of the body which contain the sensory *cells*. These include the *eye*, *ear*, *skin*, *tongue* and nose. The cells in these organs are sensitive to stimuli, for instance:

- the sensitive cells of the eyes, i.e. the rods and cones, respond to the stimulus of light
- the sensitive cells in the taste buds on the surface of the tongue respond to the stimulus of food or substances which enter the mouth. A taste bud is a small round structure on the surface of the tongue which contains a taste cell. When food enters the mouth it mixes with saliva and the presence of food stimulates the taste buds. There are four basic tastes – sweet, sour, salty and bitter. The related taste buds are situated on different areas of the tongue
- the sensitive cells in the ears, in the organ of Corti, respond to the stimulus of sound
- the sensitive cells in the nerve endings of the skin respond to the stimuli of touch, heat, cold and pain
- the sensitive cells in the nose respond to the stimulus of smell. The inner lining of the nose is kept moist due to the secretion of mucus. When air enters the nose, the olfactory cells send a message to the *brain* and any changes of smell are interpreted.

sensory impairments: disorders or *dysfunctions* which affect the *sense organs* and the *nervous system*, particularly the way in which the body responds to stimuli. These affect sight, hearing, taste, touch and smell.

sensory nerves are responsible for carrying sensory impulses to the *central nervous system*. In the spinal cord the sensory *nerve* links to a motor nerve which transmits the impulse to various *muscles*.

sensory skills are those skills which are necessary to help a young child develop their senses. They take the form of:
- visual skills – exploring and looking at different colours, pictures and in some cases using equipment to support vision
- hearing skills – encouraging listening to different sounds, language, and understanding of what is being heard. Special equipment may be needed to enhance or recognise sounds
- tactile skills – experimenting with different textures
- taste and smell – investigating different tastes and smells through food, and other materials, to develop smell.

separation is the state of a young child or person who has been taken from their parent or primary care giver. In the young child, this can affect the **bonding** process as the emotional bonds or **attachments** are interrupted. It can also lead to **maternal deprivation** when the child's emotional security and well-being are affected. When a young child is separated from their parents or primary care givers, they experience:
- distress, so that the child may persistently cry, scream and protest
- despair, when the child begins to feel helpless, becomes listless, loses interest in their surroundings and fears that the person they love will never return
- detachment, when the child is convinced that their parent or primary care giver will never return. They try to cope by detaching themselves from the memory of that parent/care giver. Relationships with others are difficult and the child's behaviour can be affected by regular mood swings.

Different researchers such as James and Joyce Robertson, and **John Bowlby**, have worked on theories of attachment and separation and have made recommendations, especially with regard to children in **hospital**.

services are provisions or settings which provide care and are designed to meet the individual needs of service users, clients or patients, e.g. day care centres, hospitals, community care, pre-school groups. Services provide practitioners who are available to meet holistic needs and basic physical needs. Different approaches are used to meet these needs. These include the:
- behavioural approach – methods used to influence **behaviour** through shaping and modifying, using selective reinforcers
- empowerment approach – gives service users the ability to have more control over their own health care by making informed choices and decisions
- holistic approach – looks at strategies to treat the whole person including psychological and social factors rather than just exploring the symptoms of the disease (see **life quality factors**).

service users are clients or patients, who use the health and social care services provided for them. They are also described as those in receipt of direct care.

Sex Discrimination Acts 1975 and 1986: Acts of Parliament which made recommendations with regard to **discrimination**. The Acts make it unlawful to discriminate on the basis of **gender** or marital status in the areas of employment, trade union membership, education, the provision of goods and services, housing and in advertising. Sex discrimination can be unfair treatment of women or men, and of single or married people. In employment, the Acts apply to recruitment, day-to-day work activities and to dismissal.

As with the Race Relations Act, discrimination may be direct or indirect. The Sex Discrimination Regulations 2008 made amendments regarding harassment and discrimination on the grounds of pregnancy or maternity leave.

Sex Discrimination Act (Northern Ireland) 1970 (Amended) 1988 makes it illegal to discriminate against a person on the grounds of his or her sex with regard to employment, training, education, the provision of goods and facilities, and the disposal and management of premises. It also makes it illegal to discriminate against married people with regard to employment and training.

Sex Offenders Act 2003: an Act of Parliament which provides an updated framework to protect members of the public from sexual crimes. It replaces previous sexual offence legislation with more specific and explicit wording which includes new offences such as causing a child to watch a sexual attack. It also prohibits child prostitution.

sex role stereotyping: the way in which individuals are categorised according to their *gender*. For example, it might be suggested that car mechanics are always male and that cooking, cleaning and washing-up are always carried out by females, or that boys should play football and girls should play with their dolls. Sex role stereotyping is often learned in the home from parents who are their children's role models. Rigid and inflexible attitudes are formed and individuals are expected to play out these roles. These can be reinforced by books, magazines and television programmes. *Equal opportunities policies* are a means whereby these stereotypical roles can be challenged.

sexism is *discrimination* or unfair treatment of an individual on the basis of their gender group. It involves *attitudes, behaviour* and procedures in society which maintain the belief that one gender group is more important in society than the other. It also reinforces *stereotypical* roles and responsibilities of men and women in society. This can take the form of female applicants for jobs not gaining employment in male-dominated sectors. Men and women are still exposed to stereotyping in society as they are expected to behave in a particular way and fulfil certain social roles, although more liberal attitudes have developed in recent years.

sexual intercourse is the sexual contact between two individuals involving insertion of the penis into the vagina. This is how human beings reproduce.

sexual maturity: a stage in physical development that results in the ability to reproduce. This is due to different physical changes in the body resulting from the release of *hormones* in both the male and female. (See *adolescence*.)

sexual orientation: a person's identified sexual preference. It is part of anti-discriminatory policies not to discriminate on the basis of sexual preference, i.e. against gays, lesbians or heterosexuals and it is unlawful to discriminate against any person because of sexual orientation. This is underpinned by the Employment Equality (Sexual Orientation) Regulations 2003, and is also taken into account in the *Civil Partnership Act 2004*.

sexually transmitted diseases are passed from one person to another as a result of sexual contact. Examples of such diseases are clamydia, hepatitis B, genital warts, genital herpes and *HIV*.

sheltered housing: a type of accommodation for clients. It provides an alternative to care in *residential homes* for older people and for disabled clients and includes:

- independent accommodation which is usually grouped together on one site. The accommodation has an alarm which clients can ring if they need help or feel unwell
- the employment of a resident warden who supports the clients and is available in emergencies. The client's alarm bell alerts the warden
- the provision of a degree of **independence**. The older person still lives in their own home but opportunities for social contact are available.

Many sheltered housing sites have communal facilities such as a large lounge with a television where residents can hold meetings, parties, dances, courses and keep fit, or just pop in for a chat.

shock: an adverse reaction to a situation, **accident** or disorder which causes a sudden drop in **blood pressure**. This drop in blood pressure could be due to bleeding, **heart attack**, severe **infection** in the body, reaction to medicines or even bad news of an unexpected nature which causes a physical reaction. Whatever the reason, the **signs and symptoms** are the same and they include:

- a fast but weak **pulse**
- discolouration of the **skin**, resulting in a grey/blue pallor with bluish lips
- cold and clammy skin with sweating
- weakness and dizziness
- feeling sick
- fast and shallow breathing.

During shock a person may become unconscious. It is important to call the ambulance at once and not to leave the person alone. (See **ABC of resuscitation, recovery position**.)

siblings are the brothers and sisters within a **family**. Sibling rivalry is often viewed as a feature of the relationship between brothers and sisters who compete for their parents' affection.

sickle-cell disorders are inherited **blood** conditions. These include sickle-cell disease and the carrier state, the sickle cell trait. In Britain the disorder is most common in those of African or Caribbean descent, but it may also occur in people from India, Pakistan, the Middle East or the Eastern Mediterranean. It is estimated that there are approximately 6000 adults and children with sickle-cell disease in Britain at present. Sickle-cell disorder is caused by an inherited abnormal **haemoglobin** structure. Haemoglobin is the **protein** which gives the red cells their colour and carries oxygen around the body. With sickle-cell disorders the abnormally formed haemoglobin causes the usually round and pliable cells to become rigid and sickle shaped. This is called 'sickling'. Individuals may inherit this type of haemoglobin from both their parents. There are a number of haemoglobin types usually known only by a letter of the alphabet. The most common types are called normal haemoglobin (HbA) and sickle haemoglobin (HbS). Signs and symptoms of sickle-cell disorder include painful swelling of the hands and feet, **infection** and anaemia. The illness may cause frequent episodes of pain in the **bones** and **joints**, abdomen and other parts of the body. These episodes of pain are called crises.

sign language: a method of **communication** where the hands are used to convey a message. 'Talking' with the hands is an effective means whereby people with hearing impairments can communicate with others. (See **British Sign Language, Makaton**.)

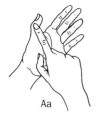
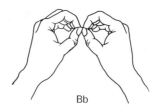
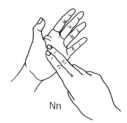

Aa   Bb   Nn

Examples of sign language

signs and symptoms are indications and features of a disease which are normally observed by a *doctor* and are used to help in the diagnosis of a disease. However, they are also those features which are noticed by the individual himself or by others such as carers and first aiders.

skeletal (striated) muscle is also known as voluntary *muscle*. This type of muscle is attached to the *bone* at a fixed point by means of a *tendon*. Contraction of the muscle results in movement of the *bone*. When viewed under a microscope, the muscle appears striped (striated). These stripes contain bundles of muscle fibres called myofibrils. They run longitudinally and are made up of thick and thin filaments. The thick filaments contain the *protein* myosin. The protein actin can be found in the thin filaments. The filaments work together to produce muscle contractions.

skeleton: the skeleton is a frame of over 200 *bones* which supports and protects the body *organs* (the viscera) and provides a solid base on which the *muscles* can work. The bones include:

- cranium or skull. A case protecting the *brain* and facial organs. It is made of cranial and facial bones. The upper jaw, for instance, consists of two fused bones called maxillae (sing. maxilla)
- rib cage. A cage of bones forming the walls of the thorax or chest area. It is made up of 12 pairs of ribs, the thoracic vertebrae and the sternum. The ribs are joined to the sternum by bands of costal cartilage, but only the first seven pairs join it directly. The last five pairs are false ribs. The top three of these join the sternum indirectly – their costal cartilage joins that of the seventh pair. The bottom two pairs are floating ribs, only attached to the thoracic vertebrae at the back
- vertebral column. Also called the spinal column, spine or backbone. It is a flexible chain of 33 *vertebrae* which protects the spinal nerves.

Dysfunctions of the skeleton cause *arthritis*, *fractures* and bone *cancer*.

skin: a protective layer which covers the body and acts as a barrier against *water* loss, *disease* and dirt. It is a waterproof covering which controls the amount of water being lost through evaporation and it also helps to regulate body *temperature*. It is sensitive to touch and contains *nerve* endings. *Vitamin* D and melanin are made here. There are two main layers to the skin, the epidermis and the dermis:

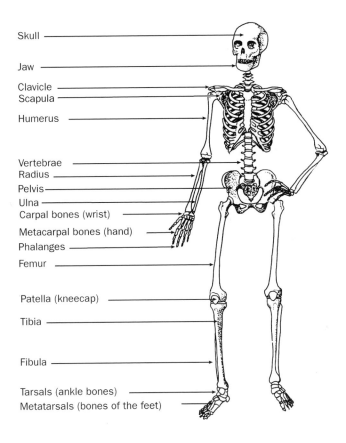

Skull

Jaw

Clavicle
Scapula

Humerus

Vertebrae
Radius
Pelvis
Ulna
Carpal bones (wrist)

Metacarpal bones (hand)

Phalanges

Femur

Patella (kneecap)

Tibia

Fibula

Tarsals (ankle bones)
Metatarsals (bones of the feet)

Skeleton

- Epidermis – the outer layer of skin which acts as a form of protection to the tissues underneath. In the epidermis there are several layers of skin cells. The lowest layer is called the germinative layer. There is continuous growth in this layer. As the cells get pushed up to the surface they die because of lack of oxygen and nutrition. The dead skin cells fill with granules of protein called keratin which forms a protective layer. In the germinative layer there are melanocytes which produce the skin pigment (melanin) giving the skin and hair their colour.
- Dermis – the inner layer which contains mainly **connective tissue** fibres, blood vessels, nerves, **glands** and hair roots. In the connective tissue there are elastic and collagen fibres which enable the skin to keep its shape. The blood vessels provide oxygen and nutrition. The sensory nerve endings are sensitive to touch, heat, cold, pain and pressure. There are five different types of sensory nerve endings in the skin. They are called receptors, and pick up information to relay through the nervous system to the **brain**. The **sweat glands** produce sweat, a watery solution of salt and some urea which evaporates on the skin thus cooling the body.

s

Hair follicles provide the means by which a shaft of hair is formed and supported. On either side of the hair follicle there are sebaceous glands which produce an oily fluid called sebum. This spreads over the hair and skin making it supple and waterproof. Excessive sebum causes oily/greasy skin, while insufficient sebum causes dry skin.

The skin regulates body temperature when it produces sweat to cool the body to prevent overheating. Other methods of controlling the skin temperature are dependent on the dilation (vasodilation) and constriction (vasoconstriction) of the blood vessels under the skin surface. During the *ageing* process the skin loses its elasticity and begins to sag and form wrinkles. Skin needs to be washed regularly to prevent a build-up of dirt, sweat and loose skin; hygiene is an essential part of caring. *Washing* and *bathing* vulnerable clients, such as older people, should be part of a regular *routine*. Young children should be encouraged to wash their hands before meals and after going to the toilet. Teaching toileting skills and *hygiene* procedures is an important aspect of working with disabled people. (See *epithelial tissues*.)

Dysfunctions of the skin cause skin *cancer*, *eczema*, scabs, blisters, spots and rashes. Rashes can be localised in one part of the body, or can be generalised covering a large part of the body, e.g. rubella or German measles.

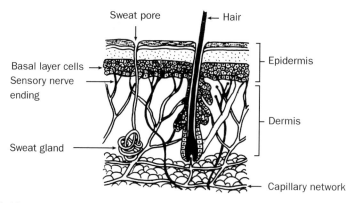

Section of skin

skin sensitivity tests are used in the identification of allergens. Suspected allergens are injected into the *skin* and the extent of the skin reaction is used to indicate sensitivity.

Skinner, Burrhus Frederic (1904–1990): a psychologist who developed a *learning theory* called operant conditioning. Skinner used an apparatus called Skinner's box to demonstrate his theory. Rats learned to press a lever to release food placed in a box. Skinner used the term 'reinforcer' which applied to anything that would produce a repeated response in either humans or animals.

skull: the structure of *bone* which protects and supports the *brain*. (See *skeleton*.)

sleep: a physiological process by which the body alters its state of consciousness within a 24-hour period. Individuals need sleep in order to function efficiently. *Babies* and young children need sleep and rest because it promotes *human growth and development*. Different individuals require varying amounts of sleep. Babies, young children and *older people* often require a short period of sleep (or nap) during the day. In hot climates there are siestas which are integrated into the daily routine. This gives people time to rest in the afternoon or during the hottest part of the day between noon and 3 pm.

smacking is physical punishment which can take many forms, such as using a hand, stick or strap. Some parents use smacking as a means of control. However, it is never appropriate for childcare workers to smack children in their care. Other strategies should be encouraged such as setting boundaries for *behaviour* with non-physical *discipline*. The *Children Act 2004* makes any punishment which leaves visible bruising, scratches, grazing, minor swelling or cuts illegal. The person responsible for inflicting the punishment can face up to five years' imprisonment.

smoking is a habit involving tobacco which contain harmful substances such as tar, nicotine and carbon monoxide. Nicotine is an addictive substance and it is this part of the cigarette that creates a dependence on smoking. It is absorbed into the bloodstream and affects the body by increasing the heart rate, *blood pressure* and *hormone* production, making smokers vulnerable to heart attack. *Carbon monoxide* combines with *haemoglobin*, the part of the *blood* which carries *oxygen* and reduces the blood's oxygen-carrying capacity. Oxygen is necessary for the healthy function of *tissues* and *organs* in the body. When the oxygen supply is reduced, this can affect growth and bodily function. In order to overcome such a reduction in oxygen, the body produces more haemoglobin. This makes the blood thicker which increases the risk of blood clot or *thrombosis*. If this condition is left untreated, it can lead to such a reduction in circulation in a limb that the only available treatment is the amputation or surgical removal of the limb. Smoking also leads to the deposit of tar on the lungs. The tar clogs up the bronchioles which leads to the narrowing of the breathing passages. This causes breathing problems, coughing and vulnerability to chest infections. For example the cilia in the ciliated epithelium in the *air passages* get clogged up so that mucus is not removed and collects, leading to 'smokers' cough'. The lining of the air passages has degenerated which causes a thickening of lining making breathing difficult.

There is also a debate about passive smoking. This takes place when a non-smoker breathes in the cigarette smoke of others, either in the form of the smoke the smoker has already breathed out or the smoke from the tip of the cigarette. Smoking is the main cause of lung cancer and is linked to heart disease, chronic bronchitis, asthma and cancers of the mouth, bladder, kidney, stomach and pancreas.

smooth muscle is the type of *muscle* found in the walls of the intestinal, genital, urinary and respiratory tracts and in *blood* vessels. Smooth muscles are controlled by the *autonomic nervous system* and *hormones*. The autonomic nervous system has a major role in controlling body movements which require no conscious thought. The muscle cells are spindle-shaped and are organised into bundles of sheets which contract rhythmically. *Peristalsis*, an example of smooth muscle movement, enables food to move through the intestinal canal.

social and economic factors are factors which affect how individuals live, work and maintain a healthy lifestyle. They are often a cause for concern because of their impact on the *health and well-being* of individuals. They include:

- poverty – people's health is affected by their circumstances, e.g. low income can make it hard to afford to keep a house warm and protect individuals and their families from fire and accidents. There is no money to pay for extras
- employment – joblessness has also been linked to poor mental and physical health.

social and economic status: the position of an individual in society in terms of *social class* and of money available to support daily living and lifestyle.

social behaviour is the way a person relates to others. Children should be taught from an early age how to behave with others. They should learn what is acceptable *behaviour* with other children and what is not. Unacceptable behaviour would include biting, swearing and hitting other children. Childcare workers are trained to develop strategies to help children deal with unacceptable behaviour. (See *discipline, tantrums*.)

social care: a type of care which is provided in domicillary, residential and day care settings. It supports the physical, intellectual, emotional, cultural and social needs of the client. Social care should extend a client's contact with others. It also involves sharing information, setting up care plans, preparing meals, shopping and some basic cleaning.

Social Care Institute of Excellence: set up in 2000 to improve the quality of social care practice and provision. It seeks out the views and experiences of users as well as producing guidelines on effective social care practice and service delivery.

social care register: a register of people who work in *social care*, who have been trained and assessed to be part of the social care workforce, i.e. social workers. It is expected that over time all social care workers from every level will be registered.

social class or socio-economic group: a way of differentiating between groups and individuals within society. (See *National Statistics Socio-economic Classification*.)

social context: a setting in which there are unspoken rules for acceptable behaviour, for example in a classroom, hospital ward, or a lounge in a residential home.

social development: the *socialisation* process of developing social relationships and learning to live in society. (See *relationships, human growth and development*.)

social diversity is diversity and variety in society and in communities such as by *social class, gender, culture* and *ethnicity*.

social exclusion: the way in which an individual or group can become isolated in society. There are a number of factors which can lead to economic and psychological isolation such as inadequate *housing, unemployment* and *inequalities in health*. Social exclusion units were set up in 1998 to work with those who are socially excluded. These include the subjects of school exclusions, pregnant teenagers and rough sleepers, i.e. homeless people on the streets.

social factors are factors which contribute to an individual's development and to their *health and well-being*. These include *social class, family structures, poverty, gender, ethnicity*, the *socialisation* process and social relationships.

social identity is how an individual develops and maintains social relationships formed through friendships. Their social *network* is developed through the different experiences that an individual will go through in a life time. It is influenced by *socialisation* as well as by other social factors such as the *mass media* and advertising. It can affect how an individual develops and maintains social relationships formed through friendships and their social network.

social inequality describes the effect of *social and economic factors* on the lives of individuals in society. These inequalities affect *health and well-being* and often result in the poor getting poorer and the rich getting richer. There are ways in which these inequalities can be addressed by the following agencies:

- government and political parties
- European Union
- pressure groups and the mass media
- national initiatives such as Sure Start, social exclusion units and community support groups for those with mental health disorders and disabilities, and for older people and children.

social issues and welfare needs in the United Kingdom are those which can affect *health and well-being* of the population, such as:

- income and wealth distribution
- poverty
- an ageing society
- disability and dysfunction
- mental health disorders and suicide.

These issues and needs are interrelated in many ways such as poverty with unemployment, unemployment with depression and mental health disorders.

social policy: the way in which a government introduces legislation and implements policy with regard to issues such as employment, education, health and social care. It also encompasses the academic study of how different policies are developed and the impact that they have on the life of individuals and society. The aims of social policy are to maintain and improve the well being of people in the population by means of an appropriate distribution of resources, including cash and services. There are many influences on social policy such as Central Government, Parliament, political parties, regional parliaments and assemblies, local government, the *European Union (EU)*, *World Health Organisation (WHO)*, the mass media, pressure groups, resource availability and *demographic* change. (See *resourcing of services*.)

social relationships: see *social support networks*, *relationships*.

social role is the way in which *social status* is represented in society. For example, a *nurse* confirms his or her position by wearing a uniform and will be expected to take on the caring nature of a nurse.

social services: see *personal social services*, *Department for Children, Schools and Families.*

social skills are those which assist in forming relationships with others.

social status: the position which people hold in society. These positions can be different in various settings or groups such as nurse, hospital doctor or care manager. (See *social role*.)

social stratification: the outcome of dividing the population into layers or strata. Society can be divided on the basis of *class*, income, *race, age* and any other characteristic or grouping by which people can be separated. (See *social class or socio-economic group*.)

social structures are systems in society such as families, education provision and health care services.

social support networks: networks including family, friends, partners, relatives and the membership of community groups which offer and provide support for an individual's *self-esteem*. Support is often provided in the context of conversation which permits *self-disclosure*, i.e. talking about oneself. (See *networks*, *relationships*.)

social trends: aspects of society which represent *demographic changes* and the effects of that change on society. Examples of this are divorce, crime, *poverty, disability* and *dysfunction*. These aspects of society are closely linked to *social and economic factors*. Social trends are measured through research and statistical information which is publicised annually as a way of monitoring aspects of society and social change. (See *demography*.)

social well-being: an attitude which reflects an individual's approach to forming relationships and developing *social support networks.*

Social Work (Scotland) Act 1986: an Act of Parliament which provides a framework for social work practice in Scotland. (See *foster care*.)

social workers are qualified professionals who operate with individuals and families with different problems within *voluntary* or *statutory organisations*. They help people to come to terms with, or to solve, their problems but their statutory responsibilities, especially in *child protection*, mean they are often viewed as agents of control. Social workers receive professional training which requires them to study all aspects of the principles of social work. Following qualification (usually the Diploma in Social Work), social workers may operate in different areas, which include:

- advice and working across the different client groups
- children and the child protection team
- youth and community service
- learning disabilities
- mental health
- older people.

They are usually employed by local authority social service departments and deal with people of all types, ages and backgrounds (see *client classification*). Some may specialise in particular areas such as:

- cases involving young children (including young offenders in the criminal justice system), *adoptions* and *foster care* arrangements
- supporting those who are mentally or physically ill
- work in *residential homes* with children and young people who cannot live with their natural families
- an increasing amount of *community care* work with older people and disabled people who might previously have lived in hospitals or residential homes.

socialisation: the lifelong process by which individuals learn about themselves, others and the world around them. It plays an important role in how *attitudes, beliefs* and *values* are developed and personalities are formed and shaped. There are three different types of socialisation:

- primary – the relationships formed in the first few years of life, i.e. within families, with parents, siblings and relatives
- secondary – the relationships formed with friends or peers outside the home
- tertiary – the relationships formed within other formal groups within society.

Socialisation within a group involves relationships between its different members. This may or may not involve rules or codes of behaviour.

society: a group of individuals living together in an organised way.

sociogram: a method used to explore how relationships are determined within group interaction. *Group* dynamics are observed and a diagram is constructed (see example below) to summarise the information gathered.

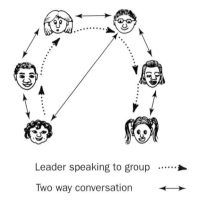

Leader speaking to group ······▶

Two way conversation ◀──▶

Example of a sociogram

sodium: a *mineral* which is required in small amounts to maintain healthy body function. It is essential for *nerve* and *muscle* development and helps maintain osmotic pressure in the *cells*. The sources of sodium are *salt*, and most other *foods*. The signs and symptoms of sodium deficiency include muscle cramp.

solubility: if the atoms, molecules or ions of a substance become evenly dispersed (dissolve) in a solute such as water, then a solution is formed. If they do not, the mixture is either a colloid, a suspension or a precipitate. Solubility is defined as how well a substance dissolves. It depends on the substance's properties, those of the liquid and other factors such as temperature and pressure.

solvents are liquids that dissolve other substances to form a solution. Some solvents can have a harmful effect on the body; these include butane gas lighter refills, text correction fluids, glues, dry cleaning fluids, aerosols like deodorants or pain-relieving sprays, paint thinners or strippers, and petrol. Solvent misuse to the point of unconsciousness can cause *death* through *choking* on vomit. Death from suffocation is a serious risk if solvents are sniffed in a plastic bag placed over the head. Regular use can be habit forming and the addiction can be difficult to break. Solvent use is not a criminal offence, but it is illegal for a shopkeeper to sell solvents to anyone under 18 if they suspect such products are intended for abuse. (See *substance abuse*.)

special care baby unit: a highly specialised team of trained *doctors* and *nurses* working with *babies* who are premature or who experience neonatal problems and therefore have specific needs such as assistance with breathing. Such babies need individual care often requiring incubators. In addition, other sophisticated equipment may be used to maintain the baby's life.

special education needs: relates to children who have specific needs which should be addressed in their education and learning (see *children with disabilities, Special*

Education Needs – Code of Practice). Legislation is in place to support these children in the following way:

- children with special needs are to be integrated into mainstream *schools* wherever possible
- special education needs must be more clearly defined. The terms mild, moderate and severe were introduced (see *statementing*)
- a child's individual and specific needs are to be part of a continuous assessment process
- a child's abilities are to be identified alongside their disabilities
- the term 'specific learning difficulties' (e.g. dyslexia) are to be introduced for any child having problems in one area of the school curriculum.

Special Education Needs – Code of Practice: this code of practice is aimed at ensuring that children with special education needs have the opportunity to release their potential. The code places the rights of children with special education needs at the centre of the approach, ensuring that they are listened to and allowed to take part in decisions affecting them. It sets out a framework to ensure early identification of children's special education needs and to ensure that they are met. It also includes a framework for developing partnership working between parents, schools, local education, health and social services and voluntary organisations. Underpinning the *code of practice* is the *Special Education Needs and Disability Act 2001*.

Special Education Needs and Disability Act 2001: an Act of Parliament which amended the Education Act 1997 with regard to children with *special education needs* and their rights. It strengthened the rights of SEN children to be educated in mainstream schools. It also protects such children against disability *discrimination* in schools and in other educational establishments.

special health authorities (SHAs) are health authorities, like the National Blood Authority, that provide a national service.

special needs: these can be temporary or permanent, short- or long-term. However, there are some special needs which are more permanent and long-term. These are categorised into the following:

- *physical disabilities* affecting *motor skills*
- chronic illness and terminal *disease*
- *communication* defects, involving speech and language impairments
- *mental health disorders*
- *learning disabilities* and difficulties
- sensory impairment or defects such as deafness, blindness and those relating to touch, taste and smell.

(See *Contact a Family*.)

specific needs: identified needs which require support, care and treatment.

speech therapists are professionals who are trained to help adults and children to overcome language and *communication* problems. Qualified therapists work in a variety of settings which include *hospitals*, *schools*, community clinics and in private practice (see *language development*). Qualifying to be a speech therapist involves completing a three- or four-year degree course or a two-year postgraduate diploma course.

spina bifida is a spinal defect which occurs in early *pregnancy*. It affects development of the unborn baby's spine when one or more of the *vertebrae* fail to close properly, leaving a gap. This means that the *spinal cord* and the *nerves* are likely to be damaged, often resulting in *paralysis* in the area below this point in the spinal cord. It can also impair the way in which the spine develops. Walking can be affected and there can be damage to the *bladder* and bowel causing incontinence. One of the side effects can be *hydrocephalus*. Others include learning and memory difficulties, spatial and perception problems and poor concentration. According to recent research on the prevention of spina bifida, women can reduce the risk by taking 5 mg folic acid daily for at least one month before *conception* and during the first 12 weeks of pregnancy.

spinal cord: the cord of neurones that extends from the *brain* down the *vertebral canal* to the second lumbar vertebra. There are 31 pairs of spinal nerves that leave the spinal cord at different levels to supply various parts of the body. Injury to the spinal cord can be serious and, in some cases, can lead to *paralysis*. (See *nervous system*.)

spiritual development: the development of an individual's *belief* system.

spiritual health: a person's religious beliefs and cultural identity contribute to his or her health and *well-being*. Spiritual health forms part of *holistic care* revolving around the physical, intellectual, emotional, spiritual, cultural and social development of the child or person.

spirometry: a test of the body's ventilation capacity with regard to respiration and breathing. A spirometer is the machine used to provide readings which are called spirometer tracings. (See *mechanism of breathing*.)

spleen: an *organ* situated high up in the *abdomen* against the *diaphragm* on the left side of the body and protected by the ribs. It is a small dark brown organ and is like a fibrous sponge which contains lymphoid *tissue*. It filters *blood* as it passes through. The spleen:

- makes *antibodies* as part of the body defence mechanism
- destroys mature or worn-out red blood cells.

It is important to mention that individuals can function without a spleen because its operations are also carried out in other organs. However, when the spleen is removed individuals are more prone to infection.

squint (strabismus): the unco-ordinated action of the *muscles* in the *eye* causing a child to have visual difficulties. A child with a squint is unable to see properly as the two eyes are not able to focus on an objective point. There are two types of squint:

- convergent squint – when the eyes turn inwards
- divergent squint – when the eyes turn outwards.

standard assessment tests are tests which assess children's performance in school.

standard mortality ratio: (SMR) a way of comparing mortality rates in different population groupings. It takes into account the different age structures of the population. The observed number of *deaths* is the actual number of deaths occurring in the geographical area or subgroup of the population. The expected number of deaths is calculated by applying the national age-specific mortality rates to the population of a health authority area or population sub-group.

star ratings are grades given to local councils based on the quality of services which they are offering to adults through their social care.

statementing: an assessment process to determine the specific needs of individual *children with disabilities*. It can be instigated by a local education authority at any time during a child's school life from 4 to 18 years of age. Any statementing before the age of four years is organised by the *strategic health authorities*. Involved in the process are parents and the education authority who negotiate and agree the relevant education needs of the child. The aims of the process are to identify areas of need and define the resulting educational requirements of the individual. This may require extra resources and facilities to be set up, for example physiotherapy, speech therapy, modification of buildings, extra teacher or adult support. In 1994, a *code of practice* was introduced to give guidance to schools with regard to the statementing process. Following this, schools were expected to identify a member of staff who would take responsibility for *special education needs* with the title of Special Educational Needs Co-ordinator (SENCO).

statistics are numerical data which are collected to provide *information*. The use of statistics and the analysis of the information collected with regard to health and social care give indications which can be used in the allocation of resources required for different target areas. Information collected includes:
- the overall state of health of the nation
- *divorce*/remarriage/*family structures*
- *mortality rates*
- the number of children under five in the United Kingdom.

status: a measure of the rank and prestige of a person or group of people. Status can define how people are treated by others and how they see themselves. (See *social class or socio-economic group*.)

statutory: a formal legal requirement agreed by Parliament and reinforced by legislation.

statutory organisations are health and social care services set up as a requirement by law. They are expected to provide a range of services. These include the National Health Service and social service departments.

stereotyping: applying a set of presumed attitudes about groups of individuals in society. This relates to the formation of positive and negative *attitudes* which can affect *behaviour* towards a particular group or individual. Stereotyping can be learned by children from their parents. In addition to this, the mass media (e.g. television, newspapers, books, films, games and comics) can reinforce stereotypical attitudes.

stillbirth: the *birth* of a baby showing no signs of life, if it occurs after 24 weeks or more in the mother's womb.

stomach: the body's reservoir for *food*. In the stomach the food is churned up by muscular action which changes it into a more liquid form called chyme. The presence of food in the stomach stimulates *glands* in its lining to secrete rennin and pepsin, which react with food and hydrochloric acid (see *digestion*). The walls of the stomach are composed of longitudinal *muscle*, circular muscle, submucosa and mucosa.

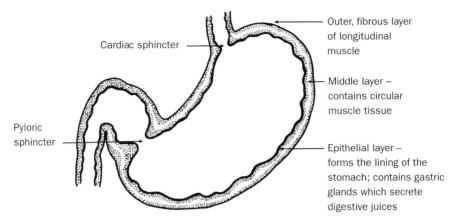

The stomach

storytelling: telling stories to stimulate interest. Books may or may not be used. Storytelling is a powerful way of influencing children's views about the society in which they live. It can be a means whereby children can develop an interest in books and reading for themselves. Guidelines for the telling of stories are as follows:

- the choice of books or stories is important and should be appropriate to the age of the child
- childcare workers should prepare stories in advance
- the seating in the storytelling area should be comfortable with enough space for numbers of children to sit comfortably
- children should be able to see any pictures being used
- stories should be told with enthusiasm, using different voice tone and pitch. *Gestures* should be encouraging and positive
- children should be encouraged to respond to the story with questioning by the storyteller to develop the children's communication skills
- the use of props such as puppets, storyboards and other visual aids can facilitate the storytelling
- songs, rhymes and creative activities should be used as a follow-up to the story using the same themes and topics. (See also *play, music and singing*.)

Storytelling is a traditional method of communicating items of interest, family news and images representing a person's culture. People can train to become storytellers enabling them to tell stories in a variety of settings to different age groups.

strategic health authorities: set up by the Department of Health to manage and improve services for patients in 10 different geographic areas. Part of their role is to ensure that local health services can provide more and better services to meet the required need.

strategies for effective communication: methods used to support good communication between carers and service users. These include:

- using technological aids and devices
- using translators, interpreters and advocates
- adapting to the care environment – helping service users cope with change
- having an understanding of cultural differences

- resolving differences between own beliefs and those of others
- checking of listening and understanding so that any issues are clarified.

stress is a term used to describe a condition being suffered by an individual who feels that they are unable to cope with demands on their time and capabilities. Most people will say that they suffer from stress at certain times in their lives. Stress levels can build up when individuals:

- feel that they do not meet the expectations of others
- feel that work or home responsibilities are increasing and that they have insufficient resources to manage
- find that they are unable to communicate how they are feeling or are in difficult relationships
- find they are in a continual and demanding role such as caring for a close relative.

stress management: strategies used by individuals to cope with the build-up of stress in their lives. (See *relaxation techniques*.)

stress-related illness is any type of illness which is brought on by or made worse by *stress*. Illnesses particularly associated with stress are *heart* disease, *diabetes*, digestive disorders, *skin* disorders and a vulnerability to colds and flu.

stress-response: physical response which supports a person's fight and flight reaction. The stress response may create problems when a person cannot fight or run away or such reactions are inappropriate. A person can become agitated because he or she cannot escape from difficult problems or situations in their lives. (See *adrenaline*.)

stroke volume: the volume of *blood* which is pumped out from a *ventricle* during each contraction of the *heart*.

strokes: see *cerebrovascular accident (CVA) or stroke*.

substance abuse is misuse of various substances including *alcohol, drugs* and *solvents*. Abuse describes the way in which the substances are taken, causing risk to *health*.

sudden infant death syndrome (cot death): the sudden and unexpected *death* of a *baby* without any obvious or apparent reason. It is a very distressing experience for parents, who need support and *bereavement* counselling to cope with their *grief*. In recent years, cigarette *smoking* in the home has been found to be a high risk factor. These days babies are laid on their back or side, not on their front, to help prevent over-heating. There is currently extensive research being undertaken to find out the reasons why babies die in this way.

sugars: the common name for a group of chemicals known as *carbohydrates*. They are made up of *carbon*, hydrogen and *oxygen*. They are classified according to the number of sugar units which make up their structure:

- monosaccharides (e.g. glucose, fructose, galactose) have one sugar unit
- disaccharides (e.g. sucrose, lactose and maltose) have two sugar units
- polysaccharides are complex carbohydrates, with many sugar molecules which are joined together.

support agencies: these are the individual organisations which offer assistance through a variety of methods such as: an *information* service, supplying leaflets, research statistics, videos and advice sessions, *counselling*, telephone helpline, immediate crisis support, local support and *self-help* groups. (See *network*.)

support groups are available to help individuals through difficult and unsettling situations. They may comprise collections of people who organise themselves to care for each other and to share mutual experiences. They are an essential link for individuals who require positive support during times of crisis.

support network: personal or professional contacts within the health and social care system. They consist of a large number of *organisations* set up to provide *information, advice, self-help* and telephone helplines, which offer individual and group support. They can either be *statutory* or *voluntary sector organisations*. Examples include social service departments, Relate and the Citizens Advice Bureaux. Informal support networks are set up within families and amongst friends and neighbours. Details of such organisations can be found in 'Yellow Pages'. The Citizens Advice Bureaux can also provide a full list of these organisations.

Sure Start: an initiative set up by the government designed to improve the health and *well-being* of families in deprived areas who suffer from poverty and under-performance in education.

surgeons: qualified *doctors* who specialise in surgery.

survey: a set of questions formulated to obtain information from people in their natural environment. It may ask individuals about their attitudes, beliefs, plans, health and work; in fact any subject can be covered in a survey. The researcher can survey a group of individuals who have undergone certain experiences. The responses obtained constitute the data upon which the research hypothesis is examined. People who are contributing to the survey are called *respondents*. A good example of a survey is the National Census which is conducted every ten years. Before setting up a survey it is necessary for the researcher to ensure the following:
- permission to carry out the study has been given
- a research *hypothesis* is in place
- the size of the *sample* of respondents is appropriate
- the type of sample is relevant
- the *research methods* are effective
- the ways in which the results will be recorded and analysed are agreed.

swallowing: the mechanism involved in the passage of food from the mouth through the back of the *throat* (the pharynx) into the *oesophagus*. The epiglottis is the flap of *cartilage* which covers the windpipe or trachea. When the swallowing reflex is activated the epiglottis automatically covers the trachea to prevent the food being inhaled into the windpipe. Food is pushed through the oesophagus in a process called *peristalsis*. Swallowing is essential for life. The reflex is controlled by the *autonomic nervous system*. The medulla oblongata, situated in the hind *brain*, is that part of the brain responsible for swallowing.

sweat glands are found in the dermis of the *skin*. They produce sweat which contains *water, minerals, salts* and *urea*. The sweat is excreted through the pores of the skin and helps to regulate *body temperature* when it evaporates.

symbolic play: type of play in which a child uses his or her *imagination*. During *play* a child may use one object as a symbol for another. A child may care for a doll, to represent a baby. A cardboard box can be used as a hat, while a saucepan and wooden spoon are used as a drum. When the child engages in symbolic play he/she is developing skills which can be used again as they grow older. (See *Piaget's theory of cognitive development*.)

symbols are signs which represent an object, route or situation and convey a message to the reader. Examples in health and social care include the symbols:

- used by equal opportunities employers
- used to indicate wheelchair access
- used to indicate that a substance is dangerous – gloves should be worn.

sympathetic nervous system: part of the *autonomic nervous system* which is activated in stressful situations. The sympathetic nervous system stimulates the *adrenal glands* to produce *adrenaline*. The effects of adrenaline are:

- an increased *heart* rate
- increased respiration affecting the breathing rate and its depth (see *mechanism of breathing*)
- increased sweating
- a dry *mouth*
- dilated pupils.

synovial joints are types of freely movable *joints* which connect one *bone* to another to form part of the human *skeleton*. Such joints are supported by a synovial capsule which is reinforced by bands of elastic fibre called *ligaments*. The ends of the bones are covered with articular *cartilage*. The joint is lined with a membrane called synovial membrane. This is filled with synovial fluid which acts as a lubricant and aids movement. There are various types of synovial joints, such as the hip joint.

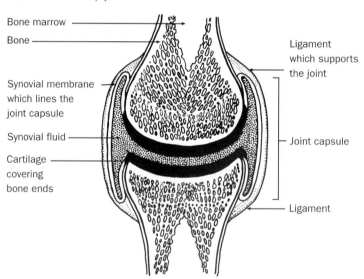

A section of a synovial joint

system of the body: a collection of *organs* which are interrelated and work together to carry out specific functions in the body.

systems of redress: procedures which are put in place in an organisation to deal with *grievances* and *complaints*.

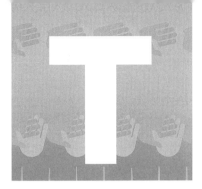

tabulation: a method using tables to display complex numerical data. A table should be as simple and unambiguous as possible. Tables are used to:

- display a distinct pattern in the figures
- summarise the figures
- provide information
- present collected data in an orderly manner.

All tables should:

- have a title
- include the source of the data
- have column or row headings as brief as possible but clearly labelled
- have units of measurement specified
- have sets of data which are to be compared with each other
- have approximations and omissions from the table explained in footnotes.

Tackling Health Inequalities – A Programme for Action 2003: This document sets out the plans to tackle *inequalities in health* and in particular to reduce the gap in *infant mortality* across social groups by the year 2010.

tantrums: outbursts of screaming, uncontrollable rage and frustration which can occur in young children. Tantrums are common between the ages of one and three years. Children aged four or five can also behave in this way. Such fits of rage are equally common in boys and girls. Behaviour includes whining, screaming, kicking and punching. A young child may have a temper tantrum because he/she wants to challenge the limits set on their behaviour, but children who are raised in an environment where no boundaries are set are just as likely to have tantrums. (See *challenging behaviour, discipline*.)

target group/audience: a large or small group of individuals who have been identified for a particular purpose. In health education a target group is a collection of individuals who are to be given a specific message. Talks about different aspects of *health promotion* would be prepared in different ways for different target groups, e.g. a talk about the advantages and disadvantages of breast feeding would be targeted at pre- and post-natal mothers. It is very important that health educators match their oral and visual presentation to the needs of the target group. A formal lecture with many tables and statistics would be unsuitable for a group of primary school children, but would be beneficial to some adults. Leaflets or activity packs which reinforce the message could be more applicable for children or the message may perhaps take the form of a story. The following indications of the nature of the group should be taken into account:

- *age* – different ages and stages of development
- *gender* – different information for men and women, i.e. 'well women' and 'well men'
- subject interest – the topic must be applicable to the group concerned
- *special needs* such as hearing, visual or disability – different methods of communication e.g. *Bliss boards*. (See *giving a talk, creating a PowerPoint presentation*.)

taste buds are found on the surface of the *tongue*.

taxation is money raised by governments by direct or indirect means to finance spending on public services:

- direct taxation is tax taken through wage packets in the form of income tax, and tax taken from the profits of companies in the form of corporation tax
- indirect taxation mainly takes the form of value added tax (VAT) that is added to consumer goods such as alcohol and petrol, and to other goods and services.

team: a group of individuals who work together for a common purpose. This may be in several ways:

- on a professional basis – a team of nurses on a ward
- on a multi-disciplinary basis – different professionals working together in the care of a client
- on a learning basis – a group of students on a research topic
- on a leisure or sporting basis – a group of people who meet for leisure pursuits such as swimming, squash, football
- on an educational basis – year groups of pupils, or students who are academically streamed
- on a competence requirement basis – groups of individuals who work together to achieve certain competencies or skills in the workplace, e.g. those studying for their *National Vocational Qualifications* in health care, community care and child care.

Teams can be formal or informal:

- formal teams are those set up within a professional context, such as a *multi-disciplinary team*
- informal teams are those set up for leisure pursuits, such as pub quizzes.

All teams have boundaries which provide a framework for behaviour within that team. Boundaries in formal teams are underpinned by professional *codes of practice.*

Teams in health and social care settings should work effectively towards meeting the needs of the service users they are responsible for by ensuring that each team member:

- has a role and responsibility within the team
- is accountable to the team for their practice
- can work collaboratively with others in the team
- is responsible for the ongoing care of the service users
- can work with other service providers and professionals (see *groups*).

Effective teamwork involves using the skills of each member and ensuring that each person has a function, role and responsibility within the team. It is usual for teams to have a leader who co-ordinates the work carried out by the group. Teams often meet regularly to share information, discuss problems and make decisions. These meetings are often minuted and an agenda or action plan prepared. Written and verbal *communication* between team members is vital, especially when it involves the health and social well-being of service users, clients or patients. (See *groups*.)

teeth are used to break up *food* in the *mouth* making it easier to swallow. There are four different types of teeth:

- incisors – situated in the front of the mouth. These teeth have chisel-like edges for biting
- canines – pointed so they can be used for tearing off pieces of food
- premolars – have a flatter surface and are used for grinding food into small pieces
- molars – similar to premolars but larger; generally, the upper molars have three roots, the lower molars only two, while the other teeth have a single root.

Teeth develop at any time during the first two years of life. The first set of teeth are called the 'milk' or 'deciduous' teeth. They usually begin to appear when the child is a few months old. There are 20 milk teeth, ten each in the lower and upper jaw, four incisors, two canines and four molars. They will usually be completely formed by the age of three years.

Between five and six years these teeth begin to fall out as permanent ones come through. There are 32 permanent teeth, 16 each in the lower and upper jaw. These consist of two incisors, one canine, two premolars and three molars on each side of the mouth. Dental caries are a result of the decaying process in teeth. This decay is often due to poor dental *hygiene* and to eating large amounts of sugar.

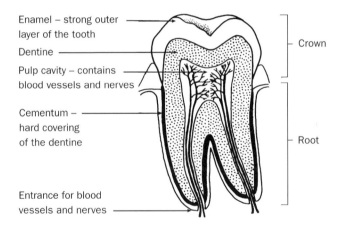

Enamel – strong outer layer of the tooth

Dentine

Pulp cavity – contains blood vessels and nerves

Cementum – hard covering of the dentine

Entrance for blood vessels and nerves

Crown

Root

A tooth

temperament governs an individual's emotional reactions to situations. (See *personality*.)

temperature: a measure of heat. Temperature is measured using a thermometer which can be calibrated to show a number of different temperature scales. (See *body temperature*.)

tendon: a cord which consists of bundles of fibres, responsible for attaching the muscles to the *bone*. Tendons assist muscle movement on a particular area of the bone.

terminal illness is a *disease* or physical disorder which results in *death*, e.g. an advanced *cancer* which has spread to different parts of the body. In terminal illness, individuals need highly specialised care. The basis for this type of caring is compassion, commitment, consistency and the necessary skills to carry out practical tasks and activities. Terminally ill people may have many needs including:

- physical needs, such as help and support with toileting, washing, bathing and feeding through the provision of nutritious meals to stimulate their diminishing appetite
- social needs, such as contact with others, conversations and outings with families and friends
- emotional needs, such as feeling that they are still loved, that they are not useless and that their lives still have purpose; this is a difficult time for *carers* who can feel helpless as there is no cure for the illness and they may observe the person struggle with pain and despair; *listening* and sharing interesting news and making the person feel that their contribution is important is essential
- spiritual needs, such as facing the issues of life and death, exploring their beliefs and talking about death
- cognitive and intellectual needs, such as information sharing; learning new skills could still be helpful to a terminally ill person and the problem-solving aspects of dealing with information should be encouraged
- pain control is an important aspect of this type of illness and adequate medical provision should be determined by the *doctor*.

(See *holistic care, palliative care*.)

tertiary care: *care* which is offered through specialist *hospital* services. Examples include cancer hospitals, hospitals offering neurosurgery, and those offering psychiatric treatment and care.

testicles: one of the two glandular bodies contained in the male scrotum. (See *male reproductive system*.)

testicular self-examination: regular self-examination of testicles is important to check for testicular cancer, as cancers that are found early are easier to treat. Self-examination of testicles should take place once a month when the scrotum is relaxed, for example after a bath or shower. The procedure is as follows:

- hold the scrotum in the palm of the hand so that fingers and thumb can be used to carry out the examination
- note the size and weight of the testicles (it is normal to have one testicle slightly larger than the other, or that hangs lower), but any notable difference requires further investigation
- gently feel each testicle, which should be smooth with no lumps or swellings
- feel for the soft tube at the top and back of the testicle, the epididymis, which is normal and not a abnormal lump
- if any abnormal swelling or lumps are found then further investigation by a GP should be sought.

tetanus (lockjaw) is a disease caused by the bacterium *Clostridium tetani*. It is found in earth and enters the body through cuts and scratches. The *incubation period* for tetanus is 4–21 days. It is a disease in which muscles of the neck, back and limbs contract and tighten. The muscles of the jaw can lock. Tetanus prevention is an integral part of any *immunisation* programme.

tetraplegia is a disorder, dysfunction or disease which causes *paralysis* of the four limbs of the body. (See *disability*.)

thalassaemia is an inherited *blood* disorder which is widespread in certain parts of the world such as Mediterranean countries, Africa and Asia. The disorder affects the protein component of *haemoglobin*. There are three classifications:

- minor – the person is a carrier but does not have any signs and symptoms themselves
- intermediate – the person has a mild form of the disease which may require the occasional *blood transfusion*
- major – the person has other signs and symptoms and the haemoglobin disorder causes *anaemia*, enlargement of the spleen and the *bone marrow* is affected.

The degree to which a person is affected depends on whether one or two parents are carriers. Where the disorder is inherited from one parent, the child usually has no signs and symptoms.

thalidomide: a *drug* which was prescribed for *pregnant* women during 1959–1961 to help their morning sickness. Side effects were found to include severe deformities in developing babies, some being born without fingers, arms or legs.

The New NHS – Modern, Dependable: a government White Paper introduced in 1997 which proposed changes to the National Health Service. One of these changes involved a review to ensure that patients would receive fair access to NHS services.

therapy: a process which is used to help individuals overcome their physical, psychological, social or cognitive difficulties. It can take the form of:

- counselling
- art/drama/music therapy
- light and sound experiences
- physical exercises
- complementary or alternative methods such as *massage* and *aromatherapy*.

throat: (pharynx) the passage which joins the mouth, nose, windpipe and the oesophagus.

thrombosis: a blood clot. It is often the result of a disorder which changes some of the liquid form of *blood* into a more solid state. This can lead to a blockage in an *artery* which restricts the *blood flow* to the *tissue* that it supplies. Examples of thrombosis are *coronary thrombosis*, stroke or *cerebrovascular accident*.

thymus: a *gland* situated in the base of the neck. It lies behind the breast bone and extends to the *thyroid gland*. It develops and grows from infancy and is at its largest during *puberty*. The function of the thymus is to support the *immune* system of the body.

thyroid gland: a *gland* situated in the neck, near the lower part of the larynx where it meets the trachea. It produces a *hormone* called thyroxine which controls the body's *basal metabolic rate (BMR)*. This is the rate at which the body releases energy and directly influences the body's level of activity. (See table overleaf.)

tidal air: the air breathed in and out of the *lungs* during each cycle of breathing.

tidal volume: the amount of air which is breathed in and out during each cycle of breathing or inspiration. It can be measured and assessed. This is particularly important where *clients* or *patients* have breathing problems such as bronchitis or asthma. (See *mechanism of breathing, spirometry*.)

Overactive and underactive thyroid

Overactive thyroid	Underactive thyroid
increased metabolic rate	reduction in metabolic rate
raised temperature/sweating	low body temperature
heart damage, fast pulse	slow pulse rate, weight gain
weight loss, increased appetite	changes in hair and skin
swelling behind the eyes	stunted growth
swelling of the thyroid gland	

tissue: a group of *cells* which carry out a particular task, e.g. muscular tissue, nervous tissue, connective tissue. Tissues have various functions:
- they act as a barrier against *infection*
- they enable other materials to be deposited in their matrix in order to carry out specific functions (in the formation of *bone*, calcium is deposited between the bone cells in order to make it strong)
- protection
- support
- they respond to stimuli
- they enable movement to take place
- they increase surface area enabling diffusion to take place
- they allow the diffusion of *nutrients*, gases, *hormones* and other substances to pass through its walls to other tissues and different parts of the body.

Examples of the various types of tissues are:
- *epithelial tissue* – cover or form lining in different parts of the body;
- *glandular tissues* which line the spaces in glands and secrete substances into these spaces
- *nervous tissue* – link together and form a network enabling messages or nerve impulses to be sent to all parts of the body
- *connective tissue* – composed of different cells and fibres which support and hold other tissues and organs together, e.g. cartilaginous tissue which supports bones
- *muscular tissue*.

tongue: a muscular *organ* attached to the floor of the *mouth*. It is covered in mucous membrane and is made up of muscle fibres which allow the tongue to move about in several directions. The tongue is covered on its upper surface with tiny projections called papillae. There are also taste buds, which are small pores, situated on the surface of the tongue. The functions of the tongue are:
- chewing food so that the food forms a *bolus* or ball
- using muscular actions to push food to the back of the *throat* enabling it to be swallowed
- sensitivity to the taste, texture and temperature of the food being eaten
- speech production.

touch: see *sensory skills*.

tranquillisers are *drugs* which are used to reduce tension, relieve *anxiety* and make a person feel relaxed and calm. The potential side effects include drowsiness and *dependence*.

transfusion: the procedures used to introduce fluid into a tissue or blood vessel in the body. Fluid is transfused when the body's own supply has been diminished due to accident or disease. An example is a *blood transfusion* where blood is pumped into the body via a blood vessel, usually in the arm.

transitions are *changes* which occur in a person's life. These changes may require a period of adjustment and can relate to many aspects of an individual's life such as *work*, *family* and *lifestyle*.

transplantation: ('transplants') the process by which an *organ* or *tissue* can be transplanted from the body of one person to that of another person. For example, *kidney* transplants, *heart* transplants.

trauma: a physical wound caused by an external force. The term can also be used in a psychological sense (see *post-traumatic stress disorder*).

treatment: methods used to cure or support a *client*, *patient* or *service user*. Methods of treatment can be either short-term or long-term depending on the condition. Short-term treatment can involve a course of antibiotics for a throat infection, for example. Long-term treatment can involve surgery, different types of *drugs* and physiotherapy for *diseases* such as rheumatoid arthritis. Treatment can be:

- conservative, where different methods are used including bed rest, drugs, alternative therapies or any other procedure which does not involve surgery
- surgical, where different operations are used to treat the condition.

Factors which affect treatment include poor underlying health, delayed *diagnosis*, previous *lifestyle* choices with regard to *diet*, *alcohol* consumption and cigarette *smoking*.

treatment and care: the provision of support and care given within a care environment which promotes the positive life qualities of the service user. Positive treatment involves meeting all the basic and holistic needs of the service user. Negative treatment involves abuse, neglect, rejection, hostility, bullying, violence or discrimination. (See *positive care environment*.)

trends in health care: ways in which aspects of health care are changing. The following examples consider various trends:

Social and demographic changes:

- *ageing* population – people are living longer. This is putting extra demands on health resources particularly as there are fewer in the working population to generate those resources
- medical advances – due to more sophisticated methods of treatment lives are being saved which would otherwise have been lost
- *health care* – responds to the requirements of society. Increased homelessness has seen *tuberculosis* return as a significant cause of ill health in the UK
- modern *lifestyles* affect *health* – *alcohol*, *diet*, *smoking*, *exercise*.

Changes in technology:

- *keyhole surgery* – available for many procedures. This has changed the nature of *hospital* care, e.g. day stay rather than a long period in hospital
- diagnostic equipment – *computed axial tomography* and *magnetic resonance imaging* scanners, *ultrasound*. Earlier detection of disease allows for more effective treatment

- computerisation has improved efficiency of different aspects of care such as *laser* treatments to treat various conditions.

Changes in practice:
- more emphasis on patient-focused care
- nursing techniques which includes *care planning*.

Care in the community:
- *mental health* – moving long-term patients from large asylums (i.e. psychiatric hospitals) into smaller units of residential care
- primary care expansion with some GPs providing *day surgery*.

triangulation: three or more methods used in one piece of research. This can improve the validity of research. For example, in exploring issues with mature women who are studying nursery nursing, a researcher may use:
- a case study of a particular training centre or college
- both structured and in-depth interviews involving students and lecturers
- questionnaires.

truancy: unauthorised absence from *school* by children of compulsory school age (5–16 years of age). Children stay away from school for a variety of reasons. Under the Education Act 1993, children do not break the law when they 'play truant'; it is the parents who are viewed as committing an offence. *Youth courts* deal with such offences and insist through legislation that parents accept responsibility for their children.

trust is the result of a positive relationship which has developed between a service user and their carer or between colleagues.

trusts: see *acute trusts, foundation trusts, care trusts, primary care trusts, mental health trusts, strategic health authorities*.

tuberculosis is an infectious disease (*notifiable disease*) caused by the tubercle bacillus (see *bacteria*).
It causes lesions in different parts of the body although in the initial stages of the *disease* the person only suffers from a debilitating cough, loss of weight and night sweats.
The person often coughs up blood which can be distressing. Treatment involves antibiotics, bed rest and isolation from others during the infectious stages. Recovery can take a number of months.

tumour: a swelling or lump which can occur in different parts of the body. It may contain abnormal *tissue* which has no useful function in the body. A tumour can be:
- benign – the tumour is in a capsule and therefore does not invade or harm the surrounding tissues and organs
- malignant – the tumour is not encapsulated and therefore can invade surrounding tissues and organs causing more tumours to grow and develop.

There are various types of *cancer* which start with one tumour but then affect other parts of the body, e.g. a cancerous tumour of the lung can spread to the ribs or the liver.

twins occur when a woman produces either two eggs at ovulation or one fertilised egg which divides in two and both become implanted in the uterus. If twin eggs are produced and both are fertilised by male sperm, the two embryos grow and develop into two individual *foetuses* with the end result of two babies at *birth*.

- Identical twins occur when the one egg divides in two. The babies are born identical with the same physical characteristics.
- Non-identical twins occur when two separate eggs are fertilised. The babies are born with some but not all features and characteristics similar, in the same way as ordinary *siblings*. For example, one baby may have blonde hair and blue eyes while the other baby may have brown hair and brown eyes.

typhoid fever: an infectious disease caused as a result of a person eating or drinking milk or *food* contaminated by *Salmonella typhi*. The disease can be contracted by drinking unclean *water*, particularly water which has been contaminated with sewage. Flies or unhealthy living conditions can also lead to the disease. The disease often thrives in conditions where there are no public health regulations or standards. It can be passed from person to person and individuals can be infected by carriers. Carriers are people who do not themselves have any *signs and symptoms* of the disease but carry the bacteria in their system. Symptoms of the disease are a high temperature or fever with diarrhoea (which may contain blood). At the end of the first week of typhoid fever, a rash may appear on the upper abdomen. The incubation period is from 10 to 14 days.

Do you need revision help and advice?

Go to pages 292–304 for a range of revision appendices that include plenty of exam advice and tips.

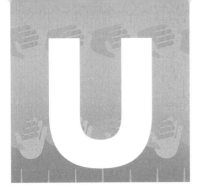

ultra-high temperature (UHT): the process of sterilisation of *food* at very high temperatures for short periods. This reduces the chemical changes in food in comparison with other traditional methods whilst extending the length of time that food can be safely kept before being eaten (see *food preservation*).

ultrasound is an imaging technique which displays the body's anatomic features. It is a non-invasive diagnostic and therapeutic process. It produces high frequency sound waves (not audible to the human *ear*) which are directed into the body and generate echoes as they bounce off structures. The resulting pattern of sound reflection is processed by a computer to produce a moving image on a screen or a photograph. Fluid conducts the ultrasound well. It is therefore useful in diagnosing cysts (which are filled with liquid), or in examining other structures which are fluid filled (e.g. observations of the *foetus* in the *amniotic sac*).

unemployment is a stage or period in an individual's life when they are without paid work. Individuals can either be viewed as short-term or long-term unemployed. The unemployed are expected to register with the local Department of Social Security. Once registered they are entitled to *jobseekers' allowance* and family credit. (See *benefits, worklessness*.)

unfair treatment: see *discrimination*.

United Nations Convention – The rights of the child: sets out a number of statements called Articles, which describe the rights of all children and young people. The rights include:

- Article 2 – all rights in the convention apply to all children whatever their race, sex, religion, language, disability, opinion or family background
- Article 3 – all decisions which are made affecting children should be in their best interests
- Article 7 – all children have a right to a name when they are born and to be able to become a citizen of a country
- Article 16 – all children have the right to personal privacy. This includes not having their personal phone calls intercepted or overheard unless the law allows it
- Article 19 – all children have the right to be protected from all forms of violence.

(See *National Children's Bureau*.)

Universal Declaration of Human Rights: declaration of the rights to which every individual in the world is entitled. It was adopted by the General Assembly of the United Nations on 10 December 1948. Parts of the declaration which apply specifically to health and social care include:

- Article 1 – all human beings are born free and equal in dignity and rights. They are endowed with reason and conscience and should act towards one another in a spirit of brotherhood

- Article 2 – everyone is entitled to all the rights and freedoms set forth in this declaration, without distinction of any kind, such as by *race*, colour, sex, language, religion, political or other opinion, national or social origin, property, birth or other status
- Article 23 – everyone has the right to *work*, to the free choice of employment, to just and favourable conditions of work and to protection against *unemployment*
- Article 23 – everyone without any discrimination has the right to equal pay for equal work.

universalism: a framework in society where policies are introduced and implemented in such a way that they are applied equally to all. Universalism was one of the intentions of the *welfare state* when it was set up in 1948 following the *Beveridge Report* in 1942.

urea: a waste product which is produced in the *liver* as a result of the breakdown of *protein*. It is removed by the *kidneys*. If the urea is allowed to accumulate in the *blood*, it can have a harmful effect on the body.

urinary system: the main system of the body involved in excretion. This is a process by which the body gets rid of unwanted substances produced as a result of cellular activity. The *alimentary canal*, *lungs* and *skin* are also involved in excretion. (See Figure on page 278.)

The urinary system is made up of:

- *kidneys* – two organs at the back of the body, just below the ribs. They are the main organs of excretion, filtering out excretory materials from the *blood* and regulating the level and contents of body fluids. Blood enters a kidney through a renal *artery* and leaves through a renal *vein*
- ureters – two tubes which carry urine from the kidneys to the bladder
- *bladder* or urinary bladder – a sac which stores urine. Its lining has many folds which flatten out as it fills up, letting it expand. Two muscular rings which are called the internal and external urinary sphincters control the opening from the bladder into the urethra. When the volume of urine gets to a certain level, nerves stimulate the internal sphincter to open, but the external sphincter is under conscious control (except in young children), and can be held closed for longer
- urethra – the tube carrying urine from the bladder out of the body (in men, it also carries sperm – see *male reproductive system*). The expulsion of urine is called urination or micturition.

urine: a watery fluid which is yellow in colour and is produced by the *kidneys*. It is a waste product formed as a result of various chemical reactions in the body. It consists of nitrogenous waste dissolved in *water*. Urine can be analysed chemically to aid the early diagnosis of *disease*. Urine contains water, urea, salt, nitrogen compounds such as uric acid and creatinine, hormones and minerals. *Drugs* or medicine may appear in urine (e.g. steroids). It can be tested to check for abnormalities or specific conditions, which include:

- sugar – if there is too much sugar in the blood it could indicate *diabetes*
- albumin/protein – when the breakdown of protein or the kidneys may be affected by some disorder or disease
- *pregnancy*.

The urinary system is shown in the diagram overleaf.

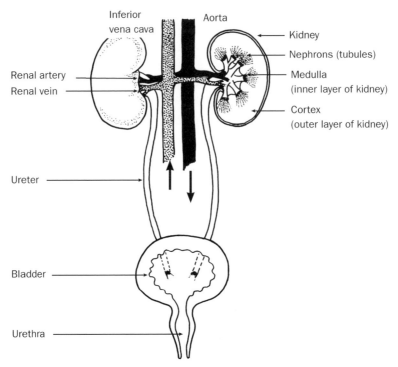

Urinary system

uterus: (womb) see *female reproductive system*.

Utting Report 1997 'People like us': a government report which reviewed the residential care of children. The committee was chaired by Sir William Utting and made recommendations which affect children's homes, boarding *schools* and foster homes. A review of the Report in 2005 found that there was still inadequate progress in bringing sex abusers to justice. The report also found that there was also inadequate support for children who have been sexually abused. It expressed concern about the lack of protection from sexual abuse for vulnerable groups such as *children with disabilities*. The report also commented on the need for increased strengthening of the provisions for safeguarding children by legislation, policies and procedures. It identified a gap between policy and practice.

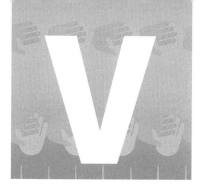

vaccination: a method of producing *immunity* by injecting dead or weakened pathogens, or closely related micro-organisms into the body in order to stimulate an immune response. It is a means whereby individuals can be protected from the disease or a fatal attack. (See *immunisation*.)

vagina: the lower part of the *female reproductive system*. It is a muscular tube which is lined with mucous membrane. The vagina connects the cervix and the womb to the outside of the body.

values form the foundation of an individual's *thoughts*, feelings, *beliefs* and *attitudes*. Values are closely related to moral principles, decision making, attitude formation and *behaviour*. Values are learned during the *socialisation* process, e.g. children learn values through the way they are reared or brought up within their families. Values can also be acquired through political beliefs, religious beliefs and secondary socialisation.

vasectomy: a surgical incision or cut through the vas deferens to prevent male sperm being ejected during ejaculation and intercourse. This is a male form of contraception and family planning.

vegans are individuals who eat no animal fats or animal derivatives. (See *vegetarians*.)

vegetarians are individuals who do not include meat in their daily *diet*. There are three types of vegetarian:

- lacto-ovo-vegetarians eat a mixed diet from both plant and animal sources. This includes dairy products and eggs
- lacto-vegetarians eat a diet of plant *food* with some milk or dairy products such as cheese. The plant food includes grain, seeds, nuts, fruit and vegetables
- vegans eat a diet containing no food from animal sources. This means they eat only plant food such as vegetables, fruit, nuts, seeds and grain.

veins are blood vessels which carry deoxygenated *blood* towards the *heart*, except in the case of pulmonary veins which carry oxygenated blood from the *lungs* to the heart. The walls of veins are much thinner and less muscular than those of *arteries*. Veins have valves to prevent the backflow of blood (see diagram overleaf).

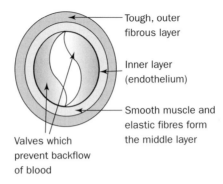

A vein

ventilation: the way in which *air* passes in and out of the respiratory tract. This includes the *gaseous exchange* in the *alveoli* of the *lungs*. Ventilation and the efficient way by which air is breathed in and out of the body are important factors in the general physical health of an individual. When there is a disorder in the ventilation system there are often signs and symptoms such as cyanosis, a bluish tinge to the skin due to the lack of sufficient *oxygen*. (See *mechanism of breathing, respiratory system*.)

ventricle: a chamber. There are several different types of ventricle in the body. The ventricles of the *heart* are its two lower chambers which pump the blood into the main vessel prior to its being distributed to different parts of the body. The ventricles of the *brain* contain cerebrospinal fluid.

vertebrae: there are 33 of these bones in the backbone. Each vertebra consists of a body and arch enclosing a cavity, which is called the neural canal. The *spinal cord* passes through this canal. The vertebrae protect the spinal cord by providing a bony framework. There are different vertebrae which include:

- seven neck or cervical vertebrae

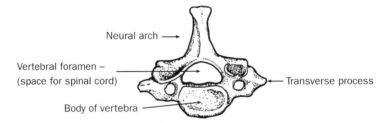

- twelve chest or thoracic vertebrae

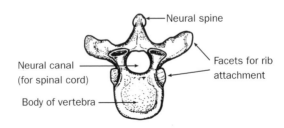

- five back or lumbar vertebrae

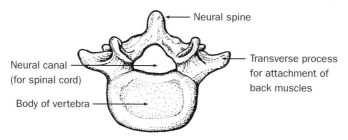

- Neural spine
- Neural canal (for spinal cord)
- Body of vertebra
- Transverse process for attachment of back muscles

- five lower back or sacral vertebrae

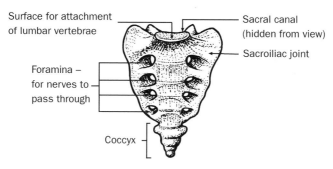

- Surface for attachment of lumbar vertebrae
- Sacral canal (hidden from view)
- Sacroiliac joint
- Foramina – for nerves to pass through
- Coccyx

- plus the coccyx (the lowest four vertebrae fused together).

Vetting and Barring Scheme – Every Child Matters: this scheme was created under the *Safeguarding Vulnerable Groups Act 2006* to replace the previous List 99, Protection of Children Act List, Protection of Vulnerable Adults and Disqualification Orders regimes. The Independent Safeguarding Agency is responsible for deciding who is unsuitable to work, or *volunteer* to work, with *vulnerable people*.

victim: a person who has been killed or injured, either in an *accident* or as a result of premeditated action, e.g. violent assault or rape. Health and social care providers are often called upon to assist victims from whatever cause.

Victim Support is a *charity* with volunteer workers who provide counselling to the victims of crime. Individuals are often referred to Victim Support by the *police*.

villi: finger-like projections from the surface of membranes. Examples include arachnoid villi in the *brain* and the villi in the lining of the *intestine*. The villi provide a greater surface area for the exchange of *oxygen*, *carbon dioxide* and *nutrients*.

violence: physical behaviour by an individual which causes hurt or damage to others. This includes physical assault, aggressive behaviour, intimidation, sexual and physical harassment. Violence is often linked with physical and sexual *abuse*.

viruses: extremely small infectious agents which are only visible under an electron *microscope*. There are many different types of virus which are harmful to the body and cause *disease*. Viruses reproduce in the body by invading a *cell*, multiplying and causing the cell to burst. An example of a virus is *HIV*.

visual impairments: disorders, dysfunctions or diseases which affect the *eyes* and the vision of an individual. (See *SeeAbility*.)

vital capacity (of lungs): the maximum volume or amount of air which can be breathed out or expelled by the *lungs* after taking a deep inward breath. It is measured on a *spirometer*. (See *respiratory system*.)

vitamins: are substances which are essential for general health and body growth. They are required in small quantities. When they are not included in a *diet*, vitamin *deficiency diseases* may become evident. (See table below.)

Examples of vitamins, their functions and deficiency disorders

Vitamin	Function	Source	Deficiency disorder
Vitamin A (retinol)	Keeps skin and bones healthy, helps to prevent infection	Carrots, milk, fish, oils, green vegetables, liver	Night blindness, lack of resistance to infection
Vitamin B1 (thiamin)	Needed for cell metabolism	Peas, beans, yeast, wholemeal bread, nuts	Beri-beri, muscle weakness
Vitamin B2 (riboflavine)	Needed for cell respiration	Liver, milk, eggs, yeast, cheese and green vegetables	Stunted growth, damage to the cornea of eye, inflamed tongue
Vitamin B6 (pyridoxine)	Needed for synthesis of amino acids	Potatoes, vegetables, meat, milk	Anaemia
Vitamin B12 (cobalamin)	Needed for formation of red blood cells, protein and fat	Liver, meat, eggs, milk, fish	Macrocytic anaemia, which is a failure to produce haemoglobin in the blood
Vitamin C (ascorbic acid)	Helps wounds to heal, necessary for healthy gums and teeth	Oranges, lemons, blackcurrants, green vegetables, tomatoes, potatoes	Scurvy – a disease which causes gum disease and affects the body's healing process
Vitamin D (calciferol)	Absorption of calcium and phosphorus which is necessary for teeth and bone growth and development	Liver, butter, cheese, eggs and fish	Weak bones – a disease called rickets in children
Vitamin E (tocopherol)	Promotes health, anti-oxidant	Vegetables, eggs, butter, fish, meat	Sterility in some animals
Vitamin K (phylloquinone)	Helps the blood clotting process	Liver, butter, cheese, eggs, fish, cabbage, spinach	Slow blood clotting

vocal cords are two folds of *tissue* which protrude from the side of the larynx and vibrate with the passage of air when stimulated by the speech centre in the *brain* to produce sounds that form the voice.

voluntary admission: a procedure which involves a *patient* agreeing that they need psychiatric care and treatment. (See *mental health*.)

voluntary sector organisations are those health and social care services set up by *charities* to provide services which are free of charge. Voluntary organisations are non-profit-making and non-statutory and depend on fund-raising and government grants for their *funding*. Workers within this sector are called *volunteers*.

volunteers: individuals who work within statutory or voluntary organisations without receiving any financial payment. They are often involved with aspects of community work such as Dial a Ride, working in charity shops and helping out in *day centres*, or the *Women's Royal Voluntary Service*.

vomiting: a reflex action in which the *stomach* ejects its contents through the mouth. Vomiting is controlled by a centre in the *brain*. Vomiting can be due to:
- stomach infection
- irritation of the stomach lining
- side effects of drugs
- travel sickness
- migraines/headaches
- inner ear disorders
- self-induced (e.g. in bulimia)
- obstruction in gastrointestinal tract.

vulnerable people are persons or groups who require support to live independently, e.g. young children, *older people* and those with disabilities.

vulva: the external opening of the *female reproductive system*.

Vygotsky, Lev (1896–1934): a psychologist who believed that a child's learning is influenced by its *social context*. He also believed that a child's memory and learning are affected by the culture in which he or she lives. One of his ideas was that a child has potential that an adult needs to 'unlock'. The gap between what the child is currently able to do and what he or she has potential to do he called the Zone of Proximal Development. Therefore the role of the adult in supporting a child's development is crucial.

Aiming for a grade A*?

Don't forget to log on to **www.philipallan.co.uk/a-zonline** for advice.

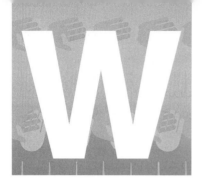

waiting lists are compiled by health and social care practitioners to control access to their services. Each *client, patient* or *service user* is given an appointment date and time. The waiting time on the day of the appointment also has a maximum limit. Most health and social care services operate a waiting list of admissions for minor and major surgical operations, treatments and therapies.

Wales (health and social care provision): the arrangements for independent health and social care in Wales is regulated by Welsh Ministers through the Health Care Inspectorate Wales, whilst the Care and Social Services Inspectorate (CSSIW) regulate the provision of social care services.

warmth (in interpersonal skills) is an important aspect of human *interaction*. It is a support skill which enables the *carer* to convey that they are interested and listening with a non-judgemental attitude to their client. It is reinforced with positive *gestures* of eye contact and facial expression. Showing warmth to a *client* can be a factor which contributes to building a positive relationship. (See *building confidence*.)

warmth (physical needs): keeping a *client*, *patient* or *service user* physically warm. Room temperature should be maintained at approximately 68°F (20°C). It is particularly important for vulnerable clients, such as older people and infants, to be kept warm as they can lose body heat very quickly.

waste disposal: the result of metabolism taking place in the body due to many chemical reactions. The body has strategies for disposing of the waste products it generates. The two types of waste disposal are termed *excretion* (getting rid of waste products as a result of metabolism) and elimination (egestion). If waste products are not removed quickly enough they have harmful side effects. Through the process of excretion the body gets rid of such substances. This is carried out by the:
- *lungs* – excrete *carbon dioxide* through respiration
- *kidneys* – excrete urea from *digestion* through urination
- *skin* – excretes *water* and *salts* through sweating
- intestines – excrete *bile salts* as a result of the breakdown of *haemoglobin*.

Through the process of elimination the body gets rid of waste such as faeces at the end of the digestion process. This is called defaecation.

water (H_2O) is a compound consisting of hydrogen and *oxygen* which is essential for all forms of life. It can exist as a gas, a liquid or a solid. It is the solvent for most body processes and can react in *cells* through hydrolysis and also condensation. The properties of water include:
- it is an excellent solvent and can dissolve more biological substances than any other fluid
- it forms 90% of the cell and is the main constituent of the cell cytoplasm

- it acts as a thermal buffer within the body, to protect it from rapid changes in temperature
- it acts as a lubricant in different parts of the body, e.g. in the air sacs (*alveoli*) which are situated in the *lungs*
- it forms part of a healthy *diet*, hydrating the body and aiding the *digestion* process.

water pollution is caused by chemical and industrial waste which contaminates water supplies, rivers and seas. This includes pollution of *water* supplies by the overuse of fertilisers in food production. The control of water pollution is supervised by the Environment Protection Act 1990, the Water Industry Act 1991 and the Water Resources Act 1991. These Acts of Parliament made recommendations which aim at:

- controlling pollution in rivers and the sea (i.e. avoiding the poisoning of water)
- ensuring that water sources are clean for domestic, industrial and agricultural use
- preventing the spread of *disease* through an effective sewage disposal system.

wealth: the total value of possessions held by an individual or a society. It is usually distinguished from income, because wealth can itself be income generating: 'money in the bank' generates interest.

welfare: the government provision for individuals on a minimum level of income, service or other support. It is also available for groups such as the poor, older people and disabled people.

welfare dependency: a situation in which personal or household income is solely dependent on welfare payments, e.g. the state retirement pension or unemployment benefit. People receiving *benefit* are likely to be the poorest in society. The term is particularly associated with the politics of the 'new right', who argue that over-generous welfare benefits have made many people too reliant on the state.

welfare provision: the provision of health and social care to all those in need; universal provision. (See *universalism*.)

welfare rights: the rights which individuals have in society in terms of access to information and support with regard to *benefits* and financial resources. *Citizens Advice Bureaux* and *social workers* in this field can also give advice and support in other areas relating to finance, such as debt counselling. The *Child Poverty Action Group* is a pressure group which publishes regular information such as an annual welfare rights handbook.

welfare services are those provided by the state. There are seven areas: *personal social services*, health*, youth services*, social services*, housing, education* and *employment*.

welfare state was set up in 1948 following the *Beveridge Report 1942*. It described a society in which the state (i.e. government) accepted responsibility for ensuring a minimum standard of living for all people. That ideal is supported by a *benefit* system and is associated with a range of *welfare services*. *New Ambitions For Our Country – A New Contract For Welfare* (1998) was a green paper produced by the government to bring in changes to the existing welfare state. It reviewed issues such as:

- encouraging people of working age to be in paid employment
- ensuring that those with disabilities receive the support which they need
- taking action against *social exclusion* and helping those in *poverty*.

well-being: a positive state of physical, intellectual, emotional and social health. It describes a feeling of being physically well and of psychological contentment. (See *health and well-being*.)

W

Welsh Office: was disbanded in 1999 when most of its powers were transferred to the National Assembly for Wales. This is the devolved *government* for Wales which has responsibility for making decisions affecting daily lives, including the economy, *health*, *education* and local government in Wales.

whistleblowing: a way in which problems and difficulties within organisations are publicised by an individual who is an employee.

white blood cells: (leucocytes) these are *cells* produced in the red *bone marrow* and the *lymph glands*. They have nuclei, are colourless and do not contain *haemoglobin*. There are two main types of white cells:

- granulocytes such as neutrophils, eosinophils and basophils. These are made up of granular cytoplasm and a lobed nucleus. They engulf bacteria and produce anti-histamine and histamine which are released by the body to deal with inflammation
- agranulocytes such as monocytes and lymphocytes. They have a spherical or bean-shaped nucleus and no granules in their cytoplasm. They engulf bacteria and produce antibodies.

The number of such cells (4000–10,000 per cubic millimetre of *blood*) is called the white cell count.

Winged Fellowship Trust: an organisation which runs holiday centres for the severely physically disabled, enabling *carers* to take a break from their duties. The centres are run by a combination of trained staff and volunteers, and 24-hour care is provided. Each centre is fully equipped for the use of disabled people. There is a shop, bar and garden. The Winged Fellowship provides an excellent opportunity for health and social care students to apply for volunteer work and develop their caring skills.

withdrawal symptoms: negative physical or psychological reactions which are experienced by individuals when they suddenly stop taking or reduce the dosage of an addictive *drug*. These include sweating, tremors, *vomiting* and abdominal pain.

womb: (uterus) see *female reproductive system*.

Women's Aid Federation: a voluntary agency in the UK for women and children experiencing physical, sexual or emotional abuse in their homes. The Women's Aid Federation of England (WAFE) is a national organisation which supports and resources a network of 214 local projects. Refuges are homes or hostels which offer a safe breathing space where decisions can be made, free from pressure and fear. There are also specialist refuges and services for women and children who face the additional pressures of racism or have specific cultural needs. National Women's Aid Federations also operate in Scotland, Wales and Northern Ireland. WAFE represents refugees as well as women and children experiencing domestic violence nationally in England. *Domestic violence* is defined as the physical, emotional or sexual abuse of women and their children in their homes by a person known to them – usually a male partner or ex-partner. Research into domestic violence shows that:

- every year over 50,000 women and children stay in refuges throughout England to escape domestic violence
- over 100,000 women use the services provided nationally and locally by Women's Aid
- 25% of all reported violent crime is 'wife assault'

- nearly 50% of female victims of homicide in England and Wales are killed by a partner or ex-partner
- recent studies have estimated that as many as one in five women experience domestic violence.

Women's Royal Voluntary Service: (WRVS) an organisation which provides practical care and support where it is needed in local *hospitals* and communities and during local emergencies. The WRVS operates in every county, region, major town and city in England, Scotland and Wales. It has three important functions:

- care in the local community – food services, family support services, home support services for older people, holidays for disadvantaged children, contact centres, tea bars in prisons and many other projects
- care in local hospitals – non-medical assistance for *patients*, enquiry and escort services for hospital visitors, tea bars, shops and the raising and donating of funds to hospitals
- care in local emergencies – WRVS emergency service volunteers are present regardless of time or location, to support the police, fire and ambulance services during incidents such as floods, fires, bomb attacks and accidents. They provide general assistance and refreshments to the rescue teams, clothing and welfare support to victims, families and friends and establish and run rest centres and enquiry points.

work is a term usually used to describe an adult form of paid employment. At the same time, offering one's services as a *volunteer* is called voluntary work. Work can also be viewed as an adult form of *play*. However, there is a need to identify the difference between work and *leisure*.

work experience: opportunities for health and social care students to practise theory, learned in the classroom, in a *care setting*. In addition to this, it gives students the opportunity to:

- apply course theory in practice
- observe experienced and professional carers as they work with clients
- meet clients, patients or service users to develop interpersonal and communication skills
- learn at first hand how to assess the different needs of clients
- use practical experience to add depth to study and research
- find out about aspects of health and social care; it is often a period when students may decide on their future career.

Work experience is a valuable aspect of any vocational course. It offers crucial features which benefit both the student and the placement organisation. The planning of work experience has the following requirements:

- the dates of the work experience to be negotiated with placements and the tutor or teacher
- students to update their *curriculum vitae (CV)*
- students to write a letter to the supervisor of the placement enclosing their CV and a supporting statement with regard to their request for work experience.

When students have obtained a placement they should:

- send their CV and supporting statement
- arrange a pre-placement visit
- co-ordinate travel plans
- prepare a *questionnaire* with regard to lunch breaks, starting/finishing time (if different from college hours)

w

287

- make sure they have a suitable set of clothes to wear. Short skirts, low-cut tops or shorts are usually not acceptable. In some work placements, students may be required to wear a uniform
- make sure that they are given suitable tasks and activities to carry out through work experience.

Guidelines – the 'P' laws for students on placement are as follows:

- be punctual – arrive on time
- be prepared – problems may arise so be as helpful as possible
- be professional – contact college and workplace if you are unwell; if you are anxious or concerned contact your teacher/tutor
- be pleasant – communicate with the clients, use your time wisely; co-operate with your colleagues
- be practical – help with all tasks and activities relating to working with clients and service users.

All students should use their work experience to:

- reflect on their own practice as well as the practice of others
- develop their **communication skills** and **observational skills**
- learn about **teams** and **group** working
- complete a work experience log or journal.

working class is the position in the social structure which is characterised by those involved in manual work or labour. The numbers in the working class have been declining because manual workers are gradually being replaced by machines. (See **social class or socio-economic group**.)

working in partnership: professionals working across their different areas of expertise to meet the needs of **service users**. (See **multi-disciplinary teams**.) An example is a physiotherapist and an occupational therapist working to support and rehabilitate a patient who has had a stroke.

Working Together to Safeguard Children 1999: a policy document which establishes **inter-agency co-operation** in **child protection** as well as promoting the welfare of children. The document was prepared jointly by the Department of Health, the Home Office, the Department of Education and Science and the Welsh Office.

Working Together to Safeguard Children 2007: an update on Working Together to Safeguard Children 1999 to take into account new **legislation**, **policies** and practice. This contains guidance on how individuals and organisations should work together **(inter-agency co-operation)** in **child protection** to promote the welfare of children.

working with parents: see **partnership with parents**.

worklessness: a term used to describe unemployment. There are various reasons for worklessness which include:

- a general rise in unemployment, particularly amongst males
- a growth in households headed by a single adult – often a single parent.

World Health Organisation (WHO) is a branch of the United Nations. It is affiliated to other worldwide organisations such as UNICEF. It is concerned with worldwide issues of health and welfare.

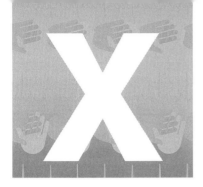

X chromosome: one of the two *chromosomes* which provide the genetic information which determines the sex of an organism. In each cell males have one X and one Y chromosome, females have two X chromosomes.

xenophobia: a fear of foreigners.

X-linked recessive gene defects: a defective *gene* which is on the X *chromosome* and affects males with certain forms of dysfunction, disease or disorder such as *haemophilia*.

X-ray examination: a method which assists in the diagnosis of a disease, disorder or dysfunction in the body. When X-rays are directed onto parts of the body they pass through *bone* and *tissue* to different extents to produce an image on a photographic film. X-ray machines are operated by *radiographers*. *Radiologists* are *doctors* who interpret the X-ray films and make a diagnosis. X-rays are used in *contrast media techniques*.

XXY syndrome: a *chromosome* disorder also known as Klinefelter's syndrome. It is a condition which affects males who are born with an extra X chromosome. Those suffering with this *disorder* are born with underdeveloped male genitalia and have pronounced female characteristics, such as *breast* development.

XYY syndrome: a *chromosome* disorder caused by there being an extra Y chromosome in each *cell*. Those who possess this *disorder* are males who grow to above average in height and have low levels of fertility.

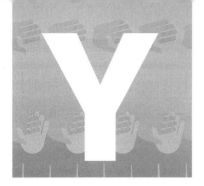

Y chromosome: a sex *chromosome* found only in males.

young carers: children and young people under the age of 16 years who take on the responsibility of caring for a parent or a close member of their *family* with a debilitating *disease* or disorder. In some cases, children forego their schooling and *education* in order to look after a sick relative. The devotion and commitment of these young carers can mean that they live restricted lives and carry heavy 'adult' responsibilities. (See *informal care, caring for the carer.*)

youth service: local authorities employ youth workers to provide a service which aims to encourage the personal development of young people in informal settings called 'youth centres'. It is an opportunity for the local authority to offer a wide range of services for children and young people which include:

- setting up community facilities and groups to provide recreational and educational input
- assisting in the organisation of youth groups and networking with other leaders and groups.

youth workers: those who are trained to work with young people in a variety of ways through the youth service. They may operate as:

- workers who may be based in a youth centre but also spend a proportion of their time talking to young people on the streets
- providers of *advice* and *support* sessions, liaising with other professionals in the care and support of young people and their families.

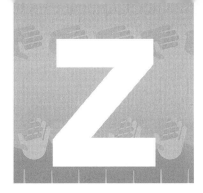

Zimmer frames are metal frames which give a person necessary support when walking. Zimmer frames have three or four feet, or wheels. Some have attachments for shopping bags and receptacles for carrying items and some fold up for easy carrying in cars and on public transport. They can be purchased or borrowed from hospitals and voluntary organisations such as *Age Concern* or the *Disabled Living Foundation*.

zygote: the product of *fertilisation*. The fusion of a male sex cell (the sperm) and the female sex cell (the ovum) produces a zygote. The zygote grows into an *embryo*, which develops into a *foetus*.

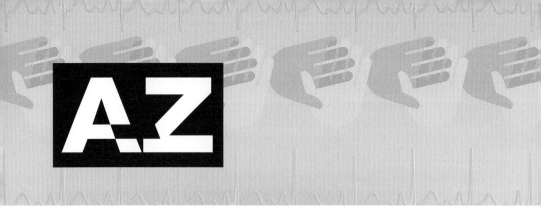

Health and social care revision lists

Using A–Z Online

On the pages that follow, we have listed revision terms for the AS and A-level examinations for the three main awarding bodies:

- AQA, see pages 293–295
- OCR, see pages 296–298
- Edexcel, see pages 299–300.

In addition to these revision lists, you can use the A–Z Online website to access revision lists specific to your exam board and the particular exam you are taking. Log on to **www.philipallan.co.uk/a-zonline** and create an account using the unique code provided on the inside front cover of this book. Once you have logged on, you can print out lists of terms together with their definitions, which will help you to focus your revision.

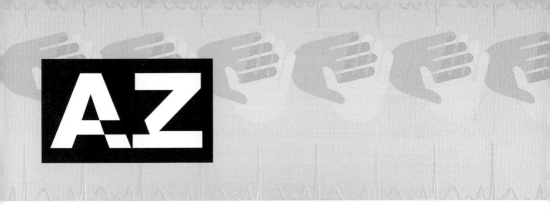

AQA revision lists

AS Unit 1 Effective caring

Acquired immune deficiency syndrome
(AIDS)

Assessment of need

Barriers to effective caring

Bullying

Caring for older people

Caring skills

Choice

Confidentiality

Day care

Dignity

Domiciliary services

Early years provisions

Effective communication

Equity

Health and safety

Hepatitis

Hygiene

Informal care

Life quality factors

MRSA

Neglect

NHS (National Health Service)

Occupation

Physical life quality factors

Psychological life quality factors

Rights and responsibilities of service users
and providers

Risk assessment

Special needs

Stereotyping

Unfair treatment

AS Unit 4 Child development

Communication

Creative play

Culture

Development

Developmental delay

Developmental norms or milestones

Education

Emotional development

Genetics

Growth

Health and safety

Housing

Infant

Intellectual development or cognitive
development

Language acquisition

Language development

Maturation

Motor skills

Nature–nurture

Physical growth and development

Physical play

Piaget's theory of cognitive development

Play

Reflex actions of the newborn

Schools

Social class or socio-economic group

Social development

Spiritual development

Symbolic play

AS Unit 5 Nutrition and dietetics

Balanced diet

Carbohydrates

Diet

Fats

Food additives

Food allergies

Food safety

Minerals

Nutrients

Proteins

Vegan

Vegetarian

Vitamins

Water

AS Unit 6 Common disease and disorders

Allergies

Disease

Dysfunctions

Ears

Eyes

Food poisoning

Headaches

Infections

Skin

Teeth

A2 Unit 12 Human development: factors and theories

Anti-social behaviour

Attachment

Behaviour

Data analysis

Freud, Sigmund (1856–1939)

Gender role

Language development

Learning theories

Piaget's theory of cognitive development

Skinner, Burrhus Frederic (1904–1990)

A2 Unit 13 The role of exercise in maintaining health and well-being

Aerobic exercise

Body mass index

Exercise

Health and safety

A2 Unit 14 Diagnosis and treatment

Biopsy

Blood tests

Computed axial tomography

Diagnosing disease

Drugs

Electrocardiogram (ECG)

Magnetic resonance imaging

Radiotherapy

Signs and symptoms

Treatment

X-ray examination

A2 Unit 15 Clients with disabilities

Aids and adaptations

Alzheimer's disease

Arthritis

Barriers to access to health and social care services

Barriers to support for service users

Disability

Care management

Care plan

Care practitioners

Cerebral palsy

Community care

Cystic fibrosis

Disability

Disability Discrimination Act 1995 and 2005

Down's syndrome

Health and social care organisations

Impairments

Multi-disciplinary teams

Multiple sclerosis

Muscular dystrophy

NHS and Community Care Act 1990

Purchasers

Personal social services

Spina bifida

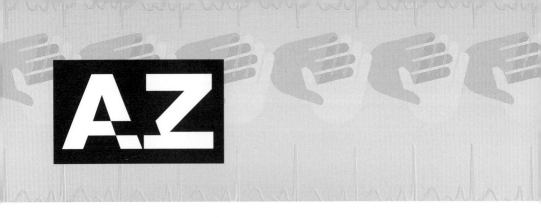

OCR revision lists

AS Unit F910 Promoting quality care

Barriers to access to health and social care services

Bullying

Care value base

Children Act 2004

Codes of practice

Confidentiality

Disability Discrimination Act 1995 and 2005

Discrimination

Every Child Matters

Harassment

Health and well-being

Human rights

Human Rights Act 1998

Needs

Organisation

Policies

Positive care environment

Protection of Vulnerable Adults

Prejudice

Race Relations Acts 1976 and 2000

Race Relations Act 2000

Reflective practice

Rights and responsibilities of service users and providers

Service user

Sex Discrimination Acts 1975 and 1986

Socialisation

AS Unit F913 Health and safety in care settings

Control of Substances Hazardous to Health (COSHH) Regulations 1999

First aid

Health and safety

Health and Safety (Signs and Signals) Regulations 1996

Health and Safety at Work Act 1974

Health and Safety Executive

Infection control

Lifting Operations and Lifting Equipment

Regulations 1998 (LOLER)

Management of Health and Safety at Work Regulations 1999

Manual Handling Operations Regulations 1992, revised 1998

Regulatory Reform (Fire Safety) Order 2005

Regulations for Reporting of Injuries, Diseases and Dangerous Occurrences (RIDDOR) 1995

Risk assessment

AS Unit F918 Caring for older people

Ageing

Aids and adaptations

Care Standards Act 2000

Care value base

Carers (Recognition and Services) Act 1995

Caring for older people

Complementary therapies

Coping

Day care

Dementia

Domiciliary services

Health Act 1999

Health and social care organisations

Health and social care workers

Individual rights

Life expectancy

Mental Health Act 1983

Mental Health Act 2007

Mental health disorder

NHS and Community Care Act 1990

Private sector

Support groups

Values

A2 Unit F920 Understanding human behaviour and development

Access to health services

Bandura, Albert (1925–)

Behaviour theories

Bonding

Bowlby, John (1907–1990)

Cognitive development

Development theories

Developmental delay

Early years provisions

Erikson, EH (1902–1994)

Freud, Sigmund (1856–1939)

Income

Language development

Learning theories

Life stages

Maslow, Abraham (1908–1970)

Nutrition

Rogers, Carl (1902–1987)

Self-concept

Social factors

Social and economic factors

A2 Unit F921 Anatomy and physiology in practice

Cardiovascular system

Diagnostic imaging techniques

Digestive system

Disease

Lifestyle

Musculoskeletal system

Nervous system

Urinary system

Reproductive system

Respiratory system

A2 Unit F924 Social trends

Bias

Biased sampling

Data analysis

Data collection

Demographic trends

Demography

Divorce

Family

Family life

Family structure

Research

Research methods

Social trends

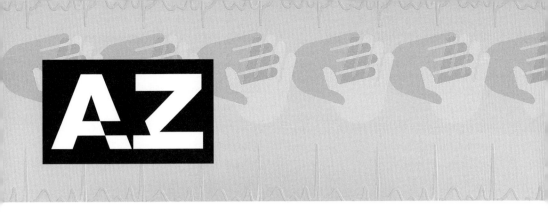

AZ

Edexcel revision lists

AS Unit 1 Human growth and development

Adolescence

Adulthood

Development

Disease

Emotional development

Environment

Genetics

Health

Health and well-being

Health promotion

Human growth and development

Ill health

Immunisation

Infancy

Intellectual development or cognitive development

Language acquisition

Language development

Later adulthood

Nature–nurture

Physical growth and development

Physical skills

Screening programmes

Social skills

Socialisation

AS Unit 4 Social aspects and lifestyle choices

Care practitioners

Care value base

Change

Effective care practice

Empowerment

Ethnicity

Gender

Health and well-being

Health and social care organisations

Income

Life course

Lifestyle

Person-centred care

P.I.E.S.

Poverty

Relationships

Self-concept

Self-esteem

Service user

Social class or socio-economic group

Social factors

Social relationships

Socialisation

Stereotyping

A2 Unit 7 Meeting individual needs

Accountability

Advocacy

Barriers to organisational culture

Care management

Care plan

Children Act 1989

Communication

Communication skills

Disability Discrimination Act 1995 and 2005

Empowerment

Enablement

Government

Human Rights Act 1998

Independent sector

Mental Health Act 1983

Mental Health Act 2007

Mixed economy of care

Networks

NHS and Community Care Act 1990

Normalisation

Organisations

Organisational culture

Positive care environment

Private sector

Provider

Purchaser

Roles and responsibilities

Safeguarding

Service user

Statutory organisations

Strategies for effective communication

A2 Unit 12 Understanding human behaviour

Behaviour

Behaviour theories

Bereavement

Bullying

Care value base

Disability

Discrimination

Empowerment

Ethnicity

Gender

Labelling

Marginalisation

Self-concept

Self-esteem

Separation

Social class or socio-economic group

Social role

Socialisation

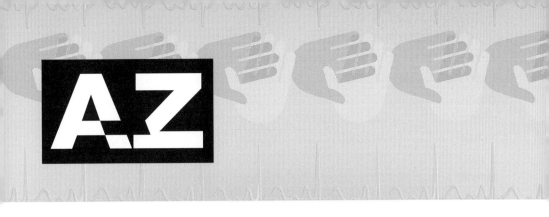

Examiners' terms

We are all familiar with the advice to 'read the question'. However, you need to understand the terminology used by examiners if you are to make the most of reading the question. In particular, there are some introductory words and phrases which, if you understand what the examiner means by them, will help you to understand what the examiner is looking for.

Here is a list of some frequently used examination terms.

Analyse: break down the topic and discuss each point in detail, explaining the relationship between them. Use point, evidence, explanation (PEE) or point, evidence, analyse (PEA) with paragraphs to back up your answer.

Apply: use knowledge learned to write into the context supplied, e.g. when you are given a scenario to read and address identified issues.

Assess: estimate the quantity, size, quality and value of evidence provided, and write up.

Compare and contrast: look for similarities and differences between two or more topics that have something in common. PEA paragraphs could be used.

Criticise: explain your judgement about an issue, backing this with evidence and research.

Define: write an accurate meaning of the word or phrase or concept. Take into account any differences or opposing definitions.

Demonstrate: show an awareness of the main points of a subject or topic.

Describe: give a detailed account of the main points of the topic in your own words.

Develop: expand or improve on a basic idea.

Discuss: write about the main arguments for and against and come to a reasoned conclusion.

Evaluate: explore the value of something. Consider its strengths and weakness and reach a balanced conclusion.

Examine: look closely at the topic. Put together an informed discussion.

Explain: describe the main points using examples to say 'how' and 'why'. A PEA paragraph could be used.

Give: write a short answer based on the facts of a subject or topic.

Identify: pick out the main points of the topic.

Justify: use evidence to back up an opinion or defend a point.

List: write down the main points on a topic, which could be in the form of a list of items or a table.

Outline: pick out the main points and write a sentence about each point, presenting the information in an organised way. You could use bullet points.

Reflect: explore or think about a subject or topic and look for strengths and weaknesses. Suggest strategies or ways of improving your own practice.

Relate: write up aspects of evidence that are associated with each other.

Review: make a critical examination of the topic and come to a reasoned judgement.

Summarise: write a shortened form of evidence using what you believe to be the main points. You do not need to go into any great detail.

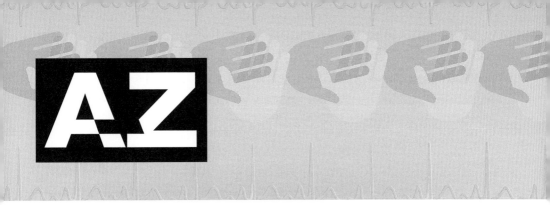

References

(Government legislation and reports are published by Her Majesty's Stationery Office (HMSO))

Government legislation

Abortion Act 1967

Anti-Social Behaviour Act 2003

Carers and Disabled Children Act 2000

Carers (Equal Opportunities) Act 2004

Carers (Recognition and Services) Act 1995

Childcare Act 2006

Children Act 1989

Children Act 2004

Child Support Act 1991

Civil Partnership Act 2004

Community Care (Direct Payments) Act 1996

Crime and Disorder Act 1998

Data Protection Act 1984, 1998

Disability Discrimination Act 1995, 2005

Domestic Violence, Crime and Victims Act 2004

Education Act 2005

Employment Equality (Age) Regulations 2006

Equal Pay Act 1970

Equal Pay (Amendment) Regulations 1983

Equality Act 2004

Food Safety Act 1990

Health Act 1999

Health Act 2006

Health and Safety at Work Act 1974

Health and Social Care Act 2001, 2008

Human Fertilisation and Embryology Act 2008

Human Rights Act 1998

Mental Capacity Act 2005

Mental Health Act 1983

Mental Health Act 2007

National Health Service and Community Care Act 1990

Northern Ireland Act 1998

Race Relations Act 1976

Race Relations (Amendment) Act 2000

Sex Discrimination Act 1975

Sex Discrimination Act 1986

Government reports and guidance

Acheson Report: Independent Inquiry into Inequalities in Health (1998)

Beveridge Report: Social Insurance and Allied Services (1942)

Black Report: Inequalities in Health (1980)

Fair access to care services – guidance on eligibility criteria for adult social care (Guidance, 2003)

Health of the Nation – A strategy for health in England (White Paper, 1992)

Our Healthier Nation – A Contract For Health (Green Paper, 1998)

The New NHS – Modern, Dependable (White Paper, 1997)

Utting Report: 'People Like Us' (1997)

Working Together to Safeguard Children (Guidance 1999, 2007)

Publications

Better Home Life: A Code of Practice for Residential Care (1996), Centre for Policy on Ageing.

First Aid Manual (1997) *St John Ambulance*, Dorling Kindersley.

Health Provision (1984), World Health Organisation.

Hungry to Be Heard (2006), Age Concern.

National Statistics Socio-economic Classifications (NS-SEC), HMSO.

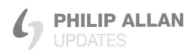
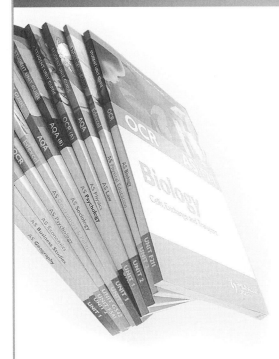

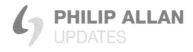
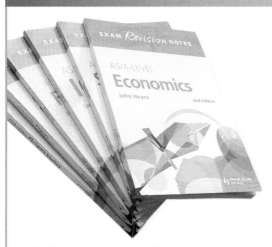